Applied Machine Learning in Healthcare

This book explores the latest advancements in machine learning techniques and their transformative applications in the healthcare domain. It delves into the use of machine learning for disease diagnosis and prognosis, showcasing its potential to enable accurate disease identification, effective risk stratification, and personalised treatment planning. The role of machine learning in enhancing clinical decision support systems (CDSS) is examined in detail, with a focus on its impact on informed decision-making, predictive modelling, and real-time patient monitoring.

- Features real-world case studies and applications that demonstrate the practical use of machine learning in healthcare, including radiology, predictive analytics, personalised medicine, and resource optimisation.
- Covers essential stages of data preprocessing and feature engineering for healthcare datasets, addressing challenges such as data cleaning, normalisation, dimensionality reduction, and feature selection.
- Provides an in-depth overview of CDSS and the integration of machine learning algorithms to improve diagnostic accuracy and clinical workflow efficiency.
- Explores machine learning-driven real-time monitoring and alert systems, underscoring their utility in promptly identifying and responding to critical medical events.
- Discusses advances in medical image analysis, including segmentation, classification, and computer-aided diagnosis techniques.

This comprehensive volume serves as a valuable resource for researchers, clinicians, healthcare professionals, data scientists, and students seeking to understand and apply machine learning for improved healthcare outcomes.

Applied Machine Learning in Healthcare
Case-Based Approach

Edited by
Dattatray G. Takale, Parikshit N. Mahalle,
Sachin S. Bere, and Piyush P. Gawali

CRC Press
Taylor & Francis Group
Boca Raton London New York

CRC Press is an imprint of the
Taylor & Francis Group, an **informa** business
A CHAPMAN & HALL BOOK

Designed cover image: ShutterStock

First edition published 2026
by CRC Press
2385 NW Executive Center Drive, Suite 320, Boca Raton FL 33431

and by CRC Press
4 Park Square, Milton Park, Abingdon, Oxon, OX14 4RN

CRC Press is an imprint of Taylor & Francis Group, LLC

ISBN: 9781032765945 (hbk)
ISBN: 9781032765969 (pbk)
ISBN: 9781003479185 (ebk)

DOI: 10.1201/9781003479185

Typeset in Times
by codeMantra

This book is dedicated to all the healthcare professionals and researchers who work tirelessly to advance medical science and improve patient lives through innovation and compassion.

We also dedicate this work to our families, whose unwavering support, patience, and encouragement made this academic journey possible.

Dr. Dattatray G. Takale
Assistant Professor,
Vishwakarma Institute of Technology, Pune

Contents

Preface

The convergence of machine learning and healthcare has opened new frontiers in medical research, diagnosis, treatment planning, and patient care. With the exponential growth of healthcare data and the rapid advancement of computational techniques, there is a growing need to understand and implement intelligent systems that can support clinicians in making data-driven decisions. This book is a response to that need.

It brings together cutting-edge research, real-world case studies, and practical applications that illustrate how machine learning can be effectively leveraged to address complex challenges in the healthcare industry. From disease diagnosis and prognosis to clinical decision support systems and medical image analysis, this volume provides a comprehensive overview of current trends, methodologies, and outcomes.

The content of this book has been carefully curated to serve as a resource for a broad audience, including researchers, clinicians, healthcare professionals, data scientists, and students. Each chapter has been contributed by domain experts and thoroughly reviewed to ensure academic rigour and practical relevance.

We hope this book will not only inform but also inspire further research and development in the field. Our sincere thanks go to all contributors for their valuable insights and to the editorial and publishing team for their support throughout this journey.

Dr. Dattatray G. Takale
Assistant Professor,
Vishwakarma Institute of Technology, Pune

Acknowledgement

We would like to express our sincere gratitude to all those who have contributed to the development and successful completion of this book.

First and foremost, we extend our heartfelt thanks to all the contributing authors whose research, insights, and dedication have enriched the content and scope of this volume. Your valuable contributions have played a pivotal role in shaping the academic quality of this work.

We are deeply grateful to the editorial and publishing team at CRC Press for their constant guidance, support, and professionalism throughout the editorial process. Your meticulous attention to detail and commitment to excellence have been instrumental in bringing this book to life.

Special thanks to our colleagues, research collaborators, and reviewers who provided critical feedback and helped refine the chapters. Your expertise and constructive suggestions added immense value to the final manuscript.

We also acknowledge the support of our respective institutions, research centres, and funding agencies for providing the resources and encouragement necessary to carry out this academic endeavour.

Finally, we extend our gratitude to our families for their unwavering support and patience during the countless hours devoted to this project.

Dr. Dattatray G. Takale
Assistant Professor,
Vishwakarma Institute of Technology, Pune

Editors

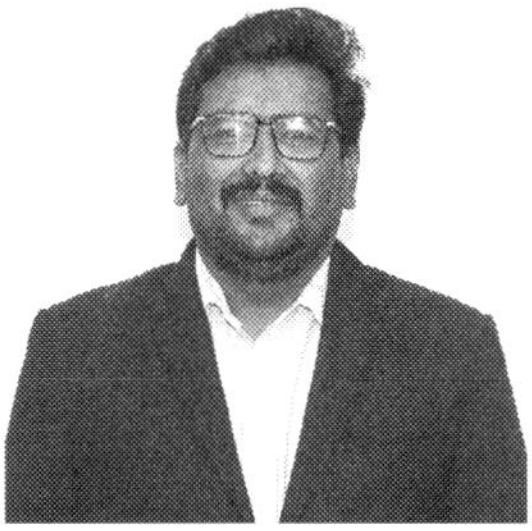

Dattatray G. Takale is an Assistant Professor in the Department of Computer Engineering at the Vishwakarma Institute of Technology, Pune, India. Dr. Dattatray G. Takale earned his Ph.D. in Computer Science and Engineering from Shri JJT University, Rajasthan. He has over 12 years of teaching and research experience. His research interests include machine learning, data science, wireless sensor networks, natural language processing, data warehousing, mining, computer networks, and network security. He is currently employed by VIIT Pune as an Assistant Professor. He has more than 9 years of teaching experience and 3 years of industry experience. He has 80 patents and 100+ research publications and has authored/edited 7+ books with reputed local and international publishers.

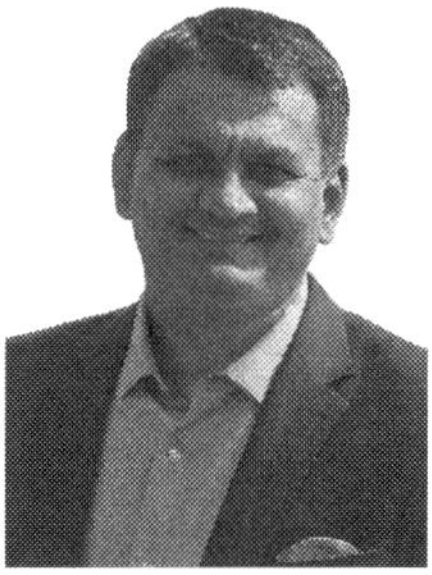

Parikshit N. Mahalle is a senior member of IEEE and currently serves as Professor and Dean of Academics at the Vishwakarma Institute of Technology, Pune, India. He previously held roles as Head of the Department of Artificial Intelligence and Data Science at the Vishwakarma Institute of Information Technology and as Professor and Head of Computer Engineering at Sinhgad Institutes. He earned his Ph.D. from Aalborg University, Denmark, and completed postdoctoral research at CMI, Copenhagen. With over 25 years of academic and research experience, Dr. Mahalle has guided eight Ph.D. scholars (seven of whom have been awarded) and mentored three postdoctoral researchers. He has authored or edited 72 books with international publishers. His scholarly output includes more than 430 publications, over 4,000 Google Scholar citations (h-index 28), and 2,200+ Scopus citations (h-index 21). Dr. Mahalle is the Editor-in-Chief of the *Research Journal of Computer Systems and Engineering* (RJCSE) and serves as Associate Editor and reviewer for several reputed journals and conferences. His research interests include machine learning, IoT, data science, identity management, and cybersecurity. He has delivered more than 400 invited talks at national and international forums and received prestigious honours, including the IEEE ICTBIG 2024 Distinguished Research Guide Award, State-Level Meritorious Teacher Award, and International Distinguished Researcher of the Year (S4DS, 2023). His textbook on design and analysis of algorithms is adopted by IIITs and NITs, and his CRC Press book on pandemic data analysis has earned two international awards. In 2024, his edited volume *Data Science: Techniques and Intelligent Applications* received the Choice Outstanding Academic Titles Award. He is also an ISO 27001:2022 Certified Lead Auditor and has served as guest faculty at institutions including National Taipei University, Taiwan, and UMA, Peru.

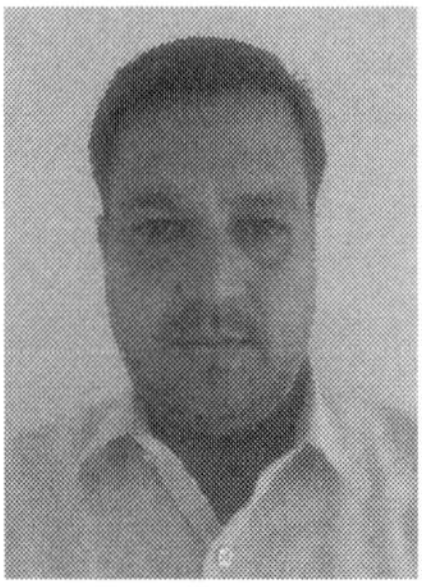

Sachin S. Bere is an Associate Professor in the Dattakala Group of Institutions, Faculty of Engineering, Bhigwan. He completed his Ph.D. in Computer Science and Engineering from the SJJT University, Rajasthan. He also completed his M.Tech. (CSE) in first class and distinction from a JNTU-Hyderabad-affiliated college. He has 18 years of teaching experience and 7 years of research experience. He has published almost 30 research articles in reputed journals and conferences. His areas of interest are machine learning, artificial intelligence, deep learning techniques, and programming languages.

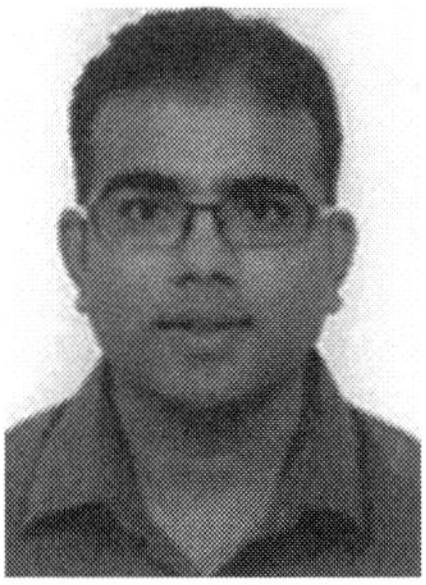

Piyush P. Gawali is an Assistant Professor in the Department of Computer Engineering at the Vishwakarma Institute of Information Technology, Pune, India. Mr. Piyush P. Gawali earned his M.E. in Computer Science and Engineering and is pursuing a Ph.D. from Savitribai Phule Pune University. He has more than 16 years of teaching experience. His research interests include quantum computing, cybersecurity, medical cyber-physical systems, machine learning, and network security. He has more than 13 years of teaching experience and two years and six months of industry experience. He has 8 patents and 14+ research publications and has authored/edited 2+ books with local and international publishers.

Contributors

Vikram Kishor Abhang
Department of Computer Engineering
MET's Institute of Engineering
Nashik, Maharashtra, India

Pankaj M. Agarkar
Department of Computer Engineering
Ajeenkya D. Y. Patil School of Engineering
Lohgaon, Pune, Maharashtra, India

Vishal Ambhore
Department of Electronics and Tele-Communication
Vishwakarma Institute of Information Technology
Pune, Maharashtra, India

Samir N. Ajani
School of Computer Science
Ramdeobaba University Nagpur, Maharashtra, India

Suruchi Bibikar
Computer Engineering Department
Bharati Vidyapeeth's College of Engineering for Women
Pune, Maharashtra, India

Amar Buchade
Department of AIDS
BRACT's Vishwakarma Institute of Information Technology
Pune, Maharashtra, India

Mayur Bahiram
Vishwakarma Institute of Information Technology
Pune, Maharashtra, India

Prasad Chaudhari
Department of CSE Internet of Things, Cyber Security including BlockChain Technology
Vishwakarma Institute of Information Technology
Pune, Maharashtra, India

Gopal B. Deshmukh
School of Engineering
Avantika University
Ujjain, Indore, India

Mrunalee Dhone
Department of Computer Science and Engineering
G H Raisoni College of Engineering
Nagpur, Maharashtra, India

Sheetal Dhande-Dandge
Computer Science and Engineering
Sipna College of Engineering and Technology
Amravati, Maharashtra, India

Pramod Dhamdhere
Department of Computer Engineering
G H Raisoni College of Engineering and Management
Wagholi, Pune, Maharashtra, India

Leena Deshpande
Department of Computer Engineering
Vishwakarma Institute of information Technology
Pune, Maharashtra, India

Devendra P. Gadekar
Mastercard Technology
Pune, Maharashtra, India

Jotiram G. Gujar
Department of Chemical Engineering
Sinhgad College of Engineering
Vadgaon, Pune, Maharashtra, India

Baisa L. Gunjal
Department of Information Technology
Amrutvahini College of Engineering
Sangamner, Maharashtra, India

Premanand Ghadekar
Department of Information Technology
Vishwakarma Institute of Technology
Pune, Maharashtra, India

Amit Gavit
Vishwakarma Institute of Information Technology
Pune, Maharashtra, India

Ali Mohammed Hendi
College of Medicine
Jazan University
Jazan, Kingdom of Saudi Arabia

Mohammad Alamgir Hossain
Department of Computer Science
College of Computer Science and Information Technology, Jazan University
Jazan, Kingdom of Saudi Arabia

Ruthik Jadhav
Vishwakarma Institute of Information Technology
Pune, Maharashtra, India

Anupama Jawale
Narsee Monjee College of Commerce and Economics
University of Mumbai
Mumbai, Maharashtra, India

Komal S. Jaisinghani
Department of Computer Engineering
St. Vincent Pallotti College of Engineering and Technology
Nagpur, Maharashtra, India

Venigalla Jithin
Department of Computer Science & Engineering
G H Raisoni College of Engineering
Nagpur, Maharashtra, India

Prashant Khobragade
Department of Computer Science and Engineering
G H Raisoni College of Engineering
Nagpur, Maharashtra, India

Amreen Khan
Department of Computer Engineering
Bajaj Institute of Technology
Wardha, Maharashtra, India

Prashant Khobragade
G H Raisoni College of Engineering
Nagpur, Maharashtra, India

Vikas K. Kolekar
Department of Computer Engineering
SMT. Kashibai Navale College of Engineering, Savitribai Phule Pune University
Pune, Maharashtra, India

Nikhila Kathirisetty
CSE (Data Science)
Vardhaman College of Engineering
Hyderabad, Telangana, India

Sonali P. Kadam
Computer Engineering Department
Bharati Vidyapeeth's College of Engineering for Women
Pune, Maharashtra, India

Masira S. Kulkarni
Computer Science and Engineering (Cyber security and Data Science)
G H Raisoni College of Engineering and Management
Wagholi, Pune, Maharashtra, India

Vinaya D. Kulkarni
Computer Engineering Department
Bharati Vidyapeeth's College of Engineering for Women
Pune, Maharashtra, India

Yash R. Kadam
Department of Artificial Intelligence and Data Science
Vishwakarma Institute of Information Technology
Pune, Maharashtra, India

Omkar R. Khade
Department of Artificial Intelligence and Data Science
Vishwakarma Institute of Information Technology
Pune, Maharashtra, India

Ketki P. Kshirsagar
Department of Electronics and Tele-Communication
Vishwakarma Institute of Information Technology
Pune, Maharashtra, India

Suresh Limkar
Department of Artificial Intelligence and Data Science
AISSMS Institute of Information Technology
Pune, Maharashtra, India

Parikshit N. Mahalle
Department of Artificial Intelligence and Data Science
Vishwakarma Institute of Technology
Pune, Maharashtra, India

Naif Ali Majrashi
Faculty of Applied Medical Sciences, Diagnostic Radiography Technology Department
Jazan University
Jazan, Kingdom of Saudi Arabia

Ashish Mahalle
Department of Information Technology
Vardhaman College of Engineering
Hyderabad, Telangana, India

Madhavi P. Mahajan
Department of Kayachikitsa
College of Ayurveda, Bharati Vidyapeeth's University
Pune, Maharashtra, India

Riddhi Mirajkar
Department of Information Technology
Vishwakarma Institute of Information Technology
Pune, Maharashtra, India

Sanah Naik
Computer Engineering Department
Bharati Vidyapeeth's College of Engineering for Women
Pune, Maharashtra, India

Ankita Ochani
Computer Engineering Department
Bharati Vidyapeeth's College of Engineering for Women
Pune, Maharashtra, India

Ruta Prabhu
Narsee Monjee College of Commerce and Economics
University of Mumbai
Mumbai, Maharashtra, India

Satyajit Pangaonkar
School of Engineering
Avantika University
Ujjain, Indore, India

Shabana S. Pathan
Department of Information Technology
St. Vincent Pallotti College of Engineering and Technology
Nagpur, Maharashtra, India

Pallavi K. Parlewar
Shri Ramdeobaba College of Engineering and Management
Nagpur, Maharashtra, India

Sakshi Pratap
Computer Engineering Department
Bharati Vidyapeeth's College of Engineering for Women
Pune, Maharashtra, India

Surendra Rahamatkar
School of Engineering
Avantika University
Ujjain, Indore, India

Vishal Shankarrao Rakh
Department of Computer Engineering
Shree Ramchandra College of Engineering
Lonikand, Pune, Maharashtra, India

Mehebubar Rahman
Department of Tropical Medicine
School of Tropical Medicine
Kolkata, West Bengal, India

Vijay U. Rathod
Department of Computer Engineering
G H Raisoni College of Engineering and Management
Wagholi, Pune, Maharashtra, India

Ganesh B. Regulwar
Department of Information Technology
Vardhaman College of Engineering
Hyderabad, Telangana, India

Katta Hartheek Reddy
Department of Information Technology
Vardhaman College of Engineering
Hyderabad, Telangana, India

Snehal Rathi
Vishwakarma Institute of Information Technology
Pune, Maharashtra, India

Mahesh Shinde
School of Engineering
Avantika University
Ujjain, Indore, India

Nilesh P. Sable
Bansilal Ramnath Agarwal Charitable Trust's
Vishwakarma Institute of Information Technology, SPPU
Pune, Maharashtra, India

Babaso Shinde
Department of Computer Engineering
Shree Ramchandra College of Engineering
Lonikand, Pune, Maharashtra, India

Sachin R Sakhare
Department of Computer Engineering
Vishwakarma Institute of Information Technology
Pune, Maharashtra, India

Vanam Prem Shanker
Department of Information Technology
Vardhaman College of Engineering
Hyderabad, Telangana, India

Dhawal Sakharwade
Department of Information Technology
Vishwakarma Institute of Technology
Pune, Maharashtra, India

Nitin Shivale
Department of Computer Engineering
JSPM's Bhivarabai Sawant Institute of Technology and Research
Wagholi, Pune, Maharashtra, India

Nitin Sakhare
Department of Computer Engineering
Vishwakarma Institute of Information Technology
Pune, Maharashtra, India

Shivam Tikone
Vishwakarma Institute of Information Technology
Pune, Maharashtra, India

Nitin Dattu Thorve
Department of Computer Engineering
BRACT's Vishwakarma Institute of Information Technology
Pune, Maharashtra, India

Shreyash Tekade
Department of Information Technology
Vishwakarma Institute of Technology
Pune, Maharashtra, India

Ankur Tripathi
Department of Information Technology
Vishwakarma Institute of Technology
Pune, Maharashtra, India

Shivam Tiwadi
Department of Information Technology
Vishwakarma Institute of Technology
Pune, Maharashtra, India

Dattatray G. Takale
Department of Computer Engineering
Vishwakarma Institute of Information Technology
Pune, Maharashtra, India

Abhijit Titarmare
Department of Electronics and Telecommunication
G H Raisoni College of Engineering
Nagpur, Maharashtra, India

Vinod S Wadne
Department of Computer Engineering
JSPM's Imperial College of Engineering and Research
Pune, Maharashtra, India

Suvarna A. Wakure
Department of Computer Engineering
Trinity Academy of Engineering
Pune, Maharashtra, India

Santosh T. Waghmode
Department of Computer Engineering
Dr. Babasaheb Ambedkar Marathwada University
Sambhajinagar, Maharashtra, India

Dnyaneshwar Natha Wavhal
Department of Computer Engineering
BRACT's Vishwakarma Institute of Information Technology
Pune, Maharashtra, India

Ashwini Yerlekar
Department of Computer Science and Engineering (AIML)
S. B. Jain Institute of Technology, Management and Research
Nagpur, Maharashtra, India

Anuradha Yenkikar
Department of CSE - Artificial Intelligence
Vishwakarma Institute of Information Technology
Pune, Maharashtra, India

Sayee Zanzane
Department of Information Technology
Vishwakarma Institute of Technology
Pune, Maharashtra, India

1 Ant Colony Optimization and Gray Wolf Optimization—A Comparative Study for Healthcare Resource Allocation during COVID-19 across States in India

Anupama Jawale and Ruta Prabhu

1.1 INTRODUCTION

A significant obstacle for any health institution dealing with COVID-19 was distributing limited resources efficiently and fairly. Even health systems with ample resources found it difficult to promptly deploy staff and beds, two essential healthcare resources, to the areas most in need. The development of vaccinations and treatments raises the importance of resource allocation; despite high-income environments being initially the most afflicted, nations like Mexico, Russia, and India top the world in the number of new cases reported every day.

Artificial intelligence (AI) is a talk-of-the-town tool widely employed in COVID-19 to aid in creating medications and vaccines, patient monitoring, contact tracing, and early illness diagnosis. A branch of AI called machine learning (ML) allows computers to automatically learn from experience and be better at making predictions and judgments without having to be rewritten again for a similar situation to handle programmatically. The viral contamination of COVID-19's unpredictable and unstable nature and the existence of asymptomatic patients' transmission have made computer-based systems that utilize real-time data evolve with time and offered adaptive reactions essential for reducing the virus's impact. Given the strain on health systems and worries over COVID-19 vaccine independence, ML provided a significant chance to inform choices about the distribution of limited resources, such as hospital beds, personnel, and vaccines, in nations with low and moderate incomes (LMICs).

DOI: 10.1201/9781003479185-1

Workforce planning can also be guided by ML. Medical professionals played a crucial role in the COVID-19 response. Rural and urban impoverished areas generally have lower health professional populations; this issue is especially severe in LMICs, which has sparked worries about the coverage of COVID-19 in these areas. ML-based risk monitoring systems can forecast future clinical and public health staffing needs by analyzing hospital patients' electronic health records or cases found through COVID-19 testing. Since occurrences are now extensively dispersed across several countries and are evolving quickly, policymakers would benefit from knowing the geographic areas where staff shortages are most likely to occur. In response, several nations have increased the size of their current public health and medical workforces. Authorities in India started looking for epidemiologists immediately because more than 25% of the country's 736 districts lacked district-level epidemiologists.

India offers a fantastic illustration of how locally generated data can enhance systems. Over 1.2 billion people have been registered on the Aadhaar program's biometric database since its nationwide launch in 2011. Data availability now ranges from smartphones, credit card histories, and bank accounts to insurance policies, income taxes, pensions, and several welfare programs. To help with the COVID-19 comeback in some LMICs, the digital infrastructure and data availability and connectivity with resources like Aadhaar, which are used to support the expansion of ML systems in healthcare, were a realistic next step.

1.2 BACKGROUND

The Indian Government Ministry of Health and Family Welfare has provided the Rural Health Statistics for 2021–2022 (dated January 12, 2023). This yearly publication, which started with its first release in 1992, offers information on the infrastructure of the public healthcare system in each nation's state and union territory at different levels. Data from subcenters (SCs), hospitals in various districts across states, community health centers (CHCs) and sub-divisional hospitals, primary health centers (PHCs), and medical colleges are included, with data collected through March 31, 2022. The report indicates notable deficiencies in the infrastructure that provided specialized care at CHCs compared to last year's data. CHCs were deficient in 83.2% of necessary surgeons, 74.2% of essential obstetricians and gynecologists, 79.1% of required physicians, and 81.6% of pediatricians needed. According to the report, "there is a shortage of 79.5% specialists." Below are the facts and numbers about available health resources in India as of March 31, 2022 (Rural Health Statistics, 2021–22, 2023).

The total number of SCs in India is 161,829, of which 157,935 operate in rural areas.

A total of 31,053 PHCs were operational in India, both in rural and urban areas.

There were roughly 6,118 PHCs in urban areas and 24,935 PHCs in rural areas.

As of March 31, 2022, there were 6,064 operational CHCs nationwide, 5,480 of which were located in rural areas and 584 in urban areas.

From 2005 to the present, there have been 11,909 more SCs. There was a discernible rise in the number of SCs in Rajasthan, with 3,011 SCs; Gujarat, with 1,858 SCs;

Madhya Pradesh, with 1,413 SCs; and Chhattisgarh with 1,306 SCs. According to the report, the average number of rural residents served by one SC was 5,691 people. In rural areas, one PHC and one CHC covered, on average, 36,049 and 164,027 people, respectively.

The report finds a 3.1% deficit in the total number of allopathic doctors required in rural PHCs across the country. A significant shortage of doctors in PHCs (the difference between the number required and the number currently employed) was observed in Odisha (298), Chhattisgarh (279), and Karnataka (60). This was true even though there were 30,640 allopathic doctors in PHCs in rural areas in 2022 compared to 20,308 in 2005, an increase of about 51%.

According to the report, as of March 31, 2022, 8,473 AYUSH doctors were employed in PHCs across the country. Between 2005 and 2022, the number of Nurses and Midwives in SCs and PHCs in rural areas expanded from 133,194 to 207,587, an increase of 55.9%. There is a 3.5% overall shortfall in the number of posts for ANMs and female health workers. The Indian Public Health Standards stipulate that each SC and PHC must have one Health Worker (Female)/ANM.

One thousand two hundred seventy-five sub-divisional hospitals in rural areas were operational, employing roughly 45,992 paramedical staff members and 18,643 doctors. Of the district hospitals in the nation, 767 were operational in rural areas. There were 29,817 physicians and approximately 95,444 paramedics working in these hospitals. In urban CHCs, there were approximately 6,121 nurses, 840 pharmacists, 902 lab technicians, 358 radiologists, and 1,568 general duty medical officers (GDMOs). In urban CHCs, there were many open positions for lab technicians (19.1%), radiographers (32.2%), pharmacists (18%), and nursing staff (19.3%). This discrepancy was between the number of filled and sanctioned posts (Rural Health Statistics, 2021–22, 2023).

Healthcare professionals, policymakers, and domain experts must work together to implement the theoretically promising optimization techniques for healthcare resource allocation in practice. Feedback from individuals familiar with the complexities of healthcare delivery in India is essential to improving the model and guaranteeing its applicability. The allocation of healthcare resources is being revolutionized by swarm intelligence (SI)-based optimization, which provides a flexible and dynamic method to deal with the intricacies of the Indian healthcare system. This optimization technique can improve the overall quality of healthcare services, reduce waiting times, and increase efficiency by utilizing the collective intelligence principles found in ant colonies.

1.2.1 Why Swarm

Let us now think of a scenario where SI might be applied. Think of yourself as Team X's captain. A team of five people needs lunch, which you must order. You have a choice from five various cuisines on the menu today, including Indian, Chinese, Mexican, Italian, and Lebanese. You choose to hold a vote because you must decide on behalf of the entire team. Let us assume two people choose Indian, while one chooses Chinese, Mexican, Italian, and Lebanese. If you choose the food that earned the most votes, you ultimately choose Indian. However, since three people were upset, most were unsatisfied, and Indian food was not the best option.

SI enters the scene in this situation. It produces an ideal solution after examining a group's collective behaviors. It is a real-time system that relies on feedback and influences how the study subjects behave, respond to, and engage with environmental changes. SI is most frequently used when the most preferred and popular solutions do not agree.

SI is one of the innovative approaches that offer hope for a more responsive and optimized healthcare system as India continues to grapple with the demands of a growing population and diverse healthcare needs (Deep *et al.*, 2013; Jeevan & Nair, 2022; Sasaki, 2022; Xia *et al.*, 2014; Yap *et al.*, 2011; Yusof *et al.*, 2021).

1.2.2 Swarm Intelligence

SI is applied to a group of objects' collective behavior to find the best possible solution to a problem. It is a natural or AI technique. It is grounded in studies of human behavior in decentralized, self-organizing networks. Many researchers have applied these techniques in AI (Mishra *et al.*, 2021; Sharma *et al.*, 2021; Hassanien & Darwish, 2020). Gerardo Benny and Joon Wang created SI for the first time in 1989 while working on cellular robotics systems. SI is the collective behavior of autonomous, decentralized systems, whether artificial or natural. Analyzing the collective behaviors of a group generates the optimal solution. It is a real-time feedback-based system that is impacted by the actions, reactions, and interactions of the research subjects in a changing environment (Bozorg-Haddad, 2018). When the most popular and favored solutions disagree, SI is often employed. The aging population has resulted in a constant rise in social demands for surgical services. The operating room (OR) division is an essential hospital component that generates over 40% of a hospital's total revenue and expenses. Therefore, it is imperative to enhance patient flow and optimize OR management to treat patients promptly and best use the resources at hand. Scheduling surgery is essential in OR management (Xiang *et al.*, 2015).

The start time of each operation is to be performed in separate operation groups, and the operation planning determines the resources allocated to each operation over a planned period. Numerous tasks are performed before, during, and after a surgical procedure, referred to as the preoperative, perioperative, and postoperative phases of the entire surgical process. Surgical scheduling is a complex problem because many hospitals use open scheduling, and surgeries are no longer assigned to specific departments. To (1) maximize the efficiency of the OR, (2) increase the number of operations performed daily, and (3) implement various optimization techniques to achieve appropriate resource allocation. Both allocation planning (surgeries are performed in an appropriate order) and advanced scheduling (patients are assigned to ORs, also known as OR planning) are used. Separate combinatorial optimization models are typically used to formulate the two subproblems. The complexity of the problem increases when multiple surgical specialties and all types of resources are considered for each of the three surgical stages in the models.

1.2.3 Research Question

Therefore, "How can we apply optimization techniques for resource allocation like hospital beds, ORs, medical equipment, doctors, and nurses in the healthcare industry of India?" is the problem formulated for the use case of resource allocation optimization for healthcare services.

1.3 SWARM-BASED OPTIMIZATION TECHNIQUES

SWARM-based optimization techniques for resource allocation are suggested in this chapter and are summarized as given below.

1.3.1 Optimization Techniques

1.3.1.1 Ant Colony Optimization

Jing and Gerardo Beni first talked about SI in the context of cellular robotic systems in 1989. It falls under the umbrella of AI and optimization. "Intelligence can be found in the masses." SI calculations aim to utilize this intelligence to determine the optimal configuration. SI is the application of group behavior to find the best possible solution to a particular problem. These collections of items, often called systems, exhibit decentralized control and self-organization. Individuals within a decentralized control system operate independently of one another. The process by which local interactions among initially disorderly components of a system result in some overall order is known as self-organization. The term originated from much research and experimentation on populations of different natural animals, such as termites, ants, fish, birds, and many more. SI can be applied to various real-world issues, such as minimization and maximization. This chapter focuses on SI, which mimics biological swarms as inspiration. Pheromone-based communication, one of the most effective forms of communication, is widespread. Pheromones are used by social insects such as termites, ants, and bees to communicate with individual agents and within swarms. Due to their viability, artificial pheromones are used in multi-robot and swarm robot systems.

There are various applications for pheromone-based communication, such as chemical and physical (Radio Frequency Identification (RFID) tags, light, and sound) approaches. These attempts, meanwhile, were unable to faithfully replicate every characteristic of pheromones present in the natural world. However, these experiments could not faithfully recreate the properties of pheromones found in the natural world. Garnier described projected light, which used as an experimental setup. Another study described a system in which the robots moved on a horizontal LCD screen controlled by pheromones. The robots had downward-facing light sensors to record the patterns they encountered.

1.3.1.1.1 Understanding Ant Colony Optimization

Fundamentally, ant colony optimization (ACO) search for the shortest route between their nest and a food source by imitating the foraging behavior of ants. Artificial ants are used in a computational method to navigate a graph representing potential solutions to an optimization problem, drawing inspiration from biology. Nodes in the graph could represent various healthcare facilities, and edges would indicate connections or potential resource allocations in the context of healthcare resource allocation. The optimization problem must first be formulated in order for ACO to effectively allocate healthcare resources. The goal may be to reduce patient wait times, maximize resource use, or guarantee equitable distribution of healthcare resources in the Indian healthcare system, which is distinguished by a diverse population and a range of regional healthcare needs. Applying the ACO model to healthcare resource allocation requires careful consideration of multiple parameters.

- **Nodes (Locations)**: These are the various locations of healthcare facilities in India, including clinics, hospitals, and health centers.
- **Edges (Connections)**: Indicate possible routes or allocation paths between medical facilities. Factors like patient flow, transportation infrastructure, and geographic distance may impact these.
- **Levels of Pheromones**: Similar to the chemical trails that ants leave behind to communicate, pheromone levels on edges represent the quality or attractiveness of a specific resource allocation path.
- **Ants**: Artificial ants symbolize resources in the healthcare industry, such as ORs, hospital beds, medical equipment, physicians, and nurses. As they travel through the network, these "ants" explore and take advantage of routes determined by heuristic data and pheromone levels.

1.3.1.1.2 Initialization and Pheromone Update

The first step of the ACO algorithm is to scatter artificial ants, which represent healthcare resources, across various areas. As these ants travel through the network, the pheromone levels on edges are updated in response to the quality of the solution. Better resource allocations result in higher pheromone levels, which affect the choices made by the ants that follow.

1.3.1.1.3 Ant Mobility and Local Search

Ants explore and exploit paths iteratively, striking a balance between discovering new solutions and using what they already know. Pheromone levels and heuristic data, like the distance between facilities and the resources' current availability, are combined to make decisions. Local search mechanisms can be added to improve the optimization process by fine-tuning resource allocations according to each healthcare facility's unique local context.

1.3.1.1.4 Considerations for Healthcare in India

The special difficulties and dynamics of the Indian healthcare system must be carefully considered when applying ACO to the distribution of healthcare resources in that country.

- **Dynamic Nature**: An adaptable ACO model that can adjust to changing conditions is required due to the dynamic nature of healthcare demands in India, which are driven by factors like population density, seasonal fluctuations, and disease outbreaks.

- **Regional Variations**: India's healthcare infrastructure and requirements may differ in various regions. The ACO model must be modified to consider these regional differences for it to be effective.
- **Capacity Planning**: An effective model for allocating healthcare resources must consider the current healthcare infrastructure and account for capacity expansions and constraints. ACO can help optimize these processes by adapting quickly to the needs that change.
- **Regulatory Compliance**: Adhering to ethical and regulatory requirements is crucial in the healthcare industry. The ACO model ought to be created with adherence to Indian healthcare laws and moral principles in mind.

1.3.2 Gray Wolf Optimization

Gray wolf optimization (GWO) is a population-based metaheuristic optimization technique inspired by the social behaviors of gray wolves. The method was introduced by the three main stages of a gray wolf's hunting behavior—finding prey, circling prey, and attacking are replicated by GWO. The method is similar in that it consists of three main stages: exploration, convergence, and exploitation. During the exploration step, the gray wolves search the search space randomly to locate the global optimum. Gray wolves modify their placements during the exploitation stage to converge toward the global optimum based on their personal and the pack's best solutions. In order to converge toward the global optimum. The convergence stage is when the gray wolves move their locations to converge on the global optimum (Hassanien & Oliva, 2018).

In the first step of the GWO algorithm, a pack of gray wolves is initially placed in the search space at random. Then, it adjusts their placements according to the gray wolves' fitness values, which are determined by an objective function. The algorithm ends when one or more stopping requirements are met, like a certain number of iterations or a high fitness value. The convergence stage is when the gray wolves move their locations to converge on the global optimum. In the first step of the GWO algorithm, a pack of gray wolves is randomly placed in the search space. Then, the algorithm adjusts their placements according to the gray wolves' fitness values, which are determined by an objective function. The algorithm ends when one or more stopping requirements are met, like a certain number of iterations or a high fitness value.

1.3.2.1 Social Hierarchy

A hierarchical structure with distinct roles and responsibilities characterizes the gray wolf (*Canis lupus*) social organization. The pack is stratified into four primary ranks: A (α), β (β), Δ (δ), and Omega (Ω). Leadership, held by αs, involves decision-making on hunting, resting locations, and waking times. Both male and female individuals can assume α roles, with their directives being obligatory for the entire pack. Notably, α wolves have been observed exhibiting democratic behaviors, occasionally following the lead of other pack members.

During communal gatherings, the entire pack exhibits a submissive gesture, with tails lowered in deference to the α. The term "dominant wolf" is ascribed to the α, emphasizing the expectation that the pack follows the leader's instructions. Exclusive mating privileges are granted to α wolves, underscoring their reproductive significance.

Significantly, selecting the α is based on leadership qualities rather than physical prowess, highlighting the importance of discipline and organization within the pack.

The β rank encompasses wolves that assist the α in decision-making and participate in various pack activities. In the absence or demise of an α, a β, male or female, is a likely candidate for succession. β wolves relay orders from the α and assume disciplinary and advisory roles within the pack.

Wolves falling outside the α, β, and Ω designations are classified as δs. This group includes scouts, guards, seniors, hunters, and caregivers. Scouts monitor territorial boundaries and warn of potential threats, while guards ensure the pack's safety. Seniors, who were previously β or α wolves, contribute their experience, acting as advisors. Hunters, collaborating with αs and βs, provide sustenance for the pack, and caregivers attend to the needs of weak, sick, or injured pack members.

The Ω, the lowest rank, serves as a scapegoat and is subject to all other dominant wolves. Ω wolves have the last priority in accessing food, and their disappearance can induce internal turmoil within the pack. This phenomenon is attributed to the unleashed frustration and discontent of the other wolves, contributing to the maintenance of the dominance hierarchy and overall pack stability. Caretakers may occasionally assume Ω roles in the interest of the pack's well-being.

1.3.2.2 Hunting Mechanism

Beyond their social hierarchy, group hunting is another intriguing facet of gray wolf social behavior. The following are the main phases of gray wolf hunting (Ojala *et al.*, 2002)

- Locating, pursuing, and approaching the victim up close to encircle, harass, and eventually stop it from moving.
- There is an attack on the prey.

1.3.2.3 Strategy

- We have specified our goal, which is the healthcare optimization function.
- The first stage in the GWO method is to initialize a population of gray wolves, each representing a possible resolution.
- The four wolf categories have been applied to the top four solutions. The α wolf symbolizes the best course of action, and the other wolves try to go forward based on this.
- The wolves of the algorithm always aim for the best result obtained thus far in each iteration.
- To help with this, the approach also adds randomization to explore new areas of the search space.

1.4 PROPOSED FRAMEWORK FOR ACO AND GWO IMPLEMENTATION FOR HEALTHCARE RESOURCE ALLOCATION

The graphical representation of the proposed framework is shown in Figure 1.1, followed by the specification of optimization techniques.

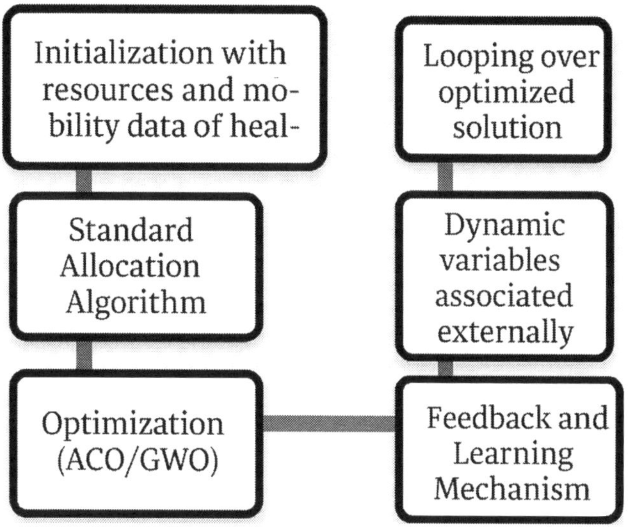

FIGURE 1.1 Framework for the proposed solution.

1.4.1 Ant Colony Optimization Implementation Flowchart

See Figure 1.2

1.4.2 Stages of Ant Colony Optimization (Tan *et al.*, 2012)

- **Initialization**: At this stage, the parameters of the algorithm are set and the problem is defined. These factors include heuristic data, the number of ants, and the rate at which pheromones dissipate. The starting pheromone levels of paths can also be specified.
- **Ant Mobility**: Ants move around the solution space, solving problems through iterative path selection based on pheromone levels and heuristic knowledge. The probability of choosing a particular path depends on the amount of pheromone on the path and the quality of the answer based on heuristic knowledge.
- **Construction of Solutions**: By continually selecting parts or components, ants construct solutions as they go. Depending on the kind of optimization problem being handled, different details apply. For example, in a traveling salesman problem, ants might be creating pathways through cities.
- **Pheromone Update**: After they have constructed solutions, the ants update the pheromone concentrations on the routes. While pheromone on some paths that are a component of better solutions receives more, pheromone on other channels may disappear. This updating process is what allows the algorithm to eventually converge toward optimal solutions.
- **Termination**: The algorithm runs until a predefined number of iterations is reached or when a convergence criterion is met. When the algorithm is done executing, the best answer found by the ants is considered the output.

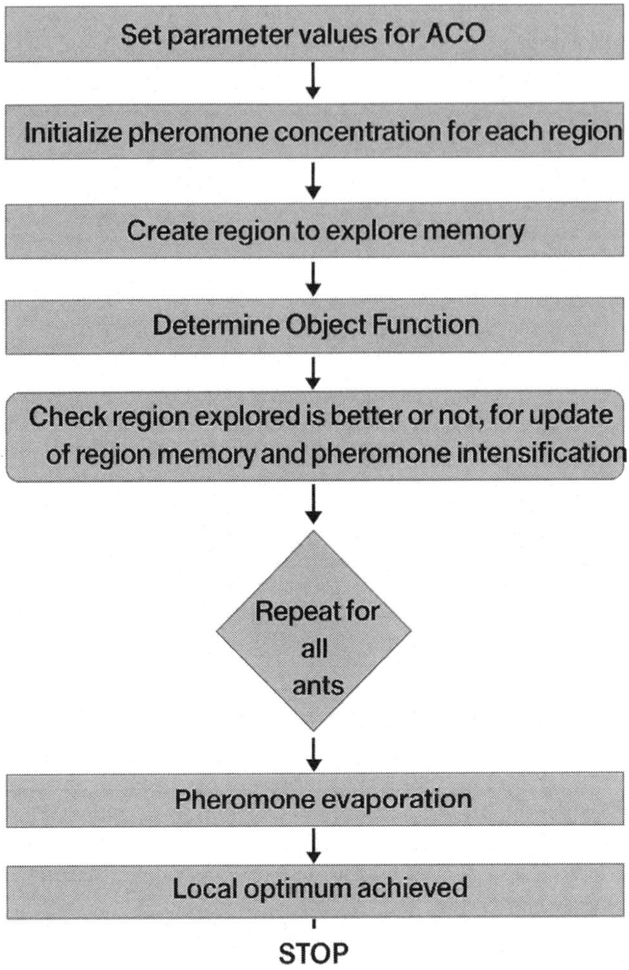

FIGURE 1.2 Flowchart for ant colony optimization.

These actions combined make up the basic building elements of the ACO method. It's crucial to keep in mind that ACO is a metaheuristic, which enables it to be applied to a variety of combinatorial optimization issues by tailoring the solution creation and updating procedures to the specific issue at hand.

1.4.3 Proposed Algorithm with Ant Colony Optimizer to Healthcare Resource Allocation

```
# Define parameters
num_states ← 5 # Number of states in India
num_ants ← 10 # Number of artificial ants
num_iterations ← 50
```

```
pheromone_decay ← 0.1
α ← 1.0 # Influence of pheromone on decision making
β ← 2.0 # Influence of heuristic information on decision
making

# Initialize pheromone levels
pheromones ← np.ones((num_states, num_states))

# Define heuristic information (e.g., healthcare
infrastructure, COVID-19 severity)
heuristic_info ← np.random.rand(num_states, num_states)

# Define constraints (e.g., maximum resource allocation for
each state)
max_allocation ← np.array([100, 150, 120, 200, 180])

# Ant Colony Optimization algorithm
for iteration in range(num_iterations):
  ant_routes ← np.zeros((num_ants, num_states), dtype←int)
  ant_costs ← np.zeros(num_ants)

  for ant in range(num_ants):
    current_state ← np.random.randint(num_states)
    visited_states ← [current_state]

    for step in range(num_states - 1):
      # Calculate probabilities for the next state based on
pheromones and heuristic information
      probabilities ← (pheromones[current_state] ** α) *
(heuristic_info[current_state] ** β)
      probabilities[visited_states] ← 0 # Avoid revisiting
already visited states
      probabilities /← np.sum(probabilities)

      # Choose the next state based on the probabilities
      next_state ← np.random.choice(num_states,
p←probabilities)
      visited_states.append(next_state)

      # Update the cost of the ant's route
      ant_costs[ant] +← heuristic_info[current_state,
next_state]

      current_state ← next_state

    # Check and enforce constraints
    if np.any(ant_routes[ant] > max_allocation):
      ant_costs[ant] ← np.inf # Penalize infeasible solutions
  # Update pheromone levels
  pheromones *← (1 - pheromone_decay)
  for ant in range(num_ants):
```

```
    for i in range(num_states - 1):
      pheromones[ant_routes[ant, i], ant_routes[ant, i + 1]]
+← 1 / ant_costs[ant]
# Obtain the best ant route and resource allocation after
optimization
best_ant ← np.argmin(ant_costs)
best_route ← ant_routes[best_ant]
# Print the best route and its cost
print('Best Ant Route:', best_route)
print('Best Cost:', ant_costs[best_ant])
```

1.4.4 Gray Wolf Optimization Implementation Flowchart

Figure 1.3 shows a flowchart for the implementation of GWO for resource allocation, followed by an illustration of the stages.

1.4.4.1 Stages of Gray Wolf Optimization

- **Establish a Population**: of wolves as a starting point, with each wolf serving as a potential solution to the optimization issue. Distribute the wolves throughout the search area at random.

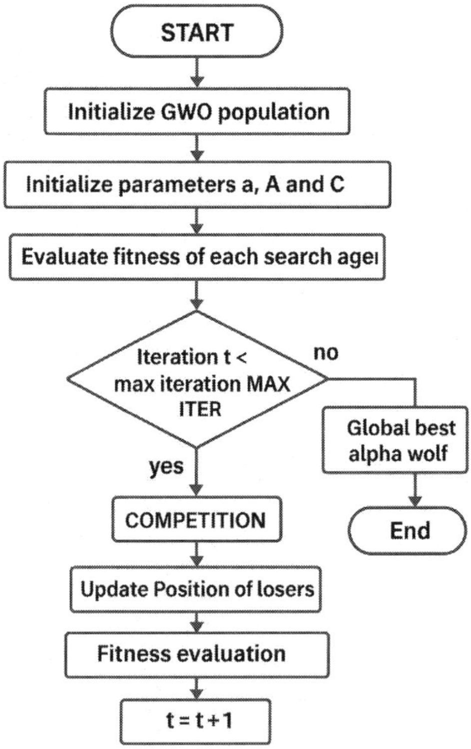

FIGURE 1.3 Flowchart for gray wolf optimization.

- **Assessment of the Objective Function**: Assess the objective function for every wolf in the population. The problem that has to be optimized is represented by the objective function.
- **The Wolves' ranking**: Sort the wolves according to the values of their objective function or fitness. The problem being solved determines the fitness: larger values are better for situations involving maximizing, whereas lower values are better for those involving minimization.
- **δ, β, and A Decision**: From the population, choose the α, β, and δ wolves. The search will be led by these wolves, who are the pack leaders. The highest fitness value belongs to the α wolf, the second-best to the β, and the third-best to the δ.
- **Update Wolves' Positions**: Using the positions of the α, β, and δ wolves as a guide, update the positions of every wolf in the population. The α, β, and δ wolf positions, as well as the present positions of the wolves, are taken into account in particular algorithms to calculate the new positions.
- **Verifying Boundaries**: Verify whether the wolves' new positions cross any boundaries or restrictions unique to the problem. If so, modify the positions to make sure they are feasible.
- **Evaluation of the Objective Function Once More**: Analyze the objective function for the wolves' revised positions.
- **Update A, β, and Δ**: Following the position update, the α, β, and δ wolves are updated according to the new fitness values.
- **Termination Criteria**: Verify if a requirement for termination is satisfied. Depending on the challenge, this could be a set number of iterations, a workable solution, or other requirements.
- **Return Outcome**: As the outcome, return the optimal solution discovered throughout the optimization process.

1.4.5 Proposed Algorithm for Gray Wolf Optimizer to Healthcare Resource Allocation

```
# Define parameters
population_size ← 20
max_iterations ← 100
a ← 2 # A
b ← 2 # β
d ← 1 # Δ
# Define the objective function to be minimized
def objective_function(state_resource_allocation):
  # Your specific objective function to be minimized (e.g.,
cost function)
  pass
# Initialize the population of wolf packs
population ← []
for _ in range(population_size):
  wolf ← {
    'state_resource_allocation': {
```

```
        'state1': random.uniform(0, 1), # Resource allocation
for state 1
        'state2': random.uniform(0, 1), # Resource allocation
for state 2
        # Add resource allocation parameters for other states
      },
      'fitness': None
    }
    population.append(wolf)
# Main optimization loop
for iteration in range(max_iterations):
    for wolf in population:
      wolf['fitness'] ←
objective_function(wolf['state_resource_allocation'])

    # Sort the wolves by fitness (minimize the objective
function)
    population.sort(key←lambda x: x['fitness'])
    α, β, δ ← population[:3]
    for wolf in population:
      a1, a2, a3 ← random.random(), random.random(), random.
random()
      # Update wolf's position
      for state in wolf['state_resource_allocation']:
          wolf['state_resource_allocation'][state] ← (
            α['state_resource_allocation'][state] - a1 * abs(2 *
a1 * α['state_resource_allocation'][state] - wolf['state_
resource_allocation'][state]) +
            β['state_resource_allocation'][state] - a2 * abs(2 *
a2 * β['state_resource_allocation'][state] - wolf['state_
resource_allocation'][state]) +
            δ['state_resource_allocation'][state] - a3 * abs(2 *
a3 * δ['state_resource_allocation'][state] - wolf['state_
resource_allocation'][state])
          )
# Obtain the best resource allocation after optimization
best_allocation ← population[0]['state_resource_allocation']
best_fitness ← population[0]['fitness']
# Print the best resource allocation and its fitness value
print('Best Resource Allocation:', best_allocation)
print('Best Fitness Value:', best_fitness)
```

1.4.6 Implementation, Analysis, and Inferences

Numerous optimization problems are tackled by metaheuristic optimization techniques such as ACO and GWO. They have several similarities, but also have several significant differences. One of the primary distinctions between GWO and ACO is their inspiration. GWO was modeled after the social behavior of gray wolves, while

ACO was modeled after the foraging behaviors of ants. Consequently, how the algorithms operate and search the search space differs (MacLean, 2013). Another noteworthy distinction is the level of collaboration and communication within the population. Ant cooperation and communication are essential for ACO to find the optimal solution. Conversely, GWO does not require the gray to collaborate and communicate as much.

In contrast, GWO does not require as much communication and collaboration among the gray wolves because each one makes their own decisions based on their own experiences and the experiences of the entire pack. The specific problem being tackled determines how effective both methods are in performance. While continuous optimization challenges have been effectively resolved with GWO, finding the shortest path and the least spanning tree problems have been successfully solved using ACO.

Although ACO's performance in resource allocation was subpar, its average improvement over GWO in terms of solution quality was 8.27. GWO's sensitivity to the starting population was a problem. Additionally, the ACO algorithm tends to become trapped at local minima. All in all, every method has benefits and drawbacks, and the optimal choice will rely on the specifics of the optimization task and the nature of the problem at hand. As shown in Figures 1.4 and 1.5, the convergence matrix for ACO and GWO techniques simplifies the decision, stating that the fastest reach of healthcare resources using the shortest path could be the possible usage of ACO. In contrast, GWO, when used for continuous improvement, can lead to better solutions when considering the inclusion of external variables.

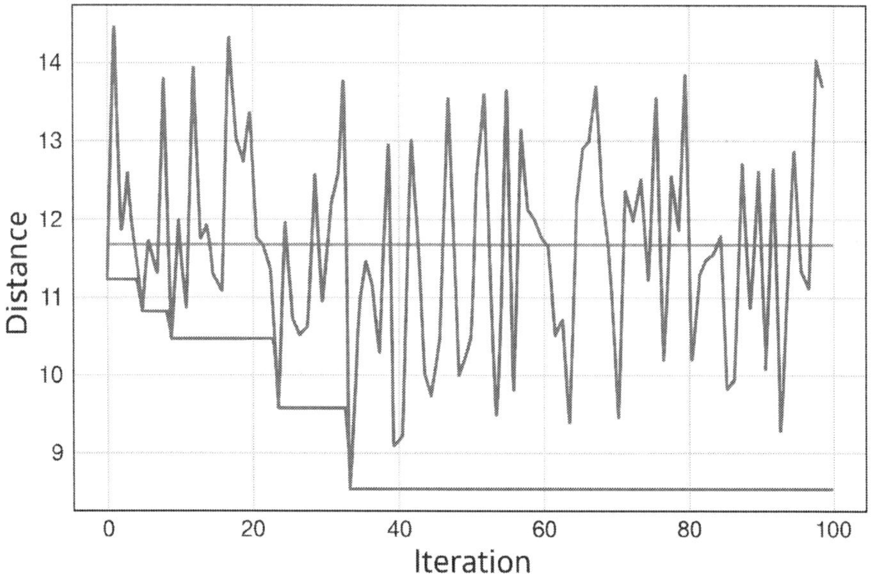

FIGURE 1.4 Convergence matrix for ACO.

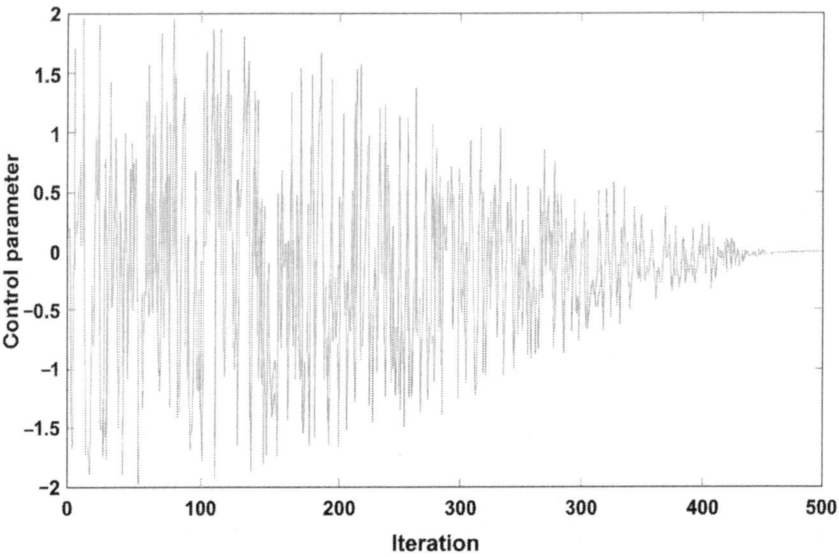

FIGURE 1.5 Convergence matrix for GWO.

1.5 CONCLUSION

ACO and GWO are metaheuristic algorithms that have proven effective in solving healthcare resource allocation problems. The foraging behavior of ants inspires ACO, while the hunting behavior of gray wolves inspires GWO. Both algorithms can find reasonable solutions to healthcare resource allocation problems relatively quickly. However, there are some key differences between the two algorithms. ACO is a stochastic algorithm, while GWO is a deterministic algorithm. This means that ACO is more likely to explore the search space, while GWO is more likely to exploit the search space. As a result, ACO is better at finding new and innovative solutions, while GWO is better at refining existing solutions. In general, ACO is a good choice for healthcare resource allocation problems that require a high level of exploration. At the same time, GWO is a good choice for healthcare resource allocation problems requiring high exploitation.

REFERENCES

Bozorg-Haddad, O. (Ed.). (2018). *Advanced Optimization by Nature-Inspired Algorithms* (Vol. 720). Springer Singapore. https://doi.org/10.1007/978-981-10-5221-7

Deep, K., Arya, M., Thakur, M., & Raman, B. (2013). Stereo camera calibration using particle swarm optimization. *Applied Artificial Intelligence*, *27*(7), 618–634. https://doi.org/10.1080/08839514.2013.813191

Hassanien, A. E., & Darwish, A. (2020). *Swarm Intelligence for Resource Management in Internet of Things*. Elsevier. https://doi.org/10.1016/C2018-0-03865-7

Hassanien, A. E., & Oliva, D. A. (Eds.). (2018). *Advances in Soft Computing and Machine Learning in Image Processing* (Vol. 730). Springer International Publishing. https://doi.org/10.1007/978-3-319-63754-9

Jeevan, J., & Nair, M. S. (2022). On the performance analysis of solving the Rubik's cube using swarm intelligence algorithms. *Applied Artificial Intelligence*, *36*(1), 2138129. https://doi.org/10.1080/08839514.2022.2138129

MacLean, D. (2013). Cutting edge: Changing the rules of the game. *eLife*, *2*, e01294. https://doi.org/10.7554/eLife.01294

Mishra, S., Sagban, R., Yakoob, A., & Gandhi, N. (2021). Swarm intelligence in anomaly detection systems: An overview. *International Journal of Computers and Applications*, *43*(2), 109–118. https://doi.org/10.1080/1206212X.2018.1521895

Ojala, T., Pietikainen, M., & Maenpaa, T. (2002). Multiresolution gray-scale and rotation invariant texture classification with local binary patterns. *IEEE Transactions on Pattern Analysis and Machine Intelligence*, *24*(7), 971–987. https://doi.org/10.1109/TPAMI.2002.1017623

Rural Health Statistics, 2021–22. (2023). https://ruralindiaonline.org/en/library/resource/rural-health-statistics-2021-22/

Sasaki, H. (2022). Emulating Heterogeneity of Individuals and Visualizing Its Influence on Ant Swarm Migration. *Applied Artificial Intelligence*, *36*(1), 2138120. https://doi.org/10.1080/08839514.2022.2138120

Sharma, A., Sharma, A., Pandey, J. K., & Ram, M. (2021). *Swarm Intelligence: Foundation, Principles, and Engineering Applications* (1st ed.). CRC Press. https://doi.org/10.1201/9781003090038

Tan, Y., Shi, Y., & Ji, Z. (Eds.). (2012). *Advances in Swarm Intelligence: Third International Conference, ICSI 2012,* Shenzhen, China, June 17–20, 2012 Proceedings, Part I (Vol. 7331). Springer Berlin Heidelberg. https://doi.org/10.1007/978-3-642-30976-2

Xia, L., Chu, J., & Geng, Z. (2014). A multiswarm competitive particle swarm algorithm for optimization control of an ethylene cracking furnace. *Applied Artificial Intelligence*, *28*(1), 30–46. https://doi.org/10.1080/08839514.2014.862772

Xiang, W., Yin, J., & Lim, G. (2015). An ant colony optimization approach for solving an operating room surgery scheduling problem. *Computers & Industrial Engineering*, *85*, 335–345. https://doi.org/10.1016/j.cie.2015.04.010

Yap, D. F. W., Koh, S. P., Tiong, S. K., & Prajindra, S. K. (2011). A Swarm-based artificial immune system for solving multimodal functions. *Applied Artificial Intelligence*, *25*(8), 693–707. https://doi.org/10.1080/08839514.2011.606662

Yusof, N. M., Muda, A. K., & Pratama, S. F. (2021). Swarm intelligence-based feature selection for Amphetamine-Type Stimulants (ATS) drug 3D molecular structure classification. *Applied Artificial Intelligence*, *35*(12), 914–932. https://doi.org/10.1080/08839514.2021.1966882

2 AI-Based Decision Support Systems for Personalized Maternal Health Management before Pregnancy

Gopal B. Deshmukh, Satyajit Pangaonkar, Parikshit N. Mahalle, Surendra Rahamatkar, Dattatray G. Takale, and Mahesh Shinde

2.1 INTRODUCTION

The conservation of prepregnancy health is essential for positive maternal and fetal outcomes. Traditionally, maternal health care was focused on the care of pregnant women. However, there is increasing awareness of the fact that many pregnancy complications depend on preconception factors. The woman's health before the pregnancy is essential to her well-being and the pregnancy [1]. The development of pregnancy outcomes depends on lifestyle, genetics, medical history, and environmental exposures. However, these can be managed before pregnancy to ensure having a healthy pregnancy and minimize risks of gestational diabetes, preeclampsia, and preterm birth, thereby having healthier pregnancies [2].

Prepregnancy health has been changed because of a paradigm change due to the growing demand for personalized healthcare. Unlike general medical advice, where fit medical advice is given, the healthcare systems have turned to a woman-specific risk assessment and risk-based treatment recommendations based on a unique woman's health profile. This has also paved the way for these new technologies to be embraced in prepregnancy care, like artificial intelligence (AI) and machine learning (ML). These technologies enable healthcare providers to use large, complex datasets to identify a mother's health more accurately and individually, giving women more personal information to choose when they have prepregnancy care [3].

At the most forward end of this technological transformation are AI-based decision support systems (DSS). DSS is a computerized tool to aid healthcare providers in making clinical decisions based on call evidence, recommendations, and predictions. In prepregnancy health, AI-based DSS can analyze multifaceted data, including medical history and genetics, lifestyle and environmental factors, and make

 DOI: 10.1201/9781003479185-2

predictions and recommendations for the packaged patient by patient. These systems can be used to view prepregnancy health from another angle, searching for chances to identify health problems they can't spot by regular clinical screening.

One of AI and ML's strongest suits is efficiently processing massive datasets with many variables, and even if clinicians can't see a pattern or relationship, AI and ML algorithms can. These systems use complex, multicomponent data from multiple sources to deliver highly accurate risk assessments and personalized health recommendations. For example, AI systems can use a woman's electronic medical health records, information about medical history, previous pregnancies, and any preexisting conditions to predict their chances of complications in future pregnancies. Data from wearable health devices that track real-time metrics like activity levels, heart rates, and sleep patterns can also be incorporated to get a more holistic picture of a woman's health status [4].

This includes genetic data, as several medical records are being used to predict the risk of certain potentially dangerous diseases during pregnancy. Genomic medicine has developed to the level of having genetic screening for conditions such as cystic fibrosis, sickle cell anemia, and other hereditary conditions that might disrupt pregnancy. In addition, these genetic markers can be amalgamated with other health data to create a more precise and targeted risk profile if AI systems can do this [5].

Another essential component of prepregnancy health is the toxic and other harmful substances and pollutants one has been exposed to in the environment. Several of these environmental factors can have a long-term impact on a woman's fertility and pregnancy outcomes. One example is that exposure to certain chemicals, such as pesticides or endocrine disrupters, increases the risk of infertility and pregnancy complications. Environmental data feeds to the AI, along with patient-specific data, which allows it to quantify how associated exposures affect health before conception [6].

In addition, factors within a woman's lifestyle, such as diet, exercise, smoking, alcohol consumption, and stress levels, are essential determinants of a woman's overall health and fertility. AI-based DSS can use data from health surveys, self-reported questionnaires, and wearable health devices to evaluate a woman's lifestyle, identify those who had positive/lack of lifestyle during prepregnancy, and predict the impact of lifestyle at prepregnancy. Let's assume that a woman has a sedentary lifestyle, not a very good diet, and a high stress level. She may be more at risk for complications like gestational diabetes or preeclampsia. AI systems can suggest particular changes in lifestyle, such as a change in diet, exercise routine, or stress management technique to enhance health outcomes [7].

Personalization of care is one of the most crucial advantages of DSS based on AI. In traditional healthcare models, generalized guidelines are used, which are not necessarily individualized based on health status, genetics, or lifestyle. AI systems can make recommendations tailored to each woman's particular health profile. These systems continually integrate new data into women's healthcare visits, wearables, and other sources, and their predictions and recommendations adapt over time, ensuring women receive the best and most current information on their prepregnancy path.

While the implementation of DSS based on AI in prepregnancy care has its challenges. A significant challenge is data privacy and security. As the information is sensitive, it has to be stored and transmitted securely, and in general, all of the information related to the patient has to be appropriately managed. Patient confidentiality requires strict data protection regulations such as the general data protection regulation (GDPR) and the health insurance portability and accountability act (HIPAA). Data quality is another key factor as well. The success of the AI models heavily depends on the quality of the data they are trained on; therefore, accurate, complete, and unbiased data is critical.

Another complication is the necessity for interdisciplinarity between the AI experts, the healthcare providers, and the policymakers. With the aim of AI to revolutionize prepregnancy care, it should and can be implemented with the collaboration of professionals in computer science, medicine, public health, and ethics. AI-powered DSS must be used effectively by healthcare providers, and all patients must be educated on the benefits and the trade-offs of these systems. In addition, AI models have to undergo extensive clinical trials to validate this efficacy and safety; only then can they fully integrate into the healthcare practice.

2.1.1 Contribution of This Chapter

- **Introduction to Prepregnancy Health**: This chapter emphasizes the importance of prepregnancy health management and its powerful influence on maternal and fetal outcomes.
- **Role of AI in Maternal Health**: The chapter discusses AI and ML in prepregnancy risk assessment, predicting and avoiding pregnancy complications before conception.
- **Personalized Healthcare Approach**: The chapter highlights how AI-based DSS facilitate personalized healthcare by recommending and personalizing the recommendations according to an individual's specific health profile.
- **Integration of Multidimensional Data**: It covers the integration of diverse data sources such as electronic health records (EHRs), genetic data, lifestyle factors, and environmental exposures into AI models for comprehensive prepregnancy risk assessment.
- **Future Prospects**: Finally, the chapter concludes with a discussion of the advantages and future direction of AI-enabled prepregnancy health management that can improve health outcomes and better decision-making.

This chapter develops and applies AI-based DSS to create a personalized prepregnancy risk assessment and health management system. It stresses how prepregnancy health is essential as it is related to poor pregnancy outcomes in developing the mothers and babies, effects of lifestyle, medical history, genetics, and environment, without which pregnancy outcomes can be significantly affected [8]. The chapter then discusses the application of AI for processing mixed complex health data in EHRs, wearables, genetics, and environmental factors to inform the prediction of prepregnancy risks and the generation of personalized health recommendations. It then displays the supplementary part, which features the second means of fabricating AI-based DSS, comprising data preprocessing, model selection (XGBoost, LightGBM neural network), and performance evaluation using accuracy, F1, and the area under the receiver operating characteristic curve (AUC-ROC). Additionally, it discusses the use of deep Q-network (DQN) for the development of personalized real recommendations for therapy, for example, medication, lifestyle adjustment, and follow-up schemes [9]. Exploring the system also allows us to constantly improve recommendations by adapting the system to new patient data and expert feedback. In conclusion, this chapter reveals how AI can enhance the two pillars of prepregnancy health management – risk assessment and data-driven decision-making – to allow women planning pregnancy to make more informed and data-driven health care decisions [10].

2.2 UNDERSTANDING PREPREGNANCY HEALTH MANAGEMENT

Maternal care, with a special emphasis on prepregnancy health, is a vital factor for pregnancy outcomes both for the mother and for the developing fetus. There is a close association of a woman's health status before conception with factors like birth weight, preterm birth, and development of gestational conditions such as diabetes, hypertension, and preeclampsia. There is a significant role in conditioning the course of the pregnancy and the health of the newborn delivery, and the background or underlying conditions and risk factors present before conception play that role. Addressing these factors will prevent complications, improve maternal well-being, and ensure that pregnancy proceeds smoothly [11].

2.2.1 Key Factors Influencing Prepregnancy Health

- **Maternal Age**: A woman's age is one of the significant risk factors that impact pregnancy. Although not proven with parallel trials, the risk of complications like gestational diabetes, chromosomal abnormalities, and preterm labor increases with the advancing maternal age. However, there are risks to pregnancy for women who are too young (especially under 18) because of physical and emotional immaturity, and that might affect pregnancy outcomes. Consequently, it is essential to understand maternal age in conjunction with other factors for prepregnancy health assessments [12].
- **Body Mass Index**: The risk of complications during pregnancy is strongly correlated with a woman's body mass index (BMI) before pregnancy. Women who are too thin may have trouble conceiving or have babies who are low birth weight or born too soon. On the other hand, obese or overweight women are at an increased risk of gestational diabetes, hypertension, preeclampsia, and delivery complications. To minimize these risks, managing BMI through proper diet and exercise before becoming pregnant is key [13].
- **Lifestyle Choices**: It is known that factors associated with a woman's lifestyle, such as smoking, alcohol use, poor diet, or lack of exercise, are, despite all the things above, very deleterious for mothers and pregnancy outcomes. For example, smoking causes low birth weight, preterm birth, and problems with the placenta. It also seems as though micronutrient deficiencies, poor diets, gestational diabetes, and other complications may be avoided if the connection can be linked. Nevertheless, regular physical activity is good for

health. In addition to helping manage weight, reducing stress, and enhancing cardiovascular health (which are all very important during pregnancy), it can also assist in increasing your energy levels, particularly if you have poor sleeping patterns.

- **Reproductive Health History**: Women with gestational diabetes, preeclampsia, preterm birth, or stillbirth are more likely to suffer the same in the following pregnancies. In this case, then, a proper understanding of a woman's reproductive health history is necessary to identify potential risks and an appropriate method of managing them before conception [14].
- **Chronic Conditions**: Among these conditions, pregnancy complication risk increases when the conditions need to be treated for an extended period, such as diabetes, hypertension, thyroid disorders, autoimmune diseases, etc. Such examples include the fact that women with diabetes (type 1, type 2, or gestational) have an increased risk of developing gestational diabetes in pregnancy and other complications, such as having a baby who is of higher birth weight or born preterm. Hypertension can lead to placental abruption and preeclampsia. These chronic conditions should be well-managed before pregnancy [15].
- **Environmental Factors**: Environmental exposures to toxins, pollutants, and chemical and endocrine-disrupting substances also impact prepregnancy health. An example of this type of exposure is linked to fertility issues, miscarriage, and pregnancy complications due to exposure to air pollution, pesticides, or endocrine-disrupting chemicals (found in plastics, personal care products, etc.). Women can avoid exposure before conception, considering environmental factors.

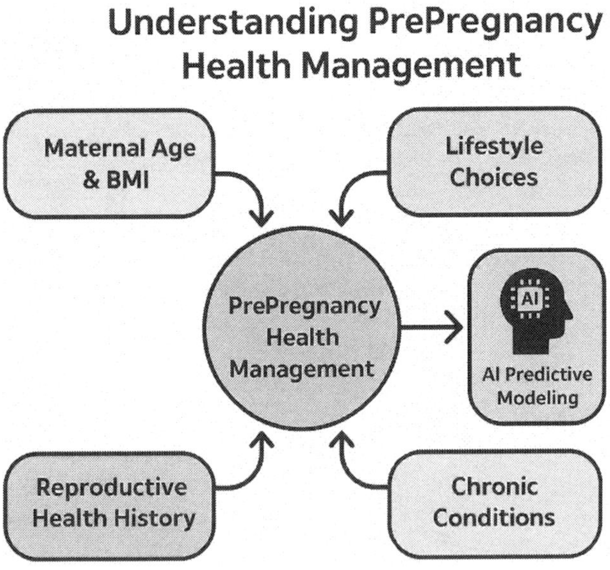

FIGURE 2.1 Parameter of prepregnancy health management.

2.3 THE ROLE OF AI IN MATERNAL HEALTH

One area where artificial intelligence (AI) technologies and their specific ML, deep learning, and, more recently, reinforcement learning (RL) applications have become a real force of nature in healthcare is in their ability to process massive multidimensional datasets, identify complex patterns perhaps impossible for clinicians to extract from, and interpret these patterns in a clinical or actionable context. Where maternal health is concerned, AI has the potential to transform how prepregnancy care takes place, with the ability to provide an accurate risk assessment, personalized health recommendations, and the support needed for medical interventions and lifestyle modification [16].

2.3.1 Predicting Health Risks

AI is particularly valuable in predicting various health risks that could affect a woman before and during pregnancy. Some of the critical risks that AI can help predict include:

- **Gestational Diabetes**: ML models can look at various factors to predict whether you'll develop gestational diabetes, including BMI, age, blood glucose levels, and family medical history. By making this early prediction, healthcare providers can recommend preventive measures (for example, lifestyle changes: diet, increased physical activity), glucose monitoring, or early screening for gestational diabetes [17].
- **Preeclampsia**: One can use deep learning algorithms to analyze variables like blood pressure, protein levels in urine, maternal age, and the previous history of preeclampsia to predict the risk of developing preeclampsia in future pregnancies. Early identification of high-risk women allows for closer monitoring, medications to lower blood pressure, and lifestyle changes to prevent the onset of preeclampsia [18].
- **Infertility**: AI systems can also predict infertility by evaluating such factors as genetic markers, the ovulation cycle, and hormonal levels. Knowing that you may have some fertility issues before pregnancy can help healthcare providers to suggest interventions, for example, to try to improve your chances of falling pregnant as fertility treatments or lifestyle changes.

2.3.2 Personalizing Health Recommendations

The biggest plus of AI is that it can give personalized healthcare recommendations based on an individual's health profile. It is prepregnancy care where AI models advise using various factors. Some examples include:

- **Dietary Modifications**: AI models can use data from health surveys, food logs, or wearable devices to identify dietary habits and suggest particular nutritional changes. For instance, a woman with high blood pressure may be advised to follow a low-sodium diet, and a woman with a history of gestational diabetes may be counseled to eat a low-carb or balanced glycemic index diet during pregnancy to avoid complications.

- **Exercise and Lifestyle Modifications**: Secondly, AI systems can also propose personalized exercise plans, including input based on factors like current activity level, BMI, and, in general, health status. The AI system can suggest low-impact exercises such as walking, swimming, or yoga for women at risk for gestational diabetes or hypertension as ways to keep their weight and their hearts healthy.
- **Mental Health Recommendations**: Physical health and mental well-being are only a part of prepregnancy health. Mental health strategies offered by AI models can include analysis of factors beyond the prescription of medicine, for instance, stress levels, emotional well-being, and history of mental health issues (anxiety and depression). These might include stress reduction techniques such as mindfulness and meditation, counseling recommendations, or therapies to reduce stress during pregnancy [19].

2.3.3 Offering Decision Support for Lifestyle Modifications and Medical Interventions

Healthcare providers use AI-based DSS to help make informed decisions concerning lifestyle shifts and medical intervention before pregnancy. These systems integrate a woman's health data and guess the most suitable actions from her health status.

- **Lifestyle Modifications**: By its design, AI systems can help clinicians make recommendations. For example, an AI system could call the attention of women with a high BMI or poor diet and suggest an individualized weight loss or dietary program consistent with the best practice evidence of improving prepregnancy-pregnancy health. To coach daily behavior, the system may suggest tracking caloric intake through mobile apps, stress, or sleep patterns, which wearable devices can track.
- **Medical Interventions**: DSS using AI can also help decide the medical interventions that can be done before pregnancy. For example, suppose a woman is at high risk for gestational diabetes. In that case, the system might suggest early screening or prescribe medication (e.g., metformin) before trying to become pregnant to reduce the risk of developing diabetes during pregnancy. It could also recommend, before conception, low-dose aspirin as a preventive measure for women with a history of preeclampsia [20].

2.3.4 AI Model Analysis: Factors and Prediction

AI systems can analyze a variety of factors to offer predictive risk assessments. These factors include:

- **BMI and Weight**: Accordingly, AI can examine a woman's BMI to forecast complications, including gestational diabetes and preterm birth.

- **Age**: Maternal age can be factored as an advanced model that weighs the effects on pregnancy risks and advises women in older age groups on possible interventions or screening protocols.
- **Family Medical History**: This helps to incorporate family history data, and thereby, identify hereditary conditions that may predispose to risks (typically genetic disorders) and inform prepregnant genetic counseling or testing.

These combined factors can be delivered in the form of tailored health advice through AI models, which is beneficial for women and healthcare providers. It allows them to make reasonable decisions on prepregnancy care, interventions, and lifestyle changes, increasing the possibility of a healthy pregnancy and reducing the risk of complications [21].

2.4 DATA COLLECTION FOR AI-BASED DSS

Data collection is the basis for building accurate and personalized predictions in the AI-based DSS context for prepregnancy risk assessment. However, the AI model should draw knowledge from multidimensional data sets, combining information from many sources to complete the load for interpreting information on each individual's highly complex health profile. The following sections detail the critical data sources needed to create an all-inclusive prepregnancy risk assessment system.

- **EHRs**: They are one of the most critical data sources, an iota of which is every individual's complete medical history. Past diagnoses of chronic conditions such as hypertension, diabetes, and thyroid disorders, which can have an impact on pregnancy outcomes, are also included. As a result, EHRs are filled with information about previous related pregnancies and, for example, having had preeclampsia, gestational diabetes, preterm birth, or a miscarriage to help estimate the future risks. EHRs also document chronic conditions, such as autoimmune diseases or heart problems that could influence pregnancy, as well as fertility drugs or insulin, both important to experience preconceptionally healthy and minimize risks.
- **Genetic Data**: It shares information about the risks of inherited conditions and inherent predispositions that may affect the successful delivery of the baby. Nevertheless, with the evolution of genomic medicine, genomic test results are now included in AI-based DSS to forecast different conditions. Identifying genetic markers can determine whether an inherited disease includes cystic fibrosis, sickle cell anemia, or thalassemia and give insight into how healthy the child is during pregnancy. Also, genetic data can indicate fertility problems to forecast conception chances or to advise assisted reproductive methods, for example, IVF or IUI. Additionally, several chromosomal abnormalities, such as Down syndrome or other trisomy disorders based on genetic predisposition, are expected, and early screening or genetic counseling is scheduled for the worsening possibility.

- **Lifestyle Data**: It allows you to determine a woman's level of preparedness for pregnancy and discover potential health threats. This includes surveys, questionnaires, or wearable devices (that measure habits of poor nutrition, high sugar consumption, vitamin deficits, absence or presence of exercise, substance use, smoking, alcohol, and pepper, etc.; and stress, anxiety, depression, etc.). These factors are directly linked to the list of poor diet and lack of physical activity, the rising risk of gestational diabetes and obesity, substance use, and stress for preterm birth and miscarriage. From this lifestyle data, it is possible to generate information that AI systems can float out to pregnant people or their partners with recommendations about reducing the risk of complications and improving maternal health before pregnancy.
- **Prepregnancy Health**: Data assists in evaluating prepregnancy health as environmental factors like toxins, pollutants, and chemicals can impact maternal and fetal health tremendously. Mainly, when PM2.5 was concerned, researchers have found that air pollution increases the risk of preterm birth, low birth weight, and gestational hypertension. Pesticides and plastics containing chemicals such as BPA that are endocrine disruptors can adversely affect fertility and pregnancy outcomes. Even in the workplace, hazards like radiation, chemicals, or high levels of stress can throw hormones out of balance and lead to fertility issues or pregnancy problems. Knowing about exposures to these substances enables us to determine risks and make recommendations to reduce known harmful environmental exposures before conception [22].
- **Wearable devices Data**: Wearable devices and health tracking technologies have a role in optimizing prepregnancy health. Key metrics of your hypertension or cardiovascular problems that can have adverse effects on pregnancy outcomes are monitored by these devices. As physical activity status, including steps, exercise routines, general activity, etc., links directly to fitness and readiness for pregnancy, tracking this information is continuous. Also, sleep patterns are tracked because disturbances in sleep can affect hormone balance and fertility. Real-time data analysis by AI systems can then recommend better cardiovascular health, better physical fitness, and more optimal sleep, all of which help you get into a healthier prepregnancy state [23].

2.5 METHODOLOGY FOR BUILDING AI-BASED DSS FOR PREPREGNANCY RISK ASSESSMENT

Figure 2.3 shows a multilayered architecture for the AI-based DSS for prepregnancy risk assessment. Data collection starts from multiple sources such as EHRs, genetic and lifestyle data, environmental exposure data, and real-time health data from wearable devices. First, the data is preprocessed so the ML models (XGBoost and random forest [RF]) can be used to predict risk. Real-time health monitoring and continuous learning with new data are integrated, and personalized treatment

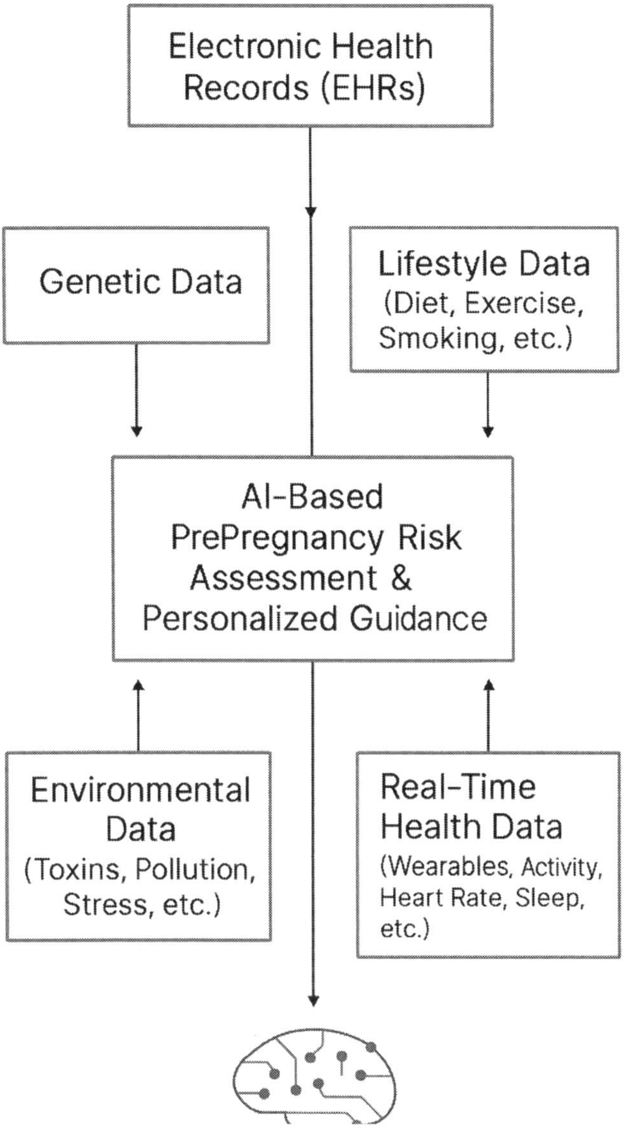

FIGURE 2.2 Different data collection methods.

recommendations are determined with DQN. The architecture allows systematic and customized health guidance to healthcare providers to make a safer choice regarding prepregnancy health management.

Data Collection: The first aspect of the system architecture is data collection from various sources. EHRs control medical histories ranging from chronic conditions to previous pregnancies to treatments. Fetal inheritance complicates pregnancy outcomes, and genetic data can provide information about inherited conditions. Diet, exercise, and substance use are captured from lifestyle data collected from surveys

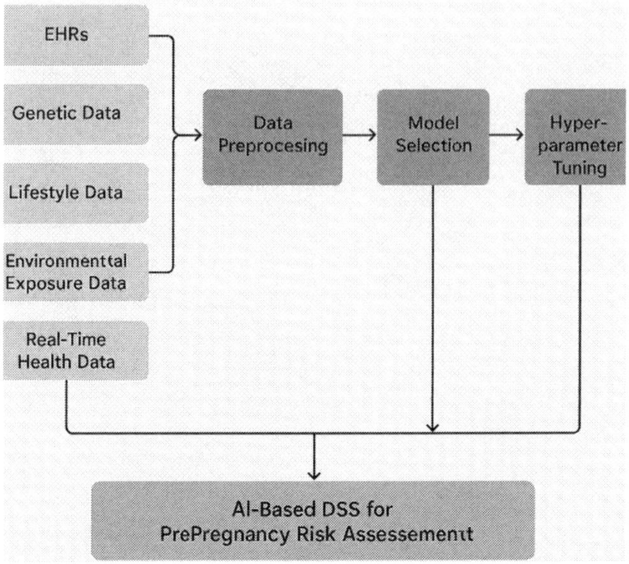

FIGURE 2.3 System architecture.

or wearable health trackers. External factors, such as environmental toxicants, pollutants, and workplace hazards, are provided as context for environmental exposure data around maternal health. The last component is real-time health data from wearable devices, which continuously update key metrics like heart rate, activity levels, and sleep patterns, allowing continuous risk assessment.

Data Preprocessing: The data then undergoes preprocessing of cleaning and standardizing data. For this step, data cleaning is done to handle the missing values or inconsistencies, feature engineering is done to have new variables that are more predictive, and normalization is done to scale the continuous variables of blood pressure and glucose levels. Also, data balancing techniques like SMOTE are used to solve class imbalance, ensuring that the model does not overstress toward the majority class (i.e., low risk) and handles high-risk cases correctly.

Model Selection: The next step after preprocessing is choosing the correct ML models according to the dataset's complexity level and nature. When it comes to complex, high-dimensional, nonlinear relationships, there is no better solution than RF and also other popular XGBoost. In addition, neural networks can be used for more sophisticated models (in terms of special cases or large, unstructured datasets, e.g., genetic or environmental). The preprocessed data will be trained on the selected models to predict the risk for the gestational patient in prepregnancy health for risk in gestational diabetes, rule of preeclampsia.

RF: In a RF, many decision trees are built and combined to get better predictive accuracy. It features a solid performance on extensive, high-dimensional data and can capture the nonlinearity of the data. It is immune to overfitting, gives feature importance practical in interpreting model results, and has a straightforward interpretation.

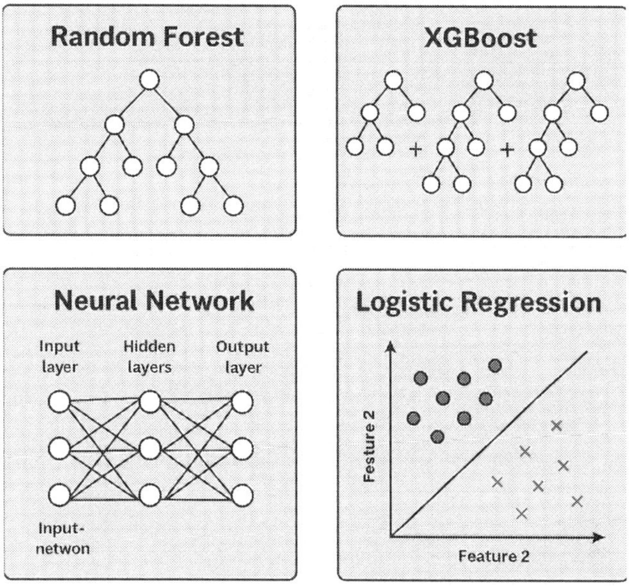

FIGURE 2.4 Architectures for random forest, XGBoost, neural network, and logistic regression.

XGBoost: XGBoost is a gradient-boosting algorithm that works. Iteratively, it gradually puts together the decision trees one after another, with one of them rectifying the errors made by the previous one. Known to be high-performance and especially good at handling imbalanced datasets, its function is handy when there are complicated interactions between features. Moreover, it is also computationally efficient compared to traditional decision trees.

Neural Networks: Deep learning models of artificial neural networks (ANNs) can learn complex nonlinear functions from large data sets. They are particularly useful when the dataset is high-dimensional or unstructured (e.g., genetic or environmental data). Traditional ML models are less flexible than deep learning models, but need less data and resources.

Logistic Regression: Logistic regression can be used for more straightforward binary classification tasks (high-risk vs. low-risk pregnancies). It's a well-understood model and not as powerful as ensemble methods nor as weak as deep learning and is, therefore, a good baseline to compare other methods against.

Model Training: ML algorithms are trained on the preprocessed data during the model training phase. Lastly, the cross-validation technique ensures the model fit is not overfitting and generalizes well to unseen data. Training models start by feeding them historical data to learn patterns and associations in the dataset. The system is trained by iteratively adjusting model parameters to predict pregnancy risks with high accuracy, given the inputs from the data collection process.

Hyperparameter Tuning: To increase performance, the model is tuned using techniques such as Bayesian optimization or grid search. These methods are used to find the best set of hyperparameters (e.g., learning rate, number of trees to use in RF) that will lead to the maximum model's predictive accuracy. Reaching these parameters better predicts high-risk pregnancies, making the recommendations more predictable.

DSS for Risk Prediction: After that, the models were trained, fine-tuned, and integrated into the DSS (associated with real-time prepregnancy risk prediction). The ML models produce predictions based on which the DSS estimates the risk of a woman developing pregnancy complications. They give insights to the health providers and provide suggestions such as medical intervention, lifestyle changes, and health screenings. The risk on model benefits healthcare providers by helping them proactively reduce the risk of diabetes, for example, dietary modifications or early gestational diabetes screening [24].

Personalized Treatment Recommendations Using DQN: The system also leverages the DQN to predict risk and provide personalized treatment recommendations based on the patient's risk profile. Using RL, the DQN makes decisions based on medications, lifestyle modifications, and follow-up schedules. The system learns an action that maximizes the effectiveness of the consequent output by receiving feedback from the treatment outcome, and the action space contains a range of possible interventions. The reward mechanism is designed to optimize patient health outcomes with minimal risk and side effects.

2.6 EVALUATION OF AI-BASED DSS PERFORMANCE

These models are trained to validate the effectiveness of these ML models for identifying high-risk and low-risk pregnancies, after which they are used to predict such pregnancies. The evaluation of the model uses key performance metrics to determine the validity, veracity, and dependability of the model. These metrics will guarantee that the AI model makes real-time, actionable predictions for the healthcare provider.

Accuracy: Measures the overall proportion of correctly classified instances in the dataset. It is defined as:

$$\text{Accuracy} = \frac{\text{True Positives } + \text{True Negatives}}{\text{Total Population}} \tag{2.1}$$

Precision: Indicates the proportion of true positive predictions out of all positive predictions made by the model. It's calculated as:

$$\text{Precision} = \frac{\text{True Positives}}{\text{True Positives } + \text{False Positives}} \tag{2.2}$$

Recall (Sensitivity): Measures the model's ability to correctly identify all the positive cases (high-risk pregnancies). It is defined as:

$$\text{Recall} = \frac{\text{True Positives}}{\text{True Positives } + \text{False Negatives}} \tag{2.3}$$

F1-Score: This is the harmonic mean of precision and recall, providing a balanced measure of the model's performance, especially useful for imbalanced datasets. It is calculated as:

$$\text{F1-Score} = 2 \times \frac{\text{Precision} \times \text{Recall}}{\text{Precision} + \text{Recall}} \tag{2.4}$$

AUC-ROC Curve: AUC-ROC provides an aggregate measure of the model's ability to distinguish between the positive and negative classes."

The experimental setup is set to evaluate the AI-based DSS by splitting the dataset into training datasets, usually 70%–80%, and test datasets 20%–30% for model training and model evaluations, respectively. Cross-validation is used to avoid overfitting and improve generalization so that the dataset (divided into k subsamples) is tested on different data points. In class imbalance problems, we apply techniques like SMOTE (synthetic minority oversampling technique) or just undersampling to have the same number of high-risk and low-risk pregnancies as part of the training dataset. Using the preprocessed data, the models (RF, XGBoost, neural networks, logistic regression) are trained, and the performance is evaluated on the test set using the metric of accuracy, precision, recall, F1-score, AUC-ROC to see if they can predict the prepregnant risks [24].

2.6.1 Comparative Model Performance

As shown in Table 2.1, different ML models, including RF, XGBoost, neural networks, and logistic regression, are compared in terms of risk assessment targeted for prepregnancy. Keys performance metrics evaluated are accuracy, precision, recall, F1-score, and AUC-ROC for the models, and the information provides a crisp portrait of each model's capacity to classify high and low-risk pregnancies. Regarding metrics, the neural networks model works best while XGBoost is closely behind, and the performance of logistic regression is relatively poor, especially for AUC-ROC and recall. In these results, we find that simpler models perform less well than ensemble methods like RF and XGBoost for predicting prepregnancy risks.

These comparative metrics are shown in Figures 2.5–2.9, where each figure corresponds to one of the performance parameters (accuracy, precision, recall, F1 score, and AUC-ROC). It also makes it easy to compare each model's strengths and weaknesses, as presented by the bar charts, which represent the model's performance

TABLE 2.1
Comparative Study of Exiting Algorithms

Model	Accuracy	Precision	Recall	F1-Score	AUC-ROC
Random forest	0.85	0.84	0.86	0.85	0.91
XGBoost	0.88	0.86	0.87	0.86	0.93
Neural Networks	0.9	0.88	0.89	0.88	0.95
Logistic Regression	0.8	0.78	0.77	0.77	0.79

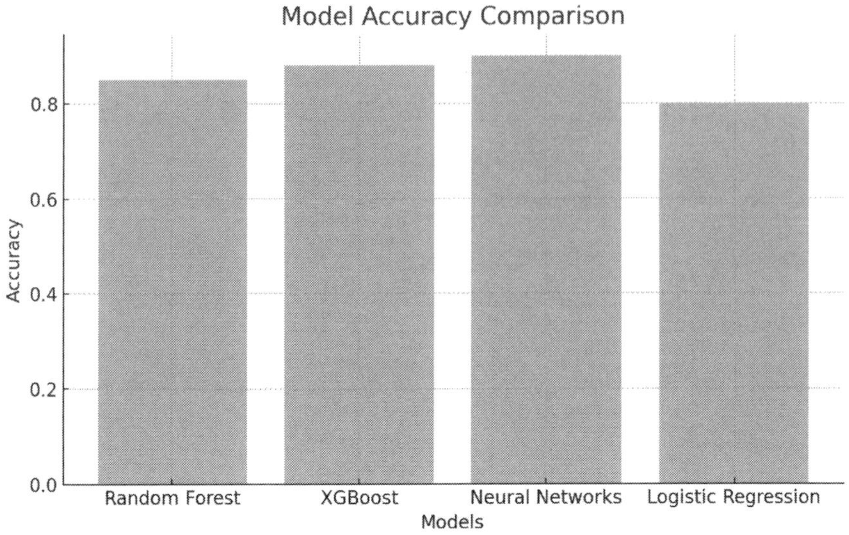

FIGURE 2.5 Model accuracy.

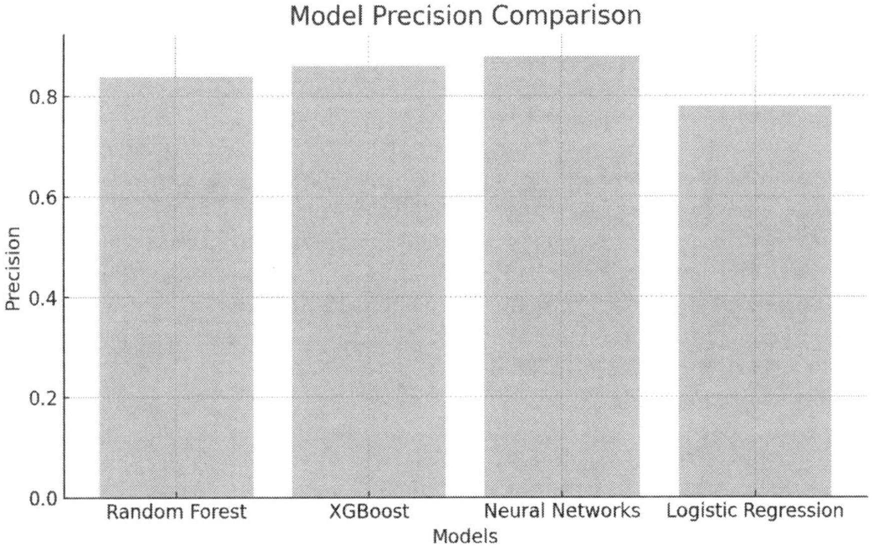

FIGURE 2.6 Model precision.

based on the various evaluation criteria. Neural network and XGBoost outperform all the graphs' parameters and prove they can accurately predict prepregnancy-prepregnancy risks. The figures and table indicate a need to select appropriate leads for proper risk prediction and decision support in prepregnancy care.

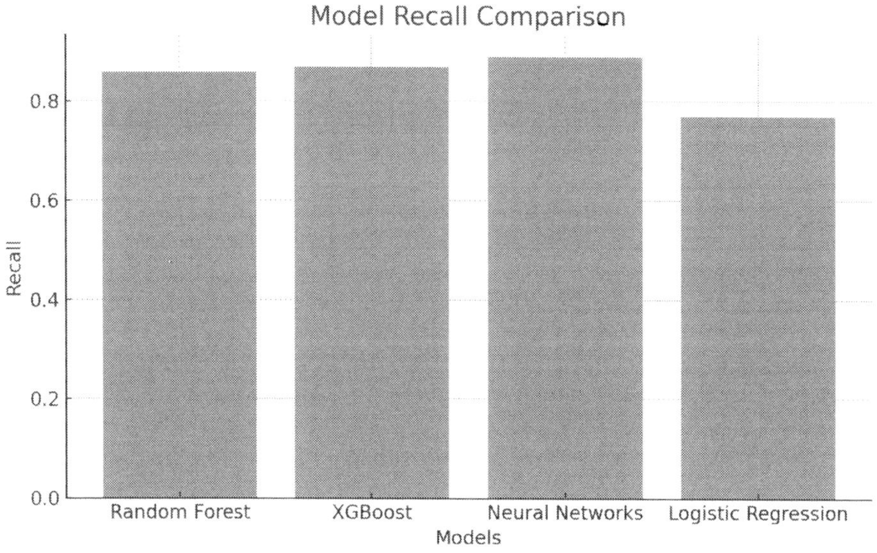

FIGURE 2.7 Model recall.

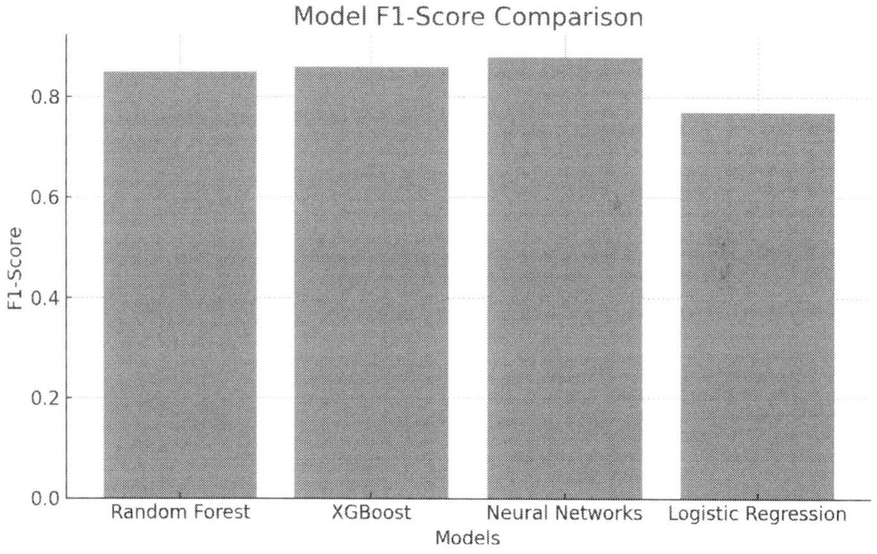

FIGURE 2.8 Model F1-score.

2.7 CONCLUSION

The AI-based DSS for prepregnancy risk assessment considers rapid changes in the DSS, and this chapter describes the continuous adaptation and expert consultation (CAEC) method. Continuously updated with real-time patient data and feedback from treatment outcomes, it will evolve the system into a forward-looking system

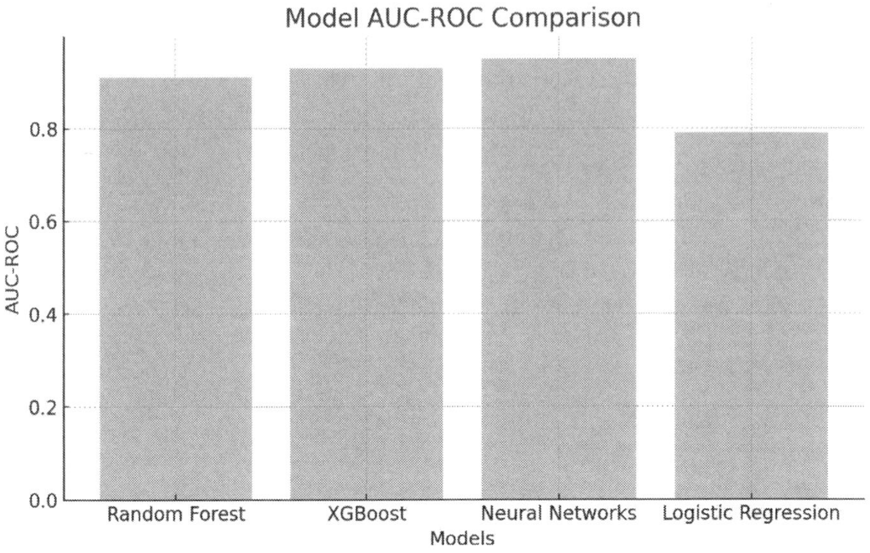

FIGURE 2.9 Model AUC-ROC.

that will continue to develop with predictions that stay accurate but always current. The model must be periodically retrained to absorb new knowledge, adjust to novel and associated patterns, and adjust its suggestions. Furthermore, expert consultations are a vital component in this process and help ensure that the AI-borne guidance makes clinical sense and is based on best medical practice. Further insights about decision-making will be offered by professors and other healthcare professionals who will review and validate the system's recommendations. This continuous adaptation and expert involvement are critical in ensuring that the system delivers relevant, reliable guidance congruent with the current medical standards.

REFERENCES

1. Berner, E. S. (2007). *Clinical Decision Support Systems* (Vol. 233). Springer.
2. Sutton, R. T., Pincock, D., Baumgart, D. C., Sadowski, D. C., Fedorak, R. N., Kroeker, K. I. (2020). An overview of clinical decision support systems: Benefits, risks, and strategies for success. *NPJ Digital Medicine*, 3(1), 1–10.
3. Cutler, D. M., Nikpay, S., Huckman, R. S. (2020). The business of medicine in the era of COVID-19. *JAMA*, 323(20), 2003–2004.
4. Wei, L., Boutouil, H., Gerbatin, R. R., Mamad, O., Heiland, M., Reschke, C. R., Del Gallo, F., Fabene, P. F., Henshall, D. C., Lowery, M., et al. (2021). Detection of spontaneous seizures in EEGs in multiple experimental mouse models of epilepsy. *Journal of Neural Engineering*, 18(5), 056060.
5. Wei, L., Ventura, S., Mathieson, S., Boylan, G. B., Lowery, M., Mooney, C. (2021). Spindle-AI: Sleep spindle number and duration estimation in infant EEG. *IEEE Transactions on Biomedical Engineering*, 69(1), 465–474.
6. Smiti, A. (2020). When machine learning meets the medical world: Current status and future challenges. *Computers in Science Review*, 37, 100280.

7. Baig, M. M., Hosseini, H. G., Lindén, M. (2016). Machine learning-based clinical decision support system for early diagnosis from real-time physiological data. *2016 IEEE Region 10 Conference (TENCON)*, Singapore: IEEE, pp. 2943–2946.
8. Holzinger, A., Biemann, C., Pattichis, C. S., Kell, D. B. (2017). What do we need to build explainable AI systems for the medical domain? arXiv:1712.09923.
9. Antoniadi, A. M., Du, Y., Guendouz, Y., Wei, L., Mazo, C., Becker, B. A., Mooney, C. (2021). Current challenges and future opportunities for XAI in machine learning-based clinical decision support systems: A systematic review. *Applied Sciences*, 11(11), 5088.
10. Adadi, A., Berrada, M. (2018). Peeking inside the black-box: A survey on explainable artificial intelligence (XAI). *IEEE Access*, 6, 52138–52160.
11. Tunçalp, Ó., Pena-Rosas, J. P., Lawrie, T., Lawrie, T., Oladapo, O. T., Portela, A., Gülmezoglu, A. M. (2017). WHO recommendations on antenatal care for a positive pregnancy experience-going beyond survival. *BJOG*, 124(6), 860–862.
12. Dalaba, M. A., Akweongo, P., Aborigo, R. A., Saronga, H. P., Williams, J., Blank, A., Kaltschmidt, J., Sauerborn, R., Loukanova, S. (2015). Cost-effectiveness of clinical decision support system in improving maternal health care in Ghana. *PLoS One*, 10(5), e0125920.
13. Usmanova, G., Lalchandani, K., Srivastava, A., Joshi, C. S., Bhatt, D. C., Bairagi, A. K., Jain, Y., Afzal, M., Dhoundiyal, R., Benawri, J., et al. (2021). The role of digital clinical decision support tool in improving quality of intrapartum and postpartum care: Experiences from two states of India. *BMC Pregnancy and Childbirth*, 21(1), 1–12.
14. Davidson, L., Boland, M. R. (2021). Towards deep phenotyping pregnancy: A systematic review on artificial intelligence and machine learning methods to improve pregnancy outcomes. *Briefings in Bioinformatics*, 22(5), bbaa369.
15. Kitchenham, B., Charters, S. (2007). Guidelines for performing systematic literature reviews in software engineering. Tech. Rep. EBSE 2007-001, Keele University and Durham University Joint Report.
16. Martín-Martín, A., Orduna-Malea, E., Thelwall, M., López-Cózar, E. D. (2018). Google Scholar, Web of Science, and Scopus: A systematic comparison of citations in 252 subject categories. *Journal of Informetrics*, 12(4), 1160–1177.
17. Gusenbauer, M. (2019). Google Scholar to overshadow them all? Comparing the sizes of 12 academic search engines and bibliographic databases. *Scientometrics*, 118(1), 177–214.
18. Damaraji, G. M., Permanasari, A. E., Hidayah, I. (2020). A review of expert system for identification of various risks in pregnancy. *2020 3rd International Conference on Information and Communications Technology (ICOIACT)*, Indonesia: IEEE, pp. 99–104.
19. Davidson, L., Boland, M. R. (2020). Enabling pregnant women and their physicians to make informed medication decisions using artificial intelligence. *Journal of Pharmacokinetics and Pharmacodynamics*, 47(4), 305–318.
20. Güvenir, H. A., Misirli, G., Dilbaz, S., Ozdegirmenci, O., Demir, B., Dilbaz, B. (2015). Estimating the chance of success in IVF treatment using a ranking algorithm. *Medical Biology and Engineering Computing*, 53(9), 911–920.
21. Van Calster, B., Timmerman, D., Kirk, E., Bourne, T., Condous, G., Van Huffel, S. (2008). Towards a clinical decision support system for pregnancies of unknown location. *21st IEEE International Symposium on Computer-Based Medical Systems*, Finland: IEEE, pp. 581–583.
22. Fernández, A. D. R., Fernández, D. R., Sánchez, M. T. P. (2019). A decision support system for predicting the treatment of ectopic pregnancies. *International Journal of Medical Informatics*, 129, 198–204.

23. Gorthi, A., Firtion, C., Vepa, J. (2009). Automated risk assessment tool for pregnancy care. *2009 Annual International Conference of the IEEE Engineering in Medicine and Biology Society*, USA: IEEE, pp. 6222–6225.
24. Paydar, K., Kalhori, S. R. N., Akbarian, M., Sheikhtaheri, A. (2017). A clinical decision support system for prediction of pregnancy outcome in pregnant women with systemic lupus erythematosus. *International Journal of Medical Informatics*, 97, 239–246.

3 Advances in Deep Neural Networks for Chronic Kidney Disease Diagnosis

A Systematic Review

Mahesh Shinde, Satyajit Pangaonkar, Parikshit N. Mahalle, Surendra Rahamatkar, Dattatray G. Takale, and Gopal B. Deshmukh

3.1 INTRODUCTION

Chronic kidney disease (CKD) is defined as a sustained decline in kidney function or structural kidney damage persisting for over 3 months, and it represents a major global health challenge. CKD affects approximately 10% of the adult population worldwide (with higher prevalence in at-risk groups) and is associated with significantly increased morbidity and mortality, particularly from cardiovascular disease. A key concern is that CKD often remains asymptomatic until its later stages, making early detection difficult. When patients experience noticeable symptoms, kidney function may already be severely compromised. If identified promptly, early-stage CKD can be managed with interventions (such as blood pressure control, glycemic management in people with diabetes, medications like ACE inhibitors, and lifestyle modifications) that slow disease progression and reduce the risk of complications. Indeed, screening and identifying CKD in its initial stages allows for treatments that may alter the disease's natural course and help prevent progression to end-stage renal disease (ESRD) and other adverse outcomes. However, current screening practices (e.g., periodic measurement of serum creatinine to estimate glomerular filtration rate (eGFR) and testing for albuminuria) have limitations in sensitivity and convenience. CKD screening rates remain suboptimal even among high-risk individuals (such as those with diabetes or hypertension), and the traditional biomarkers (creatinine, urine albumin) can be variable or insensitive in early disease. This gap highlights the need for improved methods to detect CKD earlier and more reliably (Figure 3.1).

This chapter thoroughly reviews how deep learning (DL) approaches can be used for early detection and prevention of CKD. In the first part, we introduce the background of CKD and clarify the reason for detecting it early. After that, we examine the various attempts to use DL toward CKD prediction using convolutional neural networks (CNNs), recurrent neural networks (RNNs), transformers, and ensemble techniques, showing similar representative works achieved and their outcomes.

DOI: 10.1201/9781003479185-3

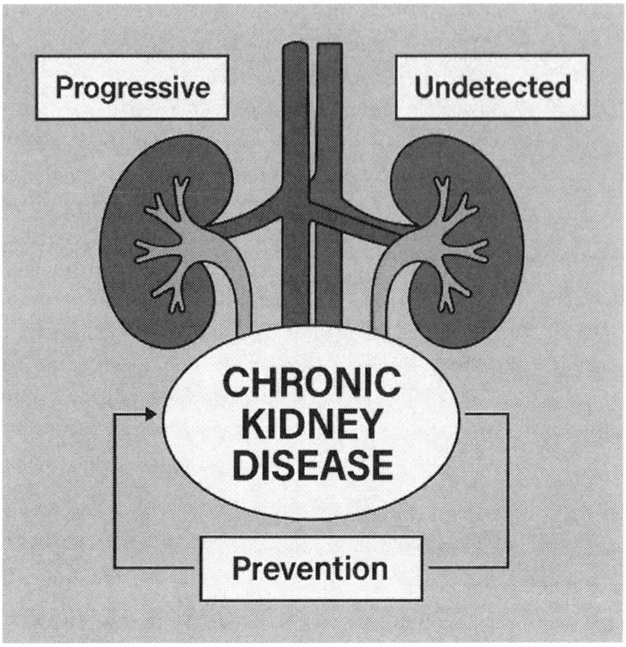

FIGURE 3.1 Chronic kidney disease (CKD).

We summarize the commonly used datasets and model performance metrics and compare the results with different modeling approaches. However, these models need to be translated into practice in the clinic where we talk, discuss the challenges related to such translation – especially regarding data, integration, and regulatory concerns – and highlight the need for interpretability and explainability of artificial intelligence (AI) in healthcare. We propose future directions and research opportunities to further develop this field, including using multimodal data, improving model generalizability, and creating clinically robust and explainable AI tools for CKD management. Through this structured review, we provide guidelines to researchers and clinicians to utilize DL to detect and prevent early CKD.

3.2 BACKGROUND: CKD AND THE IMPORTANCE OF EARLY DETECTION

CKD is a condition in which gradual loss of kidney function occurs over time and is usually measured as diminished GFR or the presence of kidney damage (i.e., proteinuria). CKD (staging from Stage 1–5) is the staging according to the level of kidney function, characterized by Stage 5, namely ESRD, where either dialysis or transplantation is required. The contribution of CKD to the global health burden is substantial as it is among the top causes of lost years of life, and prevalence has been increasing, related mainly to aging populations and rising incidence of diabetes and hypertension, both of which are major risk factors. Strange to note, in many cases, the affected person has no idea that they suffer from early CKD as symptoms start to appear only in the last stages of the disease. With this latency, opportunities for early intervention are often missed due to a lack of proactive screening.

This is important because Stage 1–3 CKD interventions can markedly slow disease progression. For instance, keeping blood pressure, using the blockers of the renin–angiotensin system, controlling blood sugar in diabetes, dietary modifications, and addressing causes (for example, relieving urinary obstructions or stopping nephrotoxic agents) can help preserve kidney function. Prevention or even delay of the progression to ESRD and reduction in the number of cardiovascular disease (CVD) events are affected by early management of CKD risk factors, as shown in the research. However, when CKD progresses to more advanced stages, patients end up developing inevitable kidney damage. They are further required for renal replacement therapy (RRT), such as dialysis or transplant and die at higher healthcare costs. There are currently no technologies for screening that test serum creatinine (to calculate eGFR) or urine albumin measurements as they are currently available. These are critical tests, but they are weaknesses as early indicators.

In some cases, eGFR estimates can be imprecise because muscle mass, diet, and medications influence serum creatinine. However, urinary albumin (albuminuria) is an important marker, which is variable day to day by 30%–50% and which has a normal level in a nontrivial fraction of CKD cases (typically in such populations as people with diabetes with low eGFR but no albuminuria). In addition, screening calls for patients to visit health facilities to undergo blood/urine tests, and follow-up can be challenging to arrange logistically, resulting in under-screening. However, these limitations lead to an impetus to find, or at the very least, complementary or alternative ways for detecting CKD earlier, preferably from noninvasive or relatively easily obtained data.

Hence, DL-based models have become a promising tool for improved early CKD detection. These models could work by training on large amounts of patient information to identify patterns for kidney function decline before clinical thresholds are crossed. For example, early renal impairment indicators include subtle changes in routine lab results or imaging features of kidneys over time. Complex, high-dimensional data is easily handled by DL algorithms that allow them to capture these patterns. Early prediction models that can identify high-risk patients for further evaluation or preventative treatment would successfully shift from reactive treatment of CKD to proactive prevention. In the following sections, we review the DL methodologies for CKD prediction and utilize different data types to enhance the early detection of the disease.

3.3 METHODOLOGY: DEEP LEARNING APPROACHES FOR CKD PREDICTION

Other than this, research on AI for CKD has explored various DL approaches to data types commonly linked to kidney diseases. In most of the methodologies, one first builds a dataset of records of patients, preprocesses the data, picks some features or modalities, and trains DL models to predict a target outcome (such as the current status of CKD or the future of CKD progress). This work describes the most common

DL techniques used in the literature: CNN, RNN, transformer, etc., and ensemble modeling strategies. Moreover, we discuss the datasets used to train these models and the performance metrics to evaluate them.

3.3.1 Data Sources and Feature Inputs

Many studies have been conducted that have used two categories of data: structured, clinical data (numeric or categorical features derived from lab tests, vital signs, demographics, etc.) and medical imaging data. Standard features of structured data include markers of kidney function (for example, serum creatinine, blood urea nitrogen, eGFR, protein in urine), other blood tests (for example, hemoglobin, electrolytes), comorbid conditions (diabetes, hypertension), and patient demographics (gender, age, etc.). For instance, based on a widely used benchmark, the CKD dataset in the University of California Irvine (UCI) ML repository contains 400 patient records accompanied by 24 features (blood pressure, specific gravity of urine, albumin level, sugar, red and white blood cell counts, hemoglobin, etc.) and a class label indicating either the presence or absence of CKD. This dataset (or a similar dataset available on Kaggle) has been the subject of many studies basing the development of the model on this dataset. However, it is small, with only a few hundred samples, so researchers have also looked for more expansive datasets.

Thus, larger structured datasets have been constructed from electronic health records (EHRs) or longitudinal cohort studies. For example, these include patient registries of numerous lab results from hospitals or health systems over time. Some studies use national health insurance databases (such as Taiwan's National Health Insurance Research Database) or population studies (NHANES or CKD cohort studies) to collect thousands of patient records. However, researchers who are trying to predict CKD progression often use a dataset of patients with early-stage CKD and their follow-up lab results to identify who goes on to get worse stages. A recent study trained models from longitudinal EHR data processed for over 1,000 CKD stage 2/3 patients (laboratory, vital signs at multiple points) who progressed to stage 4/5. One used a claims/EHR database of 130,000 patients with stage 3 CKD to predict the time to onset of stage 5 kidney failure. By supplying examples of outcome events, these large datasets enable to train complex models like deep neural networks (DNNs) and transformers.

Medical images regarding kidney health have been used with DL for early detection of CKD through noninvasive screening. We observe two imaging modalities: renal ultrasound images and retinal fundus images. Structural changes (i.e., kidney size, cortical thickness, and echogenicity) in the kidneys can be seen on kidney ultrasounds and correlate with chronic disease. While not direct images of the kidney, retinal images capture the body's microvascular health and, surprisingly, have been quite good at predicting systemic conditions like diabetic kidney disease since retinal microvascular changes usually reflect kidney microvascular changes. The hypothesis that retina signs can act as biomarkers of kidney dysfunction has motivated some innovative studies of retinal fundus photographs as input to DL models of CKD detection. For example, retinal images (tens of thousands of them) from diabetes screening programs and general population studies have been labeled as to whether or not the individual with the retinal image had CKD (defined by eGFR). Often, they are combined with matching clinical data (i.e., age or blood pressure) to improve model performance further.

3.3.2 Data Preprocessing and Feature Selection Are Essential Steps in the Methodology

Missing values are common in clinical datasets, particularly in the UCI CKD and EHR data. Alternatives include common strategies (e.g., imputation, such as replacing missing labs with the mean or k-NN imputation for bigger gaps) or more sophisticated strategies when the numbers are larger (like expectation-maximization). Feature selection techniques are applied to some studies to identify the most informative variables for CKD prediction to decrease noise and dimensionality. For instance, the data was filtered using chi-square tests, mutual information, recursive feature elimination (RFE), or genetic algorithms before feeding data into the model.

Alsekait *et al.* (2023) applied filter, wrapper, and embedded methods of multiple feature selection on the 24-feature CKD dataset. They identified that the best model performance was obtained via a subset selected using mutual information maximizing. An ant colony optimization was proposed to enhance CKD classification in another study, and a density-based feature selection was used in another study. DL models all have the potential to learn from all features, but judicious feature selection can reasonably speed up training and possibly generalization when data is limited.

3.3.3 Deep Learning Models (CNNs, RNNs, and Transformers)

Several types of DNN architectures have been applied to CKD prediction tasks:

Convolutional Neural Networks: CNNs are mainly used for image recognition tasks, and CNNs have been applied in CKD research to analyze medical images. Kuo *et al.* (2019) attempted a pioneering work by training a CNN (with ResNet-34 architecture pretrained on ImageNet) to classify CKD for a given kidney ultrasound image. In the case of recognizing the images of kidneys for CKD (eGFR < 60) and non-CKD cases, their model learned visual features like kidney texture and size (accuracy of 85.6%) better than nephrologists (accuracy between 60.3% and 80.1%), in distinguishing the images of kidneys of the patients suffering from CKD and those of patients without CKD. Second, CNNs have been applied to retinal fundus photographs; for example, Sabanayagam *et al.* (2020) employed a compact CNN (cCondenseNet architecture) for retinal images to predict reduced eGFR. There, the CNN's AUC to detect CKD was impressively 0.91 on an internal test set but dropped to 0.73–0.83 on external validation cohorts, indicating a difficulty in generalizing to out-of-population. Other groups have subsequently followed up with subsequent studies using fundus images and CNN models (e.g., VGG-19, InEfficientNet) and have similarly shown that retinal imaging contains a signal for any CKD status. Using these CNN-based image models for screening is a noninvasive approach, for example, a patient's routine diabetes retinal scan could also be used to predict CKD risk. CNNs are also sometimes used on tabular or one-dimensional (1D) clinical data beyond imaging. While lab values are a sequence of items, researchers have created

1D CNN models to ingest sequences of lab values or even the static feature vector of labs as treated as a temporal, spatial sequence. For example, one study suggests a 1D CNN model for CKD prediction designed to sift through patient feature vectors for interactions between labs and symptoms. Although a less common choice than other modeling approaches for tabular data, such CNN models will automatically learn feature combinations. In general, CNNs are very good at pattern recognition, and they have worked well when there are enough training images or structured patterns to work with (Figure 3.2).

Recurrent Neural Networks: RNNs (especially long short-term memory networks (LSTMs)) are data and mathematical neural networks for sequential data and temporal patterns. RNN is leveraged to use patients' time series data, for example, longitudinal lab test results or vital signs trends in the CKD applications. An obvious example is the study of Yuan *et al.* (2023), who built an LSTM model to predict the progression of CKD based on patients' time series in EHR. For example, they concentrated on people with moderate CKD (stage 2/3) to identify those who would develop severe CKD (stage 4/5) within a specific time. By including a wider set of features (demographic, other lab tests, blood pressure, comorbidities, etc.) in addition to eGFR, the AUROC of the model went up to 0.967. RNNs can develop accurate risk predictions by understanding the dynamic trajectory of kidney function. Even though the RNN outperformed traditional models such as Cox proportional hazards and random forests on the same task, it performed similarly to them in modeling the occurrence of the event variable. Other EHR-based studies have also used LSTMs or gated recurrent units (GRUs) for CKD onset or renal failure prediction with similar strong performance (0.85–0.95 AUROC). In cases with such a predictive signal for CKD, which would include temporal trends such as a constant decrease in hemoglobin or rise in creatinine, RNNs are well-suited. By maintaining an internal state, these networks learn how earlier patient states affect future outcomes. However, one difficulty with such data is that EHR data are often irregularly sampled, so some researchers aggregate observations into visit sequences or use time interval encoding. Despite such intricacies, recurrent models have made their way into the scene of early warning systems in CKD, learning from each patient's longitudinal "story" to make predictions (Figure 3.3).

Transformer Models: Recently, transformer architectures with self-attention mechanisms have been brought to healthcare and have been shown to surpass RNNs

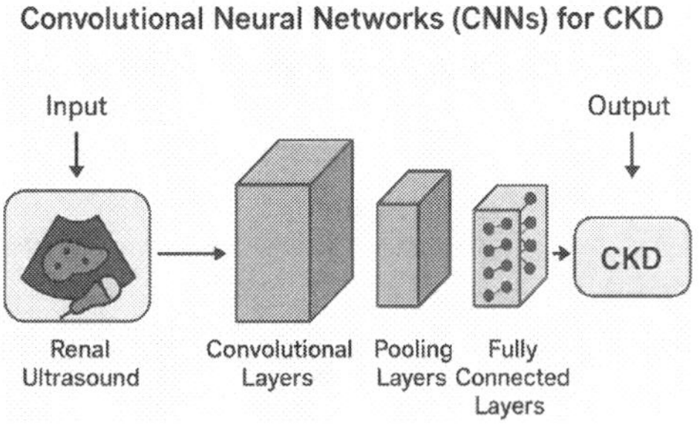

FIGURE 3.2 CNN for CDK.

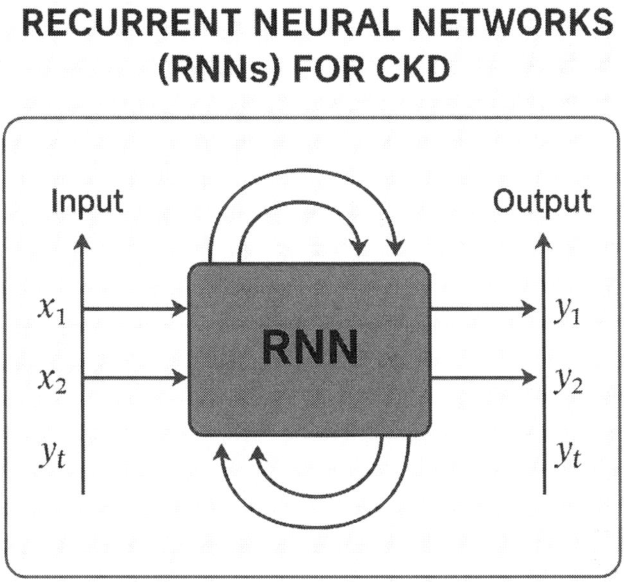

FIGURE 3.3 RNN for CDK.

in cases of massive datasets. Compared to RNNs, transformers can take advantage of long-range dependencies without the need for sequential processing; they are, therefore, very applicable to longitudinal or multimodal data in the CKD research domain. An example of one cutting-edge model is the STRAFE model (transformer-based survival analysis for EHR) proposed by Zisser *et al.* (2024). For a given sequence of patient visit codes (diagnoses, procedures, etc.), STRAFE predicts the probability of CKD deterioration over the next 48 months. STRAFE was compared to the traditional time-to-event models using a claims dataset of over 130k stage 3 CKD patients, showing that it has a lower error in time prediction and higher discriminative ability (AUC) than baseline models. Another study used transformer-based models pretrained on clinical text (e.g., Med-BERT, HERBERT) named HERBERT to learn to predict which CKD patients will progress to ESRD, and another study demonstrated transfer learning on EHR data.

Additionally, transformers have been combined with imaging, including a multimodal transformer system with retinal imaging and clinical variables for detecting diabetic kidney disease that outperforms single modality models. The attention mechanism can also improve interpretability in transformers, providing increased focus on which parts of a sequence (e.g., which past visits or which image regions) were critical to the prediction. In conclusion, transformer techniques form a recent trend in the prediction of CKD research, primarily due to the increase in size and complexity of datasets. The ability to develop complicated relationships in data (e.g., between comorbid conditions and labs calculated over time) has been instrumental to recent studies, pushing performance boundaries (Figure 3.4).

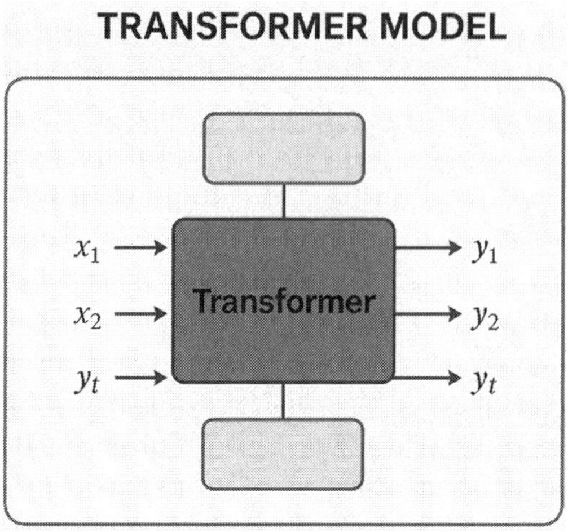

FIGURE 3.4 Transformer for CDK.

Feedforward DNNs: Many have attempted to classify CKD using specialized architectures, like CNNs, RNNs, general MLPs, or deep feedforward networks. The provided models, given a vector of input features (such as the patient's latest lab values), use these multiple dense layers to predict the probability of CKD (output). Such DNNs can be trained to learn complex nonlinear combinations of risk factors. For instance, using clinical data, Kriplani *et al.* (2019) constructed a DNN that achieved close to 97% accuracy for early-stage CKD detection, outperforming standard classifiers such as naive Bayes, logistic regression, and random forest on the same dataset. Other studies using the UCI dataset showed that achieving more than 95% accuracy is possible using a well-tuned neural network. Unfortunately, while some deeper networks did not constantly improve the performance, one referred to a DNN that only achieved ~75% accuracy due to overfitting on a small data set. In many cases, DNNs are still components of approaches but require sufficient data, regularization/feature selection, or some combination of the two to achieve their full potential. Autoencoders (unsupervised networks for feature learning) have also been integrated with DNN classifiers to uncover structure in CKD data and achieved an accuracy of ~94% in one instance (Figure 3.5).

3.4 MODEL EVALUATION METRICS

Researchers employ a range of performance metrics to evaluate DL models for CKD early detection, aligning with the binary classification nature of most CKD prediction tasks (CKD vs. no CKD or progression vs. no progression).

The key metrics reported include:

- **Accuracy**: The fraction of correct predictions (CKD and non-CKD) among all predictions. The classes might be imbalanced, and the accuracy might be misleading to understand. If the number of non-CKD cases exceeds that of

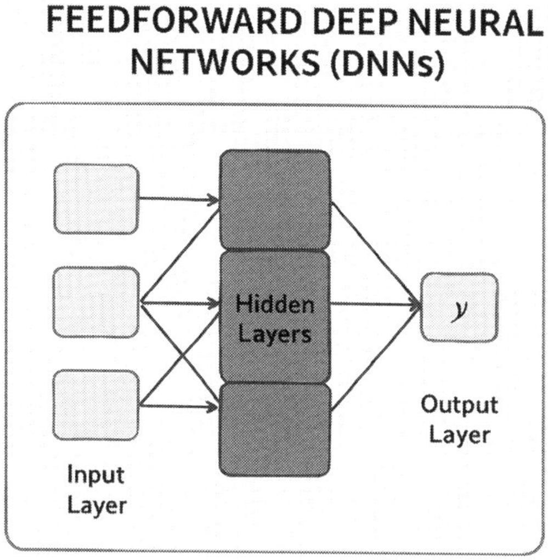

FIGURE 3.5 Feedforward deep neural networks (DNNs) for CDK.

CKD cases, a model saying "no CKD" for everybody will be highly accurate but useless in CKD datasets. However, accuracy and very high values (90%–99%) are achieved in many studies with their test sets.

- **Precision (Positive Predictive Value)**: This is the proportion of predicted CKD cases that are truly CKD. By how often the model is correct when it raises the alarm for CKD, we mean the precision. Fewer false positives result in a higher precision. This is important to keep patients with low risks from unnecessary anxiety or further follow-up when they are treated incorrectly as high risk.
- **Recall (Sensitivity or True Positive Rate)**: That is the proportion of the actual cases of CKD that the model correctly identifies. Among the properties highly desirable for a screening tool, high recall (sensitivity) means the model catches most patients that have or will develop CKD – a lost chance for early intervention if a patient is missed (false negative). Usually, precision and recall are in opposition to one another, so it is combined with a metric like F1.
- **F1-Score**: That is the proportion of the actual cases of CKD that the model correctly identifies. High recall (sensitivity) is a highly desirable property for a screening tool. It means the model catches most patients who have or will develop CKD – a lost chance for early intervention if a patient is missed (false negative). Usually, precision and recall are in opposition to one another, so they are combined with a metric like F1.
- **Area under the Receiver Operating Characteristic Curve (AUC-ROC)**: AUC represents the model's ability to discriminate between classes at any classification threshold. Values of 1.0 for an AUC represent perfect discrimination; 0.5 is no better than chance. Because AUC is threshold-independent, it is also widely used for medical prediction model evaluation: the AUC

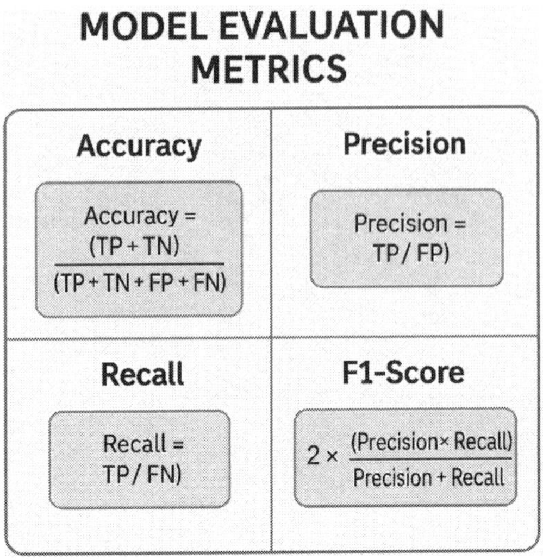

FIGURE 3.6 Evaluation model for CDK.

gives insight into how the model performs across sensitivity-specificity trade-offs. Many DL CKD models report an AUC value. In the image case, internal AUCs were ~0.85–0.93 for image-based models and ~0.96 for RNN models for progression. For models dealing with class imbalance, the area under the precision-recall curve (AUPRC) is a more informative related metric, and some of these sequence models report very high AUPRC (>0.8).

- **Others**: Depending on the task formulation, other metrics might appear. For progression or survival predictions, mean absolute error (MAE) in predicting time-to-event or concordance index (c-index) for risk rankings are used. For regression tasks like directly predicting eGFR value, root mean squared error (RMSE), or Pearson correlation coefficient (PCC) with actual values are reported (e.g., Kuo's ultrasound CNN had a PCC of 0.741 for eGFR prediction). However, classification metrics (sensitivity, specificity, etc.) remain central for early detection models (Figure 3.6).

Researchers generally evaluate the model on a held out test set or using cross-validation. An 80/20 or 70/30 train test split is often used, with sometimes a separate validation set for hyperparameter tuning. They also employ k-fold cross-validation (k = 5, 10, or even 15) to more robustly and better estimate performance. Metrics should include results on validation or test data not seen during training for generalization. Others use their DL model to compare to baseline classifiers (logistic regression, support vector machine (SVM), etc.) on the same dataset in terms of accuracy etc., highlighting improvements. Finally, it is essential to note that extremely high-performance metrics (close to 100% accuracy) can be reached even on small benchmark datasets. For example, accuracies between 95% and 100% have been reported on the UCI data by various ML algorithm combinations with feature selection, such as the 400 sample. However, these results show that models can fit the data, a feat which may underestimate performance over real-world data. On the other hand, external cohort models or larger, more diverse set-tuned models typically evaluate with more modest metrics (e.g., external AUC in the 0.75–0.85 range for image models). Therefore, it is essential to remember how much we are willing to trust a metric before we start interpreting its meaning, hence considering dataset characteristics and validation strategies when looking at metrics in this field.

3.5 CURRENT RESEARCH TRENDS AND RESULTS

In recent years, there has been tremendous progress in applying DL to CKD prediction, with several discernible trends in the research. The first trend is moving away from conventional machine learning models to exploring deep architectures to work with intricate data such as images and longitudinal records. Many previous works used traditional decision trees, SVMs, or logistic regression. Still, more recent efforts show that CNNs, RNNs, and even transformers can exceed such methods when enough data is available. To illustrate, the RNN model proposed by Yuan *et al.* (2023) achieved an AUROC of ~0.96 on progression prediction. However, simple classical approaches such as Cox regression and random forests outperformed them regarding head-to-head comparison. Likewise, some experiments have found deep CNNs to match or beat the accuracy of clinical risk score models on image data.

A second trend is the expansion of modalities and the scale of data. Early studies varied from investigating the small UCI CKD dataset or a single-center data to more recent studies using larger cohorts and often multimodal data. Around 2019–2021, retinal images were also used as a screening approach for CKD, mainly based on the successful use of retinal images in other fields, such as diabetic retinopathy screening. Zhang *et al.* (2021) used a CNN on over 86,000 fundus images from 43,000 patients and combined those image features with patient metadata (age, etc.) to help improve CKD detection; in testing the combined model outside, AUC was 0.87 compared with 0.85 when using images alone. It suggests a trend toward multifeature integration; combining deep-learned image features with clinical variables can improve performance. This is the case, such that what we call multi-input models (sometimes called hybrid models) are growing more and more frequent: one study created a hybrid CNN that takes input from retinal images as well as traditional risk factors to detect diabetic kidney disease; this hybrid model yielded better AUC performance compared to either input alone. There is also a notable trend in ensemble modeling. Above, it is discussed that many of the authors report that the best results on their dataset come from an ensemble of models. As a case study, in one study, an ensemble that combined predictions from CNN, LSTM and bi LSTM (voting majority) could predict CKD 6 months ahead with a prediction of 99.3% accuracy and 12 months ahead with 99.2% accuracy. Like Alsekait *et al.* (2023), found that a stacked ensemble had the highest accuracy (nearly 100 %) than any single model. Bearing in mind the current trend of machine learning novels, ensemble methods are frequently utilized when there exists very powerful competition to achieve the highest accuracy. Nevertheless, it should be pointed out that implementing such complex ensembles might be unfeasible in clinical deployment, and some work also seeks simpler models achieving high accuracy to support interpretability and ease of implementation.

The collective literature suggests that DL models can have excellent discriminatory ability in performance trends for relation prediction of CKD under suitable conditions. They report many studies with accuracy, precision, and recall, all over 90% on their internal test sets. For example, Precision and Recall in some studies are very high (perc = 0.95, rec = 98), particularly when we apply data balancing techniques (as in the case of SMOTE and oversampling of minority class). In these scenarios, the derived F1-scores, being high, indicate balanced performance in the case of many different studies (AUC-ROC values from 0.85 to 0.99). More complex tasks tend to yield AUC in the mid-0.7s to 0, for example, prediction of future onset among somewhat healthy people and generalization to outside datasets. For instance, AUC ~0.91 was achieved for RetiCKD (Sabanayagam *et al.* 2020), but internal AUC ~0.79 and AUC ~0.758 for CKD in the UK Biobank fundus image study by An *et al.* (2023). This is significant because it emphasizes a key point: performance is bloated on training or internally validated data while declining on external validation. This gap has been noticed for some time, and recently, there have been concrete works that explicitly include external validations or cross-institution testing in their evaluation.

A second growing field of research is forecasting CKD progression and outcomes from static detection (beyond static detection). Rather than simply defining a current CKD, these models also predict clinically significant consequences such as acceleration in the rate of decline in eGFR, development of ESRD, or need for dialysis. One thing mentioned about the RNN and the transformer models is that some researchers pinpointed specific subproblems, such as predicting the RRT requirement. As such, a DL model was developed to predict progression to dialysis from labs integrated with medication history and comorbid conditions. However, most of these are survival analysis metrics-based models evaluated on longitudinal cohorts. Furthermore, the time-to-event modeling trend (something like survival forests, Cox models, and now DL survival models) matches clinical needs – it is essential to know that a patient will deteriorate as much as to see that they won't.

It further introduces the trend of incorporating domain-specific pretraining and transfer learning. All the CNN models in image-based CKD detection begin from image net pretrained weights (transfer learning) to define the basic knowledge of object classes. Models such as Med-BERT (BERT pretrained on millions of EHR notes or structured records) have been fine-tuned for CKD tasks in the EHR space. Increasingly, this reuse of pretrained networks trained on large datasets (in general, images or large health record corpora) is standard because it is not bad for performance and convergence speed. In addition, the current interest in federated learning approaches (training models across institutions without having to gather data centrally), which would allow access to more training data than one location would restrict admissibility and preserve privacy, is also a methodological approach to the outsourcing of data vulnerabilities and parsimony expressed within the current research debates.

The research shows that DL can perform well in predicting CKD and its progression with high accuracy, provided abundant data and modern architectures are available. Still, however, it also shows that model generalizability and clinical applicability require attention. More diverse datasets are being used to validate such models in the community, and the community is increasingly validating models on external datasets. The community is increasingly seeing how these AI tools could be integrated into real clinical workflows. This naturally brings us to a discussion of challenges in deployment and model interpretability, which we address next.

3.6 CHALLENGES IN DEPLOYING DEEP LEARNING MODELS FOR CKD

Despite the promising performance of DL models in research settings, several challenges must be addressed before these systems can be widely deployed in clinical practice for CKD screening or prediction. These challenges can be broadly categorized into technical issues related to the models and data, and practical issues related to clinical integration and user acceptance.

- **Data Quality, Quantity, and Generalizability**: A central problem is the sheer lack of good, high-quality data. However, most published models are trained on small or homogeneous datasets. However, as mentioned before, some of the works were based on only a few hundred samples, a case of overfitting and limited capacity to generalize. A model trained on one population may perform poorly in a different population due to the heterogeneity of CKD, a disease influenced by patient demographics, comorbidities, and healthcare access. We had examples where accuracy dropped on external validation. To avoid algorithmic bias and ensure that a broader range of people can use the resulting model, it is essential to ensure diversity in the training data (e.g., across age groups, ethnicities, geographies, etc.) Nevertheless, large, diverse datasets are nontrivial to gather, as privacy issues and data silos between institutions make data collation difficult. Furthermore, model training is further complicated by data quality issues arising from missing values, measurement errors, and inconsistent coding in EHRs. Because of these technical hurdles, more effort is required to harmonize and share data. Even with access to federated learning databases proposed to overcome data access obstacles, models can be trained across several institutions without sharing raw patients data. This can improve generalization and still respect privacy. In addition, prospective data collection and monitoring of a model's performance in new situations will identify where the model could fail and where it needs retraining.
- **Integration into Clinical Workflow**: Besides being highly accurate, a model is of minimal value if it cannot be easily integrated into the clinical workflow. Suppose a CKD prediction model is to be deployed. In that case, it should ideally be put inside EHR systems or lab reporting systems so clinicians are alerted or even have a risk score in real-time, without downloading per software. It is very costly to implement in terms of IT infrastructure and interoperability. Also, the designed workflow should handle the false positives/negatives gracefully – for instance, what happens when the model declares a patient as high risk? Is there an explicit follow-up action for the care team (e.g., scheduling confirmatory tests or nephrologist referrals)? Clinicians may become overwhelmed by the alerts and stop ignoring the

tool altogether when models produce too many alarms (particularly false alarms). As a result, tuning model sensitivity and defining thresholds that make sense from the clinical standpoint are needed. Additionally, models may be required to produce meaningful output in context (e.g., "Patient X has 30% predicted risk of developing CKD within 5 years") for outputs to be actionable. Such a tool could work only embedded into routine practice, which, in turn, requires a degree of workflow modifications, such as the fact that staff will need time to monitor the predictions and act on the recommendations. A current challenge in AI deployment is the lack of clear pathways to act on AI predictions.

- **User Trust and Training**: Algorithmic predictions, especially from "black box" DL models, may contradict what clinicians expect and won't explain how they're made. A major nontechnical challenge is to gain the trust of physicians and healthcare providers. A nephrologist or first-line doctor will not accept the model's output if they do not trust it. Demonstrating the model's performance (its sensitivity/specificity trade-off) in clinical terms and explaining to what extent it predicted (the next section of interpretability). In addition, it also involves user training – clinicians and nurses will need training on what the model does, how to read its output, and what limitations there are. A user without understanding might ignore or abuse the tool to the extent that it does not serve its actual value. To accommodate AI usage, healthcare professionals need to be educated about AI, and there are also easy-to-use interfaces (e.g., risk dashboards in the EHR). Early pilot studies with end-user feedback allow for identifying what information clinical needs to embed model predictions within care comfortably.
- **Regulatory and Ethical Hurdles**: A predictive model in healthcare must be introduced through regulatory and ethical considerations. For example, in many jurisdictions, an AI tool for disease prediction may be viewed as a medical device or clinical decision-support tool that must be reviewed (for example, by the FDA in the US and EMA in Europe). They will search for proof of safety and efficacy: Does the model change clinical outcomes? Is it thoroughly validated? It behaves as expected in several subgroups. However, regulatory approval for most of these devices can take a long time, and current regulatory frameworks are still developing to address the regulation of machine learning-based devices. In addition, patient consent for AI-guided care may raise ethical issues, such as where there will be liability if errors (missing a patient's CKD seen by the AI), and what protection of patient privacy should be ensured during the model development process. Fairness issues also arise: If the model has a known bias in gender (in the example, the model underpredicts risk for young women because test and train data were sparsely populated with such cases), then running it could perpetuate healthcare disparities. Because of this, rigorous bias testing and fair metrics are demanded before deployment. To address these regulatory and ethical issues, a joint effort by clinicians, data scientists, ethicists, and legal experts is needed to help develop

guidelines and standards for using AI in CKD care. The past few proposals aim to simplify the approval process of the AI while maintaining strict evaluation rules.

- **Technical Robustness and Maintenance**: Some DL models are brittle, small changes to input (e.g., slight lab unit variations, or out of range values) can cause erratic outputs unless properly handled. In a clinical setting, this model will have to work with data that does not necessarily come from the distribution of its training set (e.g., different lab machines, different populations of patients). The robustness (the model should behave reasonably under slightly unexpected inputs) is not trivial. This could involve extensive testing and adding fail-safes like suggesting that things should "be uncertain" in case inputs go wild, instead of bluffing out a guess, which might be wrong. Furthermore, it will require models to be constantly updated and maintained. The model should be updated to reflect current standards in clinical guidelines, levels of biomarkers, and definitions of CKD, which may change (e.g., new thresholds or new biomarkers may be adopted). Furthermore, if more data is available or if the outcomes of using the model occur, the model may need to be retrained or updated. One essential part of setting up an ongoing system to monitor model performance after they have been deployed (often called "AI model surveillance") is to catch when the model's performance drifts or degrades over time.

3.7 FUTURE DIRECTIONS AND RESEARCH OPPORTUNITIES

DL and nephrology for early CKD detection is an emerging field. Several future directions and research opportunities have evolved from the progress and challenges identified.

Multimodal and Integrated Models: In the future, combining multiple data sources – multimodal DL will likely improve prediction accuracy and robustness. In that case, this could be integrating EHR data (labs, vitals, medications), imaging data (retinal photos or kidney ultrasounds), and genomic or proteomic data (genetic risk scores and biomarkers) to build a comprehensive risk model. CKD is a complex disease based on genetics, lifestyle, and environment, and a multimodal model could capture risk factors for all these fronts. For instance, a future model may, as input, include a patient's genome sequencing data (which provides for known nephropathy risk alleles), lab trends, and an eye exam image to estimate a highly personalized CKD risk. While these multimodal models initially tried to combine fundus images with tabular data, they are found to help with this approach. However, obtaining well-annotated datasets containing all these data types for the same individuals will be challenging, and initiatives in biobanks and integrated health systems are progressing in that direction.

Foundation Models and Transfer Learning: Foundation models (extensive models pretrained on large datasets and can be adapted for many tasks) are a hot topic for AI in its community. Already, there are BERT-based models for EHRs and vision transformers for medical images in healthcare. It is developing the foundation models specifically related to kidney disease that will delineate a future direction.

An easy example could be for a model to be pretrained on a wide set of clinical data from millions of patients (not just CKD patients but all EHR text and codes) and then fine-tuned to predict CKD with fewer labeled examples. It can significantly increase performance, especially for sparse data. Likewise, the same vision models pretrained on massive amounts of medical data (X-rays, retinal scans, pathology slides) could be retrained to interpret kidney sonography. Lin *et al.*'s scoping review also indicates that we could implement such platforms based on foundation or large language models (LLMs). For example, an LLM reads a patient's medical history and lab results and produces a narrative risk assessment or recommendations (akin to an AI assistant for the clinician). While ChatGPT has demonstrated its capacity to speak about CKD so far, the fitness of LLMs like ChatGPT to predict every synthesis directly is unknown; however, hybrid models that bring together language understanding (for texts) and deep forecasting might arise.

Real-time Monitoring and Wearable Data: Another direction is extending CKD prediction beyond periodic lab tests by utilizing continuous monitoring data. In the future, sensors in wearable devices can track blood pressure, heart rate, and physical activity and compute the GFR. It could stream such real-time data to a DL model for real-time risk scores or alerts. For example, a wearable cuff or smartwatch with persistent high blood pressure readings could dynamically update a patient's CKD risk profile between visits to the doctor. In similar research in other fields (like acute kidney injury), they attempt to predict hours in advance when a patient will suffer kidney injury and use this information to treat them before it happens. Wearables may help monitor medication adherence or lifestyle factors in the chronic form of CKD. Here, DL models that continuously learn from an individual's data (online learning) may be relevant and could detect meaningful deviations from the person's baseline Chen & Guestrin (2016).

Explainability and User-Centric Design: As such, future work will likely involve making AI tools more interpretable and user-friendly to clinicians. It covers developing standard ways to report model explanations, such as a "CKD risk report" for each patient that identifies the key factors and incorporates clinician feedback into model refinement. Models could be designed where clinicians can decide in some sense what parameters to give what significance place more weight on a specific lab if they suspect it's essential for a patient, and see what that idea looks like in terms of the concept risk, an interactive AI system rather than a static one. Visual analytics might also have a role: Would a dashboard with a doctor be able to visualize a patient's risk trajectory with a possible what-if scenario: "If we improve this patient's blood pressure by 10 mmHg, how does the model change the 5-year CKD risk?" Only through research into such decision-support interfaces can these models' preventive potential be realized.

Prospective Clinical Trials and Impact Assessment: These models must be tested in prospective settings to truly move the needle in CKD outcomes. The next step is designing a clinical trial in which one group of patients are seen under care provided by AI risk predictions (with clinicians intervening earlier for those flagged high risk) versus with standard care for the control group. This will address the question of whether early detection of CKD by an AI, coupled with an action such as early nephrologist referral or tighter BP control, results in slower CKD progression as well as other benefits. To gain clinical and regulatory acceptance of such trials, while having logistical challenges, is a key goal. This is also important to make continuous assessment of deployed models in the real world so that unintended consequences (e.g., do the AI end up encoding a policy to over test in low-risk patients?) are caught upfront and can be iterated.

Addressing Bias and Equity: Another point for future research would be to ensure that these models work equitably across all populations. On the other hand, it might involve bias mitigation techniques like re-weighting the training data or adding fairness constraints in the model training process. Validait is part of training models in underserved populations or low-resource settings. For example, an AI tool could solve the specificity problems inherent in remote areas, such as rural areas where rural patients with CKD are often underdiagnosed; however, this tool will have to be tested there. This is an opportunity for fair and inclusive AI – and if so, separate models or calibration for different demographic groups may be required. Further, in improving the handling of efficient methods for treatment in individual healthcare systems, localized models for varied healthcare systems that consider local practice patterns will prove beneficial.

Expansion to Related Renal Problems: This chapter is on CKD, but some future extensions of this could be using this DL approach to predict acute kidney injury (AKI) in hospitals or to detect specific nephropathies, such as finding patients who are likely to have IgA nephropathy or polycystic disease from some subtle clues. Adapting the tools and models developed for CKD to these related tasks may result in building an integrated AI-based kidney health platform. Another advanced direction involves using reinforcement learning (RL) not only to predict risk but also to provide optimal intervention recommendations for CKD patients over time. For instance, an RL agent can assume different treatment strategieswhen to start certain meds and refer you to the specialist while trying to learn policies that maximize kidney health outcomes. They propose that real-time treatment recommendations in CKD management could further advance AI through RL, as described by Lin *et al.* (2024). In the future, this AI could warn that the patient is at high risk and suggest changing their treatment plan accordingly. However, this would have to be extensively validated and under clinician oversight, and that's a start for AI-enabled personalized treatment.

3.8 CONCLUSION

CKD is a huge healthcare challenge that persists despite late detection and progression of the disease. Specifically, this chapter demonstrates how data from lab tests, EHRs, and medical images enable CKD prediction to be revolutionized by DL techniques, including CNNs, RNNs, transformers, and ensemble models. The high predictive accuracy of these models was demonstrated as a potential basis for early intervention and disease management. Nevertheless, issues remain, including lack of data interpretability and integration into clinical workflows. The field has been going in that direction toward multimodal modeling, explainable AI, federated learning, and real-world validations. The promise of DL is in the potential of DL to enable proactive, personalized care for CKD and to improve long-term outcomes.

REFERENCES

Alsekait, R., Kaabouch, N., & Misra, S. (2023). An efficient stacking-based ensemble deep learning model for the prediction of chronic kidney disease. *Computers in Biology and Medicine*, *158*, 106824.

An, J., Lee, H., Kim, K., & Lee, S. (2023). Predicting chronic kidney disease using deep learning on retinal fundus photographs. *NPJ Digital Medicine*, *6*, 21. https://doi.org/10.1038/s41746-023-00752-2

Chen, T., & Guestrin, C. (2016). XGBoost: A scalable tree boosting system. In *Proceedings of the 22nd ACM SIGKDD International Conference on Knowledge Discovery and Data Mining* (pp. 785–794). ACM. https://arxiv.org/pdf/1603.02754.pdf

Jongbo, O. (2019). Predicting chronic kidney disease using machine learning algorithms. *International Journal of Engineering and Advanced Technology, 8*(6), 4028–4033. https://doi.org/10.35940/ijeat.F9125.088619

Khalid, H., Khan, A., Zahid Khan, M., Mehmood, G., & Shuaib Qureshi, M. (2023). Machine learning hybrid model for the prediction of chronic kidney disease. *Computational Intelligence and Neuroscience*, *2023*(1), 9266889.

Kriplani, R., Rathi, R., & Bhatia, A. (2019). Prediction of chronic kidney disease using deep learning and machine learning models. *International Journal of Scientific & Technology Research*, *8*(10), 1092–1095.

Kuo, C. C., Chang, C. C., Liu, M. L., & Lin, M. C. (2019). Diagnosis of CKD using ultrasound images and convolutional neural networks. *Journal of Healthcare Engineering*, *2019*, Article ID 2139574. https://doi.org/10.1155/2019/2139574.

Lin, W. C., Tseng, C. H., Chen, H. H., & Hwang, S. J. (2023). Applications of machine learning in nephrology: A scoping review of the literature. *Kidney International Reports*, *8*(1), 75–84. https://doi.org/10.1016/j.ekir.2022.09.014

Lin, Y. F., Chen, H. H., & Hwang, S. J. (2024). Artificial intelligence in kidney disease: A scoping review and practical roadmap. *Kidney International Reports*, *9*(3), 443–454. https://doi.org/10.1016/j.ekir.2024.02.002

Lundberg, S. M., & Lee, S. I. (2017). A unified approach to interpreting model predictions. In *Proceedings of the 31st International Conference on Neural Information Processing Systems* (NIPS '17), California, United States, 4765–4774.

RAHMAN, M. H., Rahaman, M., Arafat, Y., Rahat, S. R. U. I., Hasan, R., RIMON, S. T. H., & Dipa, S. A. (2025). Artificial intelligence for chronic kidney disease risk stratification in the USA: Ensemble vs. deep learning methods. *British Journal of Nursing Studies*, *5*(2), 20–32.

Ribeiro, M. T., Singh, S., & Guestrin, C. (2016). "Why Should I Trust You?": Explaining the predictions of any classifier. In *Proceedings of the 22nd ACM SIGKDD International Conference on Knowledge Discovery and Data Mining* (pp. 1135–1144). ACM. https://doi.org/10.1145/2939672.2939778

Sabanayagam, C., Xu, D., Ting, D. S. W., Nusinovici, S., Banu, R., Hamzah, H., Lim, C., Wong, T. Y., & Cheng, C. Y. (2020). A deep learning algorithm to detect chronic kidney disease from retinal photographs in community-based populations. *The Lancet Digital Health*, *2*(6), e295–e302. https://doi.org/10.1016/S2589-7500(20)30058-4

Song, J., & Kim, H. (2020). Hybrid ensemble model for chronic kidney disease prediction. *Journal of Biomedical Research, 34*(3), 182–189. https://doi.org/10.7555/JBR.33.20200073

Yuan, Q., Zhang, J., Wang, X., Chen, Z., Li, Z., & Xu, Z. (2023). Predicting progression of chronic kidney disease using recurrent neural networks with longitudinal electronic health records. *BMC Medical Informatics and Decision Making, 23*, 156. https://doi.org/10.1186/s12911-023-02170-2

Zhang, K., Liu, X., Xu, J., Yuan, J., Dong, C., Liu, Z., & Wang, H. (2021). Deep learning predicts CKD from retinal photographs in a large population-based cohort. *Journal of Clinical Investigation, 131*(14), e142319. https://doi.org/10.1172/JCI142319

Zhu, Y., Bi, D., Saunders, M., & Ji, Y. (2023). Prediction of chronic kidney disease progression using recurrent neural network and electronic health records. *Scientific Reports, 13*(1), 22091.

Zisser, H., Kundu, S., Yang, Q., & Lei, L. (2024). STRAFE: Transformer-based survival model for end-stage renal disease prediction from longitudinal claims data. *Artificial Intelligence in Medicine, 143*, 102529. https://doi.org/10.1016/j.artmed.2023.102529

4 Beyond Crystal Balls

Machine Learning's Role in Proactive Healthcare – Predicting and Preventing Disease Outcomes

Samir N. Ajani, Prashant Khobragade, Komal S. Jaisinghani, Mrunalee Dhone, and Amreen Khan

4.1 INTRODUCTION

The integration of machine learning (ML) has significantly transformed healthcare in ways, where optimal well-being and preventing illness are paramount. This integration has allowed the field to move beyond outdate reactive models. In the past, medicine focused on treating illnesses after symptoms appeared. Currently, there is an increased focus on being proactive and predicting or preventing disease before it arise. This change [1] in how healthcare works is major, not minor. The future of healthcare uses advanced tools and patterns to try to foresee and avoid potential health problems. This new approach may supersede the traditional way of reviewing past issues to diagnose and manage existingillnesses. Healthcare is adapting because keeping people well, not just treatingillness, is the real goal. ML is key in this change and helps healthcare go beyond guessing to bring very exact care [2] (Figure 4.1).

For a long time, the usual way has been reacting after problems start. But as costs rise with more chronic illnesses and patients wanting more say, just reacting isn't enough. So being proactive is becoming more popular [3]. This means finding issues early, doing things to preventillness, and making plans for each person based on their health risks. This proactive way focuses on seeing problems before they happen and stopping them. It moves from just putting out fires to plans that are ready for what could happen later. These new models, shown in picture one, can predict future health dangers using how people live, genes, and their surroundings [4]. This lets help start before illnesses get really bad.

In terms of predictive abilities, ML is at the forefront of this evolution in healthcare. ML algorithms take in large and varied facts and extract valuable insights

 DOI: 10.1201/9781003479185-4

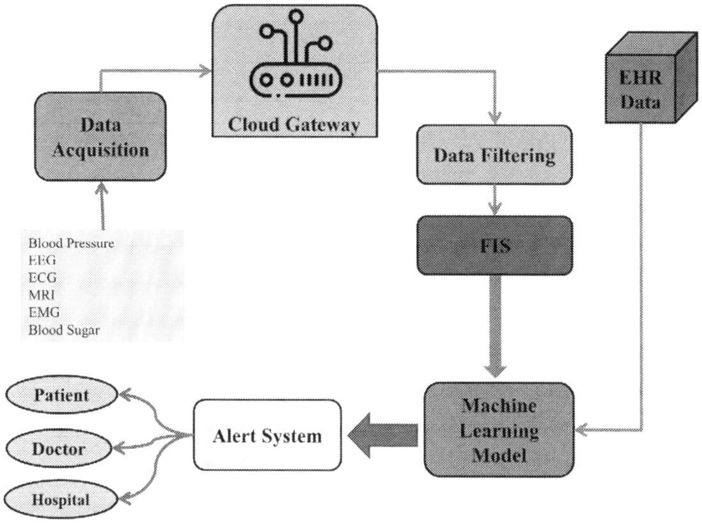

FIGURE 4.1 Representation of cloud-based health assessment system.

to guide medical decisions, surpassing crystal ball comparisons. These information-driven algorithms are able to navigate the complex network of factors affecting health results and offer a sophisticated thought that goes over human instinct. As a result, there is a greater focus on prevention, personalization, and the health of both individuals and communities within a more effective healthcare system [5]. As we outpace crystal balls, ML plays an increasingly important role in providing healthcare professionals with the capacity to anticipate and prevent potential health problems [6]. This introduction lays the foundation for a more thorough examination of the numerous ways that ML is changing the healthcare industry and bringing in a new era when algorithms will replace the crystal ball and show the way to a healthier and more resilient future [7].

4.1.1 Overview of Healthcare Landscape

In the past, healthcare focused on reacting to problems after they started. Doctors waited for people to get sick before helping. Now things have changed. Technology helps doctors learn more about staying healthy. They can find ways to stop illness before it gets bad. This is better for keeping people well. The doctors use big amounts of health info to help figure out how to prevent diseases [8].

4.1.2 Role of Machine Learning in Healthcare Transformation

ML examines large amounts of different medical data to find patterns and relationships connected to many health problems. The models can foresee how diseases may progress using details about surroundings, habits, and genes. Doctors can now make personalized care plans, adjust treatments, and employ targeted health advice, thanks to these predictive powers [9].

4.2 FUNDAMENTALS OF MACHINE LEARNING IN HEALTHCARE

4.2.1 Types of Machine Learning

There are generally three categories of ML that can be applied in different ways: reinforcement learning, unsupervised learning, and supervised learning. Models trained using supervised learning are shown labeled examples to recognize patterns and make predictions. This type is important for tasks like risk assessment and diagnosis in healthcare [10]. Unlike supervised learning, unsupervised learning analyses unlabeled data looking for hidden relationships and structures [11]. It helps group patient populations according to similarities, finds patterns not otherwise seen, and divides data to target specific needs better. Through trial and error with feedback as rewards or consequences, reinforcement learning enables an agent to learn via experience [12]. While not used directly for individual care as much, reinforcement learning may help improve treatment plans and use resources wisely (Figure 4.2).

The different types of ML can work together to greatly improve healthcare. Reinforcement learning allows for treatment plans that change based on a patient's needs. Supervised learning enhances the accuracy of diagnoses. Unsupervised learning finds patterns in large amounts of data that were not seen before. It is important to know how these main types function to make the most of ML's ability. This can help patients, make the delivery of care better, and lead to a future where health issues are detected early and treatment is provided in the best possible manner [13].

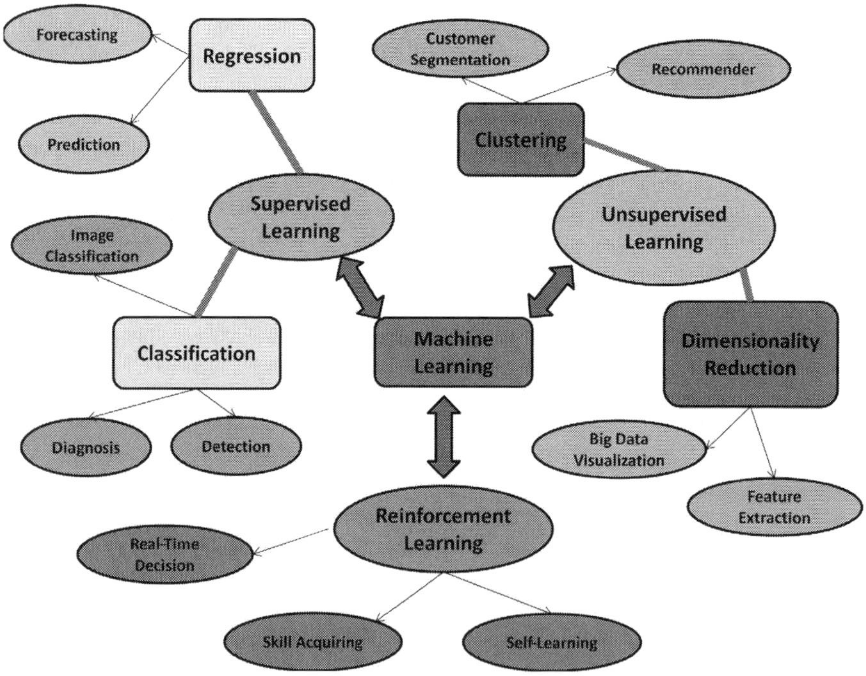

FIGURE 4.2 Different type of machine learning.

4.2.2 Data Acquisition and Preprocessing in Healthcare

Gathering data and preparation are indispensable initial phases, as shown in Figure 4.3, for employing ML in the extensive field of healthcare. Healthcare information is often intricate, diverse, and extensive, extending from medical imaging to digital health records (EHR). Effective data collection involves obtaining datasets from a variety of sources like wearable, labs, hospitals, and others to ensure a comprehensive picture of patient well-being. Once collected, data preparation is essential for transforming unprocessed information into a format that ML algorithms can use by cleansing, standardizing, and transforming it [14]. This consists of resolving data imbalances, normalizing variables, and handling missing values. To fully

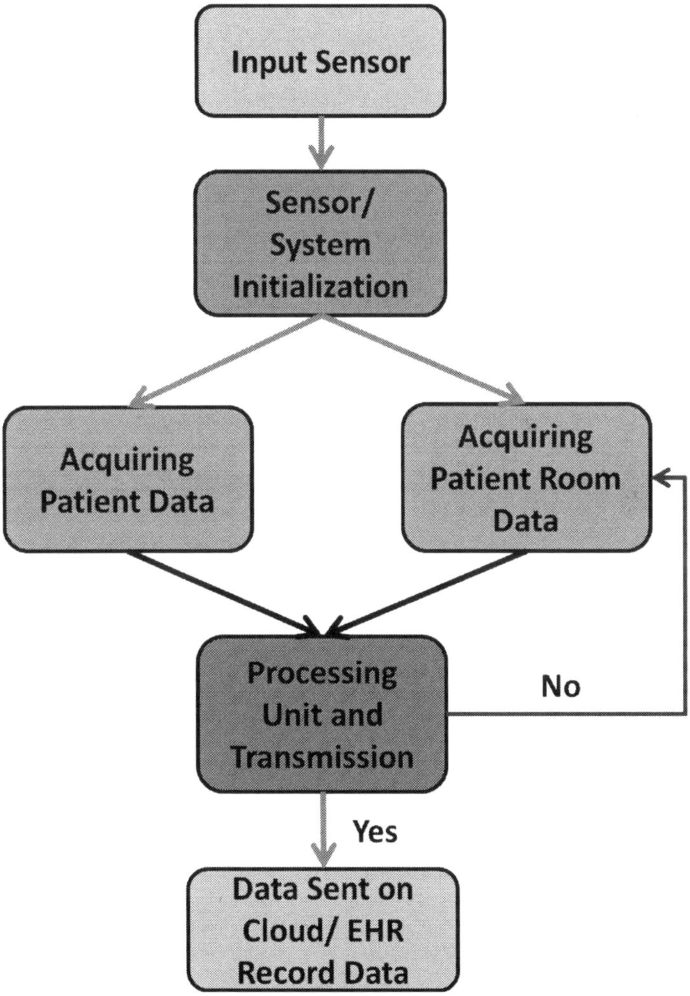

FIGURE 4.3 Flowchart of data acquisition and transmission in healthcare.

make use of predictive evaluation and pattern identification in healthcare, careful data acquisition and preparation are fundamental [15]. This is because the quality of the data directly influences how well subsequent ML models perform.

4.2.3 Supervised Learning for Predictive Modeling

In healthcare, supervised learning is critical, especially for jobs involving predictive modeling. Under this system, labeled data sets with known outcomes or goal variables are used to train the models. One important use of supervised learning is predictive modeling, which teaches models to classify or make guesses based on input features. This can be used in the healthcare industry for activities like risk assessment, treatment response evaluation, and disease diagnosis. For example, supervised learning algorithms use patterns from patient historical data that suggest how illnesses progress to forecast the chance of developing a certain condition. Decision trees, support vector machines, and group methods like random forests are examples of common algorithms (Figure 4.4).

4.2.4 Unsupervised Learning for Pattern Recognition

Unsupervised learning is essential for healthcare as it can find hidden arrangements and examples in unlabeled information without direction. Unsupervised learning equations look through information sets for intrinsic relations without predecided results, contrasting from directed learning. This enormously assists the medical services industry for undertakings, for example, discovering new comprehensions from enormous information sets, finding anomalies, and assembling patients. By sorting patients as indicated by normal qualities, conglomerating calculations permit changed consideration for explicit bunches. Calculations for anomaly location see

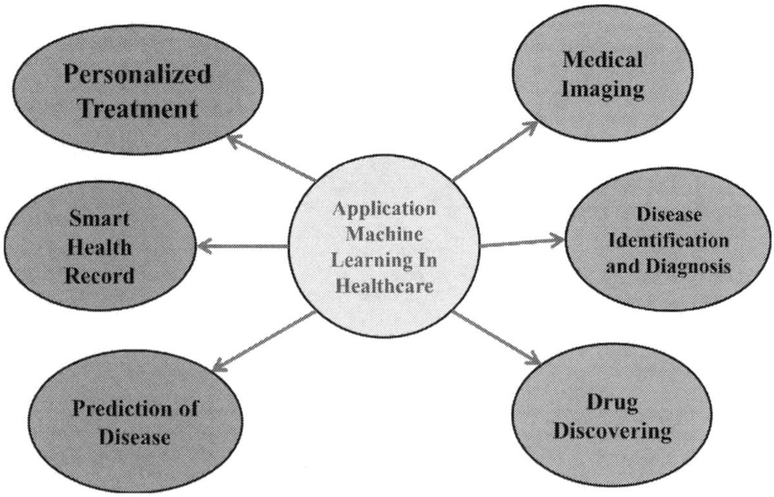

FIGURE 4.4 Overview of several keys using predictive model in healthcare.

deviations from normal, making oddities in patient information simpler to spot right on time. Unsupervised learning improves our comprehension of confused well-being occasions by uncovering fundamental structures [16]. It does this by giving a refined point of view that can point asset designation and cantered medicinal services advancement.

4.2.5 Reinforcement Learning for Adaptive Systems

Healthcare systems can benefit from the adjustable and varying decision making that reinforcement learning offers. The approach notes that an agent learns by interacting with its surroundings and getting responses through rewards or outcomes from certain behaviors. Reinforcement learning could improve how we handle treatments and distribute resources, even if it is less often used straight inpatient care now. It can help create treatment plans that adjust and develop over time based on how patients reply. Healthcare procedures could also gain from reinforcement learning, as it can maximize how work flows, where resources go, and when things are scheduled. Reinforcement learning's natural ability to change is well matched to healthcare's changing nature, as approaches and therapies need adjustments depending on real-time facts and patients' changing situations.

4.2.6 Deep Learning and Neural Networks in Healthcare

Deep learning, a kind of ML, can automatically create organized representations from intricate data. This has drawn a lot of attention in healthcare. Deep learning relies on neural systems, which are made of connected layers of nodes like the human brain. Deep learning works well for healthcare tasks like analyzing gene information, natural language processing, and inspecting medical images. Networks that repeat are great for sorting step-by-step data like patient records over time. Networks using transformation are very good at image jobs like figuring out medical pictures. By finding complicated designs and links within healthcare information, deep learning models extend how accurately we can diagnose and foreseen.

ML and healthcare are working together in new ways to change how care is given. Data and technology can help patients feel better, get the right care for each person, and use resources in better ways. Doctors and computers work as a team. Computers learn by looking at many examples. They find patterns to help doctors. Computers also learn while working with patients over time. This helps care adapt to each person's needs. Deep learning uses neural networks to find more details in data. It helps computers diagnose problems in new ways. Working together, ML and healthcare can create a system focused more on each patient. In the future, care will be proactive. It will also put patients at the center.

4.3 PREDICTIVE ANALYTICS IN HEALTHCARE

In the field of healthcare, predictive analytics is changing the field by using information from data to foresee what will happen later, particularly when it has to do with how patients will be and illnesses will advance. At its center, this different field uses a few ways, with predictive displaying being one of them [17]. In this examination, we investigate the hypothetical establishments of predictive showing and take a gander at its uses in healthcare. We likewise take a gander at instance considers that feature powerful figure models, highlighting the genuine impacts of predictive investigation on patient care and healthcare administration.

4.3.1 Predictive Modeling: Concepts and Applications

Doctors and computers both study health information to help people. Computers look at past data to see patterns and connections. This is called predictive modeling. It helps with healthcare in many ways. Predictive modeling helps doctors know who might get sick based on risk factors. It can also help figure out how well treatment works. Computers assess things like blood pressure, cholesterol, and heart disease chances to say how likely someone is to get heart disease. By doing this early, doctors can take steps to prevent problems or make personalized plans. This proactive approach reduces risks. Predictive modeling benefits diagnosis of illnesses, assessing patient risk, and predicting therapy results. It identifies patterns in a person's information that may signal certain conditions. Overall, predictive modeling and ML help healthcare professionals spot issues ahead of time and improve people's health.

Predictive modeling plays an essential role in grouping patients by risk level. Models can place people into risk groups after reviewing their complete medical profile, which includes genetic information, past health issues, and lifestyle decisions. By guaranteeing that high-risk patients get more consistent monitoring, focused care options, and quick assistance when needed, this categorization helps personalize interventions [18] and prevent unfavorable results. In addition, predicting how people will react to therapies relies heavily on predictive modeling. By studying past treatment records and patient characteristics, models can anticipate the chance of an individual responding positively or negatively to specific treatments.

4.3.2 Case Studies of Successful Predictive Models

- **Early Sepsis Detection**: This helps medical staff begin help like fluids or antibiotics at the right time. Their quick actions improve how patients feel and lower the chances someone may die.
- **Predicting Readmission Risk**: The doctors at hospitals work hard to solve a challenge that impacts how happy patients feel and how much medical care costs: some patients coming back soon after leaving [19]. To see how likely it is for people to return based on things like past hospital visits, other health problems, and their lives at home, the doctors use models that predict the chances. The doctors and nurses can decrease patients returning when not really needed by finding who faces the highest risks and giving treatments meant just for them like check-ups after leaving or help when back home.
- **Cancer Outcome Prediction**: The analysis of genetic details has assisted in envisioning cancer endings. By studying the DNA structure of growths,

designs are able to envision how the illness may progress and foresee how a specific therapy may reply to the tumor. This gift doctors the capability to tailor remedy plans, maximizing the potency of medicines, and lifting general survival rates.

The use of predictive modeling in these case studies shows clear benefits in early help, care fit for each person, and using resources wisely. The case studies show how predictive models really work in different parts of healthcare. Using predictive analytics together could make healthcare more helpful before problems start, focused more on each patient, and using resources better as healthcare keeps growing.

4.4 PREVENTIVE HEALTHCARE STRATEGIES

This examination explores how preventive healthcare techniques aim to deal with health issues before they become severeillnesses, representing an important change in the healthcare field. These answers, using ML and predictive evaluation, employ a complete strategy that includes adjusting habits, overseeing people's health overall, and finding groups at high risk. We look at each part closely in this in-depth review, shedding light on the methods and consequences that push the change to a healthcare style focusing more on people and stopping illness [20].

4.4.1 Determining Populations at High Risk

Some parts of staying healthy involve finding groups of people more likely to get sick. This needs a good understanding of what causes health problems. ML helps because it studies big collections of information to see patterns, connections, and things linked to illness [21]. It looks at past medical histories, lifestyle choices, genes, and background. Models can split people into categories by their chance of getting diseases or health troubles. They join data from all those places.

- **Genetic Risk Stratification**: Genetic data provides clues about disease likelihood. ML models detect gene patterns tied to greater chances for illnesses including diabetes, heart problems, and cancer types. Doctors can then tailor treatments and steps to avoid illness for those prone to hereditary conditions.
- **Social Aspects that Decide Health**: Besides what you inherit from family, the conditions around you significantly impact how healthy you are. This incorporates where you fit financially, if you can get treatment when you require it, and aspects of your surroundings. Machines that can learn and think can dissect this data to recognize gatherings that are in danger since they don't have similar way of life chances, homes, or admittance to therapy. Specialists can plan focal treatments that help with the fundamental reasons for well-being contrasts by considering these more extensive issues.
- **Chronic Illness Risk Prediction**: Foreseeing health problems anticipating designs are exceptionally great at anticipating the likelihood of ceaseless illnesses, which makes it conceivable to recognize gatherings in danger right

off the bat. For instance, so as to figure the danger of heart illness, these models inspect a few factors identified with cardiovascular well-being, like pulse, cholesterol, and way of life decisions. This makes it conceivable to actualize customized anticipation procedures, like medication administration and way of life adjustments, in light of each individual's exceptional danger profile.

4.4.2 Predictive Model-Based Targeted Interventions

Different types of help are needed to prevent health problems in groups with high chances of getting sick. Doctors use ways to identify individuals who are at the highest risk and develop programs for them based on things learned about what raises chances for each illness. They learn these things by studying patterns in large numbers of people.

- **Specialized Care Plans**: Starting with every individual's unique health background, computer models can generate personalized care strategies. These systems foresee how different diabetes patients may respond to specific medicines or lifestyle adjustments. This customized approach makes treatment work best, lessens unwanted reactions, and leads to better results for each person.
- **Finding Disease and Checks Early Programs**: Techniques used to find illness early are often part of planned steps. Models that foresee by looking at patient information help recognize those more likely to get some cancers. This is very useful for cancer checks. With this information, checks for people at higher risk can happen more often, allowing disease to be noticed sooner and help started when treatment works better.
- Predictive model techniques can help treat long-term illnesses like brain or immune problems. These models guess how sick someone will get and how their body will respond to different treatments by looking at patient info, like genes and body signs. This lets doctors make special plans for care, switching medicines or care based on how the person is thought to react.

4.4.3 Patient Engagement and Behavior Modification

Different types of healthcare are important beyond just medical treatments. Changing how people act and getting them involved are essential parts of preventive care. Computer programs that learn are important for understanding and changing how patients behave. This encourages people to take care of their health before problems start and to follow plans to preventillness.

- Predictive behavioral analytics looks back at past patient actions and data. Computer programs use this to predict future health steps. Models check the chances someone will stick to drug schedules or lifestyle changes. For instance, managing long-term illnesses. Doctors can leverage this foreknowledge to tailor helpful plans. Focused help addresses certain obstacles and boosts how patients get involved.

- **Customized Health Coaching**: Predictive models allow for the crafting of personalized health coaching plans. These programs leverage patient information to spotlight which habits could use adjusting most and design guidance based on each person's motivations and what inspires them. No matter the emphasis on physical activity, weight control, or stopping smoking, the success of these efforts rises when personalized for the unique qualities and challenges of each individual.
- **Digital Health Platforms**: ML algorithms allow digital health platforms to continuously communicate with patients. These systems can understand patients better by studying the information patients provide, like what they do, measurements of their body, and how they feel. Data analysis lets the systems share personalized tips with patients to prevent health issues. By predicting risks, digital health platforms empower people to take a role in staying healthy.

4.4.4 Using Machine Learning to Manage Population Health

The overall health of communities is vital, so population health management uses computers to improve medical care for many people. It finds those at great danger and makes programs to boost everyone's wellness and happiness together. By studying public health details, ML designs inspect which territories have higher rates of specific illnesses. This allows healthcare companies to better organize how they give medical services, places, and preventive plans. They can use what the designs learn to send what is needed where it is most required. As an example, some areas may soon see more individuals with diabetes. Communities in these areas can then do more to teach individuals how to stay healthy and avoid becoming ill.

- **Predictive Needs Estimation**: When managing large groups of people's health, models can recognize current illnesses and also anticipate future needs. By considering expected changes in community well-being over time, this involves estimating demand for specialized treatments, medicines, and doctor visits. Foreseeing needs allows preparing resources in advance, preventing lack and guaranteeing quick medical care when folks require it.
- Examining many types of information, like what folks say online, facts about the environment, and medical files, ML helps watch over public health better. This allows finding health risks, illnesses spreading between people, and how healthy folks are before others know. Spotting problems early leads to fast actions from health officials. Things like giving shots to certain groups or getting folks to stop illness from moving can happen soon thanks to quick discovery.

ML is helping change healthcare by focusing on prevention. These strategies spot people at high risk, provide tailored help, encourage healthier habits, and manage overall community health. Using data to predict problems and prevent illness can transform care delivery over time. It may strengthen our system and neighborhoods by using what we have more effectively and making people healthier.

4.5 DISEASE-SPECIFIC APPLICATIONS

4.5.1 Cardiovascular Diseases

New ideas to stop heart problems before they start, find them very early, and give good care fast are needed since diseases of the heart and blood vessels (CVDs) are still a big cause of illness and death around the world. When talking about ways to help with just one disease, two important parts need work to keep hearts healthy: predicting heart attacks and strokes, and watching and controlling high blood pressure (Figure 4.5).

One of the largest medical issues is foreseeing heart attacks and strokes. Computer programs using ML look at many facts about patients to foresee risk. They use things like how people live, test results, and what illnesses people had before. Doctors can lower chances of heart problems coming by finding those at high risk and doing things to help, like giving medicine or changing what people do. This helps people be healthier and costs less for healthcare. New technology helps check and handle high blood pressure, a major cause of heart issues. Devices you can wear and phone apps now let people check their pressure anytime. By giving patients and healthcare providers ongoing data, these tools help patients play an active role in their care. ML algorithms can analyze this constant stream of information to see patterns, trends, and possible problems. AI systems also assist doctors customize treatment plans based on how patients respond, optimize medicine schedules, and encourage lifestyle changes for better blood pressure management. A shift toward precision medicine is

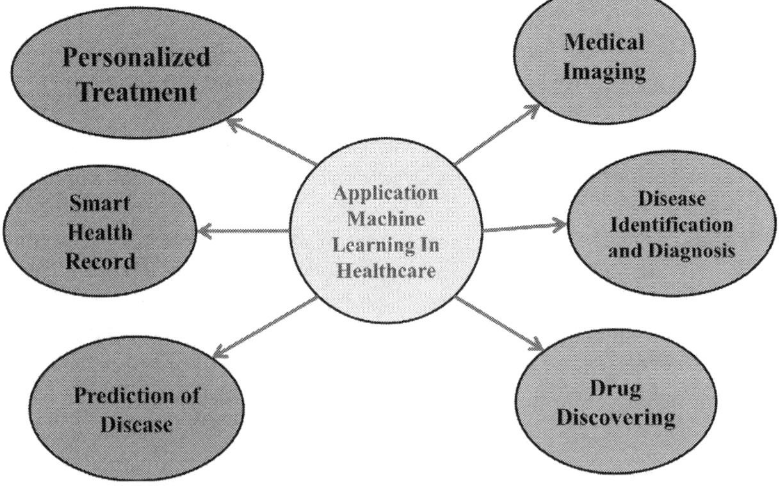

FIGURE 4.5 Application of machine leaning in healthcare.

seen in including apps for specific diseases in heart treatment. Patients can actively take part in preventive actions through these apps, which also help with early diagnosis and risk grouping. Furthermore, the ongoing monitoring of high blood pressure supports a more flexible and changing way of healthcare, moving from a model focused on one-time treatments to one that stresses care that continues and is customized for each person.

While these apps aim to help many, some issues remain. Laws are needed about AI in healthcare. People worry about privacy too. Data must move between systems, but they don't always work together well. If we want technologies to help, we must protect patient information. The easy sharing of data across devices and groups requires clear cooperation with current health setups.

4.5.2 Cancer

4.5.2.1 Early Detection and Diagnosis

Early detection and diagnosis are one of ML's most important roles in cancer care. Huge amounts of data, like genetic info, medical pictures, and patient records can be analyzed by ML programs to find tiny patterns and issues that may point to cancer. For example, ML programs can improve how doctors check medical pictures to help find problems or tumors early that human eyes could miss. Being able to act quickly and have better treatment is made possible by finding cancer soon. Furthermore, by learning from many kinds of data, ML programs can link markers to certain cancer types. This makes it possible to create blood tests and other tools that can find cancer in its beginning stages sometimes even before symptoms appear. Finding cancer early reduces needing a lot of expensive care later on, which lessens the total burden on healthcare while also upping the chance for treatment to succeed.

4.5.2.2 Customizing Treatment Plans with ML

Based on each patient's unique traits, ML helps doctors design personalized plans for cancer patients. ML algorithms find patterns that aid in predicting how a person might react to different medicines by studying huge datasets including genetic profiles, treatment responses, and outcomes. With this information, doctors can create more focused and efficient plans that maximize good results while reducing side effects. Genomics is where ML-driven precision medicine shows most clearly. ML algorithms can detect specific genetic problems or changes that may be helping cancer grow by looking at the genetic makeup of tumors. This data guides the choice of targeted treatments meant to take advantage of weaknesses in cancer cells with the least harm to healthy tissues. A big step in cancer care is the ability to customize treatment schedules at the molecular level, shifting from a one-size-fits-all approach to one that works better for each person [22].

ML helps doctors find cancer early and make treatment plans for each person. This new tech lets doctors spot illness in its first stages when it's easiest to cure. They can make care just for that patient's needs. Using ML for cancer care may help people more, make healthcare work better, and continue helping against cancer as tech improves with more information.

4.5.3 Diabetes

4.5.3.1 Predictive Models for Blood Sugar Levels

Doctors are using ML more to help predict blood sugar levels for those with diabetes. These models look at many things like what people eat, how active they are, past blood sugar readings, and other important details. ML can find patterns and trends that regular methods may miss. When guessing blood sugar highs and lows, predictive models are very useful tools for both patients and doctors deciding how much insulin to use, what to eat, and how to care for diabetes overall. For instance, you can get real-time guesses by combining glucose monitors with ML. This helps treat issues fast to avoid sugar being too high or low. By better controlling blood sugar, these preventions lower the chance of problems from poorly managed diabetes.

4.5.3.2 Personalized Dietary and Lifestyle Advice

ML can help create customized advice for diet and lifestyle for people with diabetes. Diet and activity suggestions are based on traits like age, weight, activity levels, and how foods affect blood sugar. Large amounts of data are processed using algorithms to find connections between lifestyle factors, blood sugar levels, and food choices. This permits customized recommendations for each person's needs. Diet tips may involve meal schedules, controlled portions, and tailored meal plans based on how the body functions. The suggestions can change over time as people's preferences, health, and reaction to changes are tracked. ML helps diabetics receive advice to improve choices for a healthier lifestyle. This leads to better control of blood sugar levels and overall wellness. Customized diet and lifestyle guidance as well as blood sugar predictions are part of ML's role in proactive healthcare for diabetics. Apps using these tools allow diabetics and doctors to better predict and control blood sugar highs and lows. Advanced data and insights from ML create personalized plans better than in the past. This promotes a predictive, patient centered approach to diabetes care. Applying ML to diabetes treatment can significantly improve proactive care for long-term benefits as the technology advances.

4.6 ETHICAL AND REGULATORY CONSIDERATIONS

4.6.1 Privacy and Security in Healthcare Data

When using machines that learn to preventillness, keeping private details safe and secure is vitally necessary to contemplate. Considerable amounts of sensitive health data, like what's in our genes, X-ray pictures, and records about people visiting the doctor, are frequently utilized as inputs for ML models. It is absolutely essential to protect this information's privacy to help and maintain trust among patients and those caring for their health. Adhering to rules for protecting information, like the general data protection regulation (GDPR) in Europe and the health insurance portability and accountability act (HIPAA) in America, is imperative. Making sure a patient's privacy and stopping people without authorization from attaining sensitive healthcare information can occur by using strong encryption, entry controls, and changing data so no one knows it's any one person.

4.6.2 Fairness and Bias in ML Models

The disproportionately help or disfavor of particular demographic groups may be created by models that were prepared utilizing biased or unrepresentative information sets. To ensure reasonable and equitable healthcare results, prejudices in anticipating models must be tended to and balanced. This requires consistent endeavors to diversify and improve the representativeness of preparing information, transparency in the model creation strategies, and appraisal of model execution crosswise over various subgroups. The generation and application of ML models should be directed by moral standards with the end goal of staying away from unforeseen results and advance value in the procedure of settling on healthcare choices.

4.6.3 Adherence to Healthcare Regulations (Including HIPAA, GDPR, and Others)

The healthcare rules that machines must follow are crucial. Laws such as GDPR and HIPAA protect patient information and say it can only be used with permission. Respecting what patients want and keeping their private health details private is important. This means having good rules for data, asking people if it's okay to use their data, and making certain any data use follows healthcare guidelines.

4.6.4 Guaranteeing Accountability and Transparency in Predictive Models

Using ML models in healthcare necessitates openness and duty, particularly when foreseeing illness and stopping it before it starts. Gaining the trust of patients and medical experts expects understanding how a model makes a specific figure. Direct desires and keep away from depending excessively on mechanized frameworks by being clear about the model's restrictions, uncertainties, and potential predispositions.

4.7 CASE STUDIES

4.7.1 Real-World Examples of ML Impact in Healthcare

Likewise, IBM Watson for Oncology uses ML to help medical professionals in individualizing cancer treatment plans dependent on a patient's specific situation. After thoroughly analyzing clinical trial data, patient records, and medical articles, the system provides proof-based suggestions for customized cancer care. Using ML in this way helps the system keep improving and evolving while also aiding treatment choices.

4.7.2 Testimonials from Healthcare Providers and Patients

Healthcare experts and those receiving care both emphasized how ML can help people stay healthy. Doctors found predictive models useful for deciding where to direct resources and improving how patients feel. For example, a doctor might have used an early detection system to find patients at high risk of problems, acted quickly, and stopped an illness from getting worse. People receiving care also talked about getting individualized help and suggestions based on what ML predicted. Someone could explain how a predictive model helped their healthcare team customize a treatment plan specific to them, leading to better handling of their condition and a higher quality of life. These stories showed how ML can really help healthcare focus more on each person and catching issues before they start.

4.7.3 Lessons Learned from Implementing Predictive and Preventive Models

Healthcare organizations face numerous roadblocks and chances for progress when employing predictive and preventive models. The significance of diverse and high-quality data is one critical lesson. Predictions from ML models can be considerably impacted by biases or shortfalls in the training information. As a result, maintaining representative and high-quality data sets is a constant problem and an essential factor in effective use of models. Creating a basis of trust between stakeholders is helped by regarding these factors early in the development method. Cases of thriving and troublesome technological unifications into medical practices are given by case reports, testimonies, and classes gained from applying ML in predictive and preventive healthcare designs. These useful occurrences give aware perspectives on the reforming might of ML and stress the importance of righteous, collaborative, and information-driven approaches for the continuing progression of proactive healthcare.

4.8 CONCLUSION

ML is changing how healthcare works by helping spot issues before they become big problems. Instead of just guessing what might happen, ML gives doctors better tools to study large amounts of data, see patterns, and act fast. This is clearly making a difference as real examples show how ML can predict problems coming, customize treatment plans, and generally improve patient care. To fully use this tech for helping people, we must understand the moral, legal, and practical issues. Private health information needs strong protections to keep people anonymous. Making sure the ML is fair and does not treat some people worse than others helps outcomes stay equal. Laws like HIPAA and GDPR that keep data private and used properly must be followed. Talking to patients and doctors shows moving to personalized care focused more on each person, and how ML is changing healthcare in big ways. Over time, healthcare can get better at using ML by paying attention to what works and does not from tests, like needing good and various data, teams working across fields, and always checking results. A new age of preventing illness before it starts is here thanks to predictive and preemptive ML models. As this area grows smarter, these models could completely change how care is given and be core parts of a complete healthcare system that cares for all.

REFERENCES

1. O. M. Moushi, N. Ara, M. Helaluddin and H. S. Mondal, "Enhancing the accuracy and explainability of heart disease prediction models through interpretable machine learning techniques," *2023 International Conference on Information and Communication Technology for Sustainable Development (ICICT4SD)*, Dhaka, Bangladesh, 2023, pp. 1–6, doi: 10.1109/ICICT4SD59951.2023.10303572
2. W. Baddah, H. A. Qasem, A. Alsabry, A. M. Hussein obaid, A. abdo Mohammed and F. E. Hanash, "Predicting heart disease using machine learning techniques on electronic health records data," *2023 3rd International Conference on Emerging Smart Technologies and Applications (eSmarTA)*, Taiz, Yemen, 2023, pp. 1–8, doi: 10.1109/eSmarTA59349.2023.10293622
3. Y. Galphat, L. Kithani, D. Raghani, C. Dayaramani and Y. Kriplani, "PREDICARE: Machine learning based disease diagnosis system," *2023 3rd International Conference on Pervasive Computing and Social Networking (ICPCSN)*, Salem, India, 2023, pp. 245–250, doi: 10.1109/ICPCSN58827.2023.00046
4. H. Yu, "Analysis and prediction of heart disease based on machine learning algorithms," *2023 8th International Conference on Intelligent Computing and Signal Processing (ICSP)*, Xi'an, China, 2023, pp. 1418–1423, doi: 10.1109/ICSP58490.2023.10248219
5. S. Kumar, A. Mallik, A. Kumar, J. Del Ser and G. Yang, "Fuzz-ClustNet: Coupled fuzzy clustering and deep neural networks for Arrhythmia detection from ECG signals," *Computers in Biology and Medicine*, vol. 153, pp. 106511, 2023.
6. G. Kim, M. Yang, G. -H. Kim, S. -H. Eom, T. -S. Lee and S. Park, "Predicting heart failure prognosis using deep learning based on FT-transformer," *2023 Fourteenth International Conference on Ubiquitous and Future Networks (ICUFN)*, Paris, France, 2023, pp. 932–936, doi: 10.1109/ICUFN57995.2023.10200998
7. T. Doi, A. Langsted and B. G. Nordestgaard, "Elevated remnant cholesterol reclassifies risk of ischemic heart disease and myocardial infarction," *Journal of the American College of Cardiology*, vol. 79, pp. 2383–2397, 2022.
8. A. Ali, H. V. Ramachandra, N. Ramakrishnan and G. Murtugudde, "Prognosis of chronic kidney disease using ML optimization techniques," *2023 International Conference on Advances in Electronics, Communication, Computing and Intelligent Information Systems (ICAECIS)*, Bangalore, India, 2023, pp. 459–463, doi: 10.1109/ICAECIS58353.2023.10170077
9. G. Pepera, M.-S. Tribali, L. Batalik, I. Petrov and J. Papathanasiou, "Epidemiology risk factors and prognosis of cardiovascular disease in the Coronavirus Disease 2019 (COVID-19) pandemic era: A systematic review," *Reviews in Cardiovascular Medicine*, vol. 23, pp. 28, 2022.
10. J. Kundu and S. Kundu, "Cardiovascular disease (CVD) and its associated risk factors among older adults in India: Evidence from LASI Wave 1," *Clinical Epidemiology and Global Health*, vol. 13, pp. 100937, 2022.
11. M. Ullah, A. Wahab, S. U. Khan, U. Zaman, K. urRehman, S. Hamayun et al., "Stent as a novel technology for coronary artery disease and their clinical manifestation," *Current Problems in Cardiology*, vol. 48, pp. 101415, 2023.
12. S. A. Ungerand A. M. Kucia, Diagnostic procedures. In *Cardiac Care: A Practical Guide for Nurses* (2nd ed., pp. 76–102). Edited by Angela M. Kucia & Ian D. Jones. Hoboken, NJ: Wiley-Blackwell, 2022.
13. A. Kishor and W. Jeberson, "Diagnosis of heart disease using internet of things and machine learning algorithms," *Proceedings of Second International Conference on Computing Communications and Cyber-Security: IC4S 2020*, pp. 691–702, Ghaziabad, India, 2021.

14. G. E. Shaya, T. M. Leucker, S. R. Jones, S. S. Martin and P. P. Toth, "Coronary heart disease risk: Low-density lipoprotein and beyond," *Trends in Cardiovascular Medicine*, vol. 32, pp. 181–194, 2022.
15. N. B. Amma, "Cardiovascular disease prediction system using genetic algorithm and neural network," *2012 International Conference on Computing Communication and Applications*, pp. 1–5, Tamil Nadu, India, 2012.
16. T. Münzel, O. Hahad, M. SØrensen, J. Lelieveld, G. D. Duerr, M. Nieuwenhuijsen et al., "Environmental risk factors and cardiovascular diseases: A comprehensive expert review," *Cardiovascular Research*, vol. 118, pp. 2880–2902, 2022.
17. F. Rustam, A. Ishaq, K. Munir, M. Almutairi, N. Aslam and I. Ashraf, "Incorporating CNN features for optimizing performance of ensemble classifier for cardiovascular disease prediction," *Diagnostics*, vol. 12, pp. 1474, 2022.
18. C. Gupta, A. Saha, N. S. Reddy and U. D. Acharya, "Cardiac disease prediction using supervised machine learning techniques," *Journal of Physics: Conference Series*, vol. 2161, pp. 012013, 2022.
19. E. Dritsas, S. Alexiou and K. Moustakas, "Cardiovascular disease risk prediction with supervised machine learning techniques", *ICT4AWE*, vol. 1, pp. 315–321, 2022.
20. S. Muthukaruppan and M. J. Er, "A hybrid particle swarm optimization based fuzzy expert system for the diagnosis of coronary artery disease," *Expert Systems with Applications*, vol. 39, pp. 11657–11665, 2012.
21. C. Dangare and S. Apte, "A data mining approach for prediction of heart disease using neural networks," *International Journal of Computer Engineering and Technology (IJCET)*, vol. 3, pp. 30–40, 2012.
22. I. S. F. Dessai, "Intelligent heart disease prediction system using probabilistic neural network," *International Journal on Advanced Computer Theory and Engineering (IJACTE)*, vol. 2, pp. 2319–2526, 2013.

5 Unveiling the Veil
A Comprehensive Exploration of Interpretable Machine Learning for Healthcare and Its Role in Elevating Transparency in Decision Support

Vinod S. Wadne, Suvarna A. Wakure, Devendra P. Gadekar, and Santosh T. Waghmode

5.1 INTRODUCTION

Machine learning (ML) is changing how we make choices in healthcare. This change is thrilling, but it makes us consider the complexity of these computer programs [1]. We need to learn why clear decisions in healthcare are essential as we start using ML more. What is ML in healthcare? It's when we use computer instructions and math to look at healthcare data, improve patient care, and guess what will happen with health. With lots of data, ML finds trends that help figure out diseases, plan treatments, and make medicines just for you. ML is good at looking at pictures and seeing what's abnormal, like in X-rays and MRI scans [1]. It also predicts which patients might get sick so doctors know who to help first. Plus, ML speeds up how we find and make new medicines. Despite its potential, challenges like data privacy and model interpretability require careful consideration. ML promises to revolutionize healthcare, enhancing efficiency, precision, and the overall quality of patient care [2].

5.1.1 The Need for Transparency in Healthcare Decision Support

In the healthcare field, every choice matters because it affects health and well-being. We must be open about how we can use tech in this area. If people can't see how complete systems decide, they do not trust them. As shown in Figure 5.1, there's a risk that people won't accept advice from a system they can't understand [2]. We need clear ML that's easy for everyone to get. We're working to bridge the gap. To match the power of ML in healthcare with our duty to keep it clear and trustworthy for doctors and patients alike. We focus strongly on the need for openness [3].

DOI: 10.1201/9781003479185-5

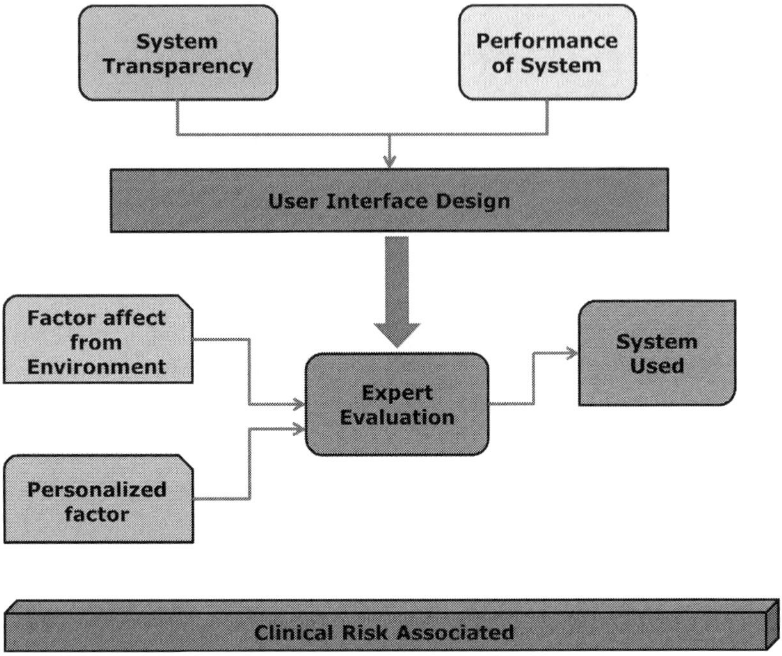

FIGURE 5.1 An examination of the level of transparency in the application of machine learning techniques.

5.1.2 Scope and Objectives

This chapter focuses on making healthcare choices clear with help from computers. We aim to explore how machines can learn in a way we can understand, including the theory, methods, and real-life uses.

The two main goals are to:

1. Explain the challenges that complex computer programs create in healthcare.
2. Describe how ML that's easy to understand could really make a difference.

5.2 FOUNDATIONS OF MACHINE LEARNING IN HEALTHCARE

5.2.1 Overview of Machine Learning in Healthcare

ML is changing healthcare in significant ways. It allows computers to learn from lots of data [4]. This way, they can discover patterns and predict things without being directly programmed. ML's role is getting even bigger as the healthcare data grows, along with advances in algorithms and more powerful computers. In healthcare, as shown in Figure 5.2, ML helps in many key areas. For instance, ML helps read medical images like X-rays, CT scans, and MRIs [5,6]. It finds tiny problems that can be signs of disease. This means doctors can identify illnesses earlier for quicker treatment. ML is also used in predictive analytics. By looking at patient data, ML

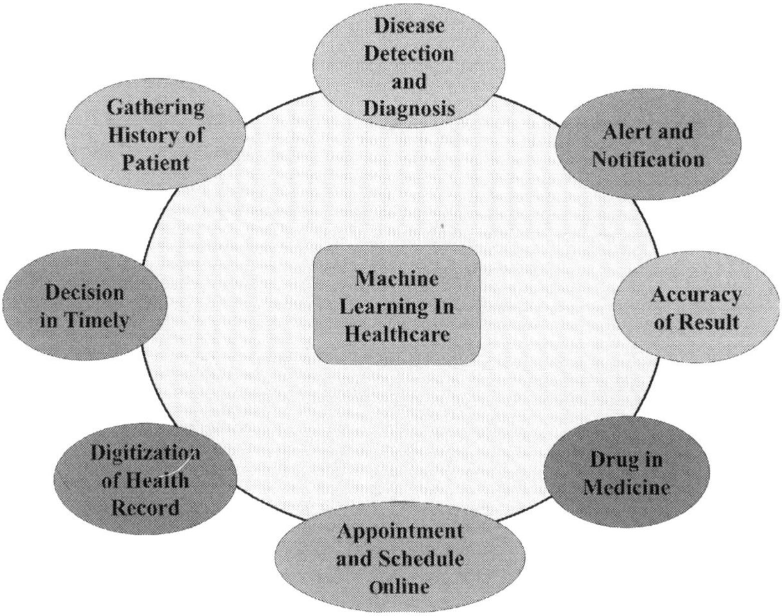

FIGURE 5.2 Machine learning in the healthcare domain.

models can guess disease risks and likely outcomes [7]. Healthcare workers then use this info to tailor care and prevention plans to each person's needs, improving health results and making healthcare more efficient.

Privacy concerns, data security, and the black-box nature of some algorithms raise ethical and regulatory questions [8]. Guaranteeing the openness and interpretability of ML models is critical to alleviating these worries and promoting patient and healthcare provider confidence.

5.2.2 Types of Machine Learning Models

Within artificial intelligence (AI), ML is a subset that includes a range of models for various data-driven activities. Comprehending the distinct categories of ML models, as illustrated in Figure 5.3, is crucial in [9] order to appreciate their extensive range of uses in the healthcare industry and beyond.

- **Supervised Learning**: Under the popular supervised learning paradigm, models are trained on labeled datasets. These datasets comprise input–output pairs, which help the algorithm figure out how inputs and matching outputs are mapped. In medicine, supervised learning is widely used for tasks like disease classification, in which models are trained on historical data to predict and categorize future cases [10].
- **Unsupervised Learning**: This method applies to datasets without labeled outputs. Unsupervised learning aims to find patterns, correlations, or structures in the data rather than making predictions about particular events.

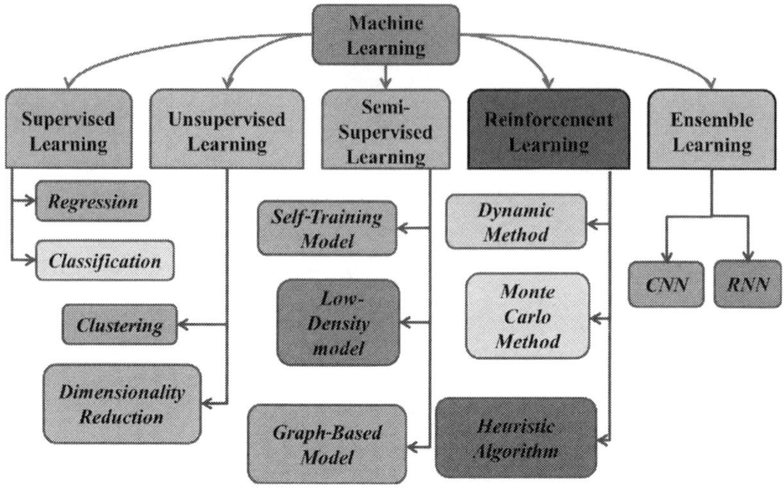

FIGURE 5.3 Different types of machine learning.

In healthcare, clustering and dimensionality reduction are often used techniques that aid in identifying patient groupings or simplifying high-dimensional datasets [11].

- **Reinforcement Learning**: This approach, which is based on behavioral psychology, involves an agent that discovers how to make decisions in a given environment via trial and error. Through feedback in the form of incentives or penalties, the agent gradually improves its approach to making decisions. Although it is not as common in clinical settings, adaptive therapies and personalized treatment plans can benefit from reinforcement learning [12].
- **Semi-supervised Learning**: Between supervised and unsupervised learning are two methods: semi-supervised and self-supervised. To take advantage of the benefits of both paradigms, models are trained on labeled and unlabeled data in semi-supervised learning. Using the available data, the model produces its labels using self-supervised learning, which promotes learning without needing explicit external annotations. These methods are becoming increasingly popular in the healthcare industry, where obtaining labeled data requires many resources [13].
- **Ensemble Learning**: Ensemble learning combines several models to increase overall performance. Boosting and bagging (bootstrap aggregating) generate multiple models and combine their forecasts. Ensemble learning improves prediction robustness, accuracy, and generalization across various patient groups in the healthcare industry [14].

Every kind of ML model has advantages and disadvantages, which make it appropriate for specific uses in the healthcare industry. While unsupervised learning can help uncover hidden patterns, supervised learning best suits tasks with well-defined objectives. Reinforcement learning presents opportunities for dynamic treatment [15] planning, and ensemble learning is a potent method for enhancing overall model performance. Understanding these model types in depth is crucial for prudent and successful implementation as the healthcare sector continues to harness the potential of ML (Table 5.1).

5.2.3 Applications in Decision Support Systems

The use of ML applications in the healthcare industry has increased dramatically, especially in decision support systems where the incorporation of cutting-edge algorithms greatly aids in clinical decision-making. These apps use data-driven insights to support medical practitioners, increase the precision of diagnoses, and improve patient outcomes. The following are essential domains where ML is significantly influencing healthcare decision support:

- **Diagnostic Imaging**: An everyday use case for ML algorithms is the analysis of medical pictures, including MRIs, CT scans, and X-rays. Radiologists can more quickly and accurately diagnose diseases like tumors [16], fractures or neurological illnesses using these algorithms to identify patterns and abnormalities.
- **Clinical Decision Support Systems (CDSS)** help doctors decide better by looking at patient info. ML makes CDSS smarter. It uses past health records and test results to suggest what might be wrong, what to do, and what medicine to give. This helps doctors make choices based on solid facts, simplifies steps, and cuts mistakes [17].
- **Predictive Analytics for Disease Risk**: ML analyzes patient information to find what causes illness. It's good for predicting health risks early on. For example, these models can tell if someone might get sick with cancer, diabetes, or heart problems. This means doctors can act sooner with special care or steps to stop the illness [18].
- **Drug Discovery and Development**: ML examines biology to find new drugs. It speeds up research, cuts costs, and might give us new treatments [19].
- **Patient Monitoring and Early Detection**: ML uses devices and health records to monitor patients around the clock [20]. It spots tiny health changes fast, helping catch illnesses early, which is essential for people with ongoing health issues.
- **Fraud Detection and Billing Optimization**: Beyond treating people, ML finds fake insurance claims and smooths billing. Noting odd patterns helps stop fraud and maintains the money side of healthcare rights.

5.3 INTERPRETABLE MACHINE LEARNING: A NECESSITY IN HEALTHCARE

5.3.1 Defining Interpretability

The ability to comprehend and provide a clear and understandable explanation for the judgments made by ML models is known as interpretable machine learning (IML). Interpretability [21] is essential in the healthcare domain to guarantee that

TABLE 5.1
Summary of Different Types of Machine Learning Models

Types of ML Algorithm	List of Algorithms	Details	Applications	Evaluation Parameters
Supervised Learning	Linear Regression	Predicts a continuous outcome based on input features	Predicting house prices, sales forecasting	Mean squared error, R-squared
	Decision Trees	Hierarchical tree-like structures for decision-making	Medical diagnosis, credit scoring	Gini impurity, information gain
	Support Vector Machines	Finds hyperplanes for classification	Image classification, fraud detection	Accuracy, precision, recall
	Random Forest	Ensemble of decision trees	Disease prediction, stock market analysis	Out-of-bag error, feature importance
	k-Nearest Neighbors	Classifies based on the majority class of nearest neighbors	Handwriting recognition, recommendation systems	Accuracy, F1-score
Unsupervised Learning	K-Means Clustering	Divide data into k-clusters based on similarity	Customer segmentation, anomaly detection	Silhouette score, Davies-Bouldin index
	Hierarchical Clustering	Forms a tree-like hierarchy of clusters	Taxonomy creation, document organization	Dendrogram analysis, cophenetic correlation coefficient
	Principal Component Analysis (PCA)	Reduces dimensionality by transforming features	Image compression, feature extraction	Explained variance, screen plot
	Gaussian Mixture Model (GMM)	Represents data as a mixture of Gaussian distributions	Image segmentation, speech recognition	Log-likelihood, Bayesian Information Criterion (BIC)
	t-Distributed Stochastic Neighbor Embedding (t-SNE)	Visualizes high-dimensional data in lower dimensions	Visualization, anomaly detection	Perplexity, KL divergence

(Continued)

TABLE 5.1 *(Continued)*
Summary of Different Types of Machine Learning Models

Types of ML Algorithm	List of Algorithms	Details	Applications	Evaluation Parameters
Semi-Supervised Learning	Self-Training	Expands labeled data by iteratively adding confidently predicted unlabeled data	Sentiment analysis, document classification	F1-score, precision
	Multi-instance Learning	Handles bags of instances where only some are labeled	Drug activity prediction, image classification	Area under ROC curve (AUC-ROC), Hamming loss
	Co-Training	Two models trained on different features collaborate	Information retrieval, part-of-speech tagging	Mutual information, confidence measure
Reinforcement Learning	Q-Learning	Learns optimal actions by updating a Q-value table	Game playing, robotic control	Reward, discount factor
	Deep Q Network (DQN)	Q-learning with neural networks for function approximation	Video game playing, robotic control	Experience replay, target networks
	Policy Gradient Methods	Directly learns policy function for decision-making	Robotics, autonomous vehicles	Policy loss, advantage function
	Actor–Critic	Combines value-based and policy-based methods	Continuous control, finance trading	Advantage function, policy gradient
Ensemble Learning	AdaBoost	Boosting algorithm combining weak learners	Face detection, text classification	Weighted votes, error rate
	Gradient Boosting	Builds trees sequentially, correcting errors of previous trees	Fraud detection, ranking algorithms	Learning rate, number of trees
	XGBoost	Scalable and efficient gradient boosting	Predictive modeling, anomaly detection	Learning rate, max depth
	LightGBM	Gradient boosting with a focus on speed and memory efficiency	Large datasets, real-time predictions	Tree depth, leaf count
	Voting Classifiers	Combines predictions from multiple models	General classification tasks	Weighted votes, probability threshold

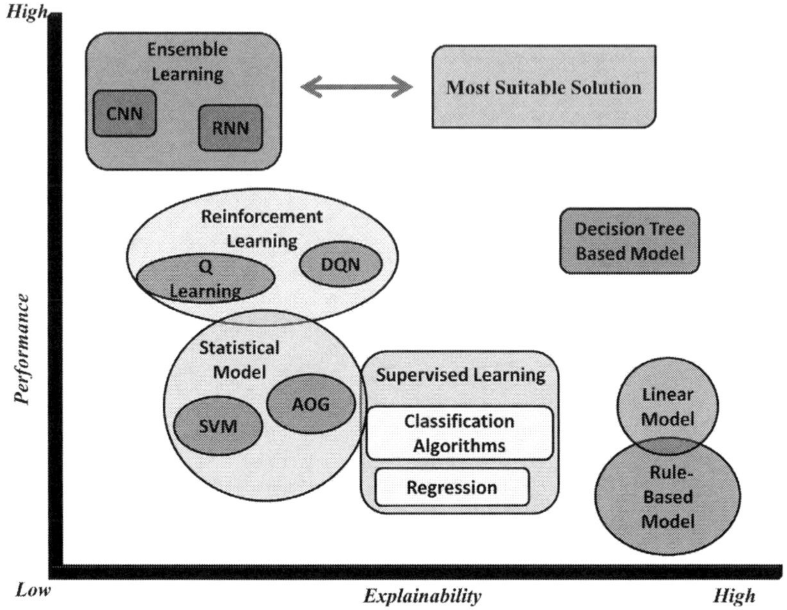

FIGURE 5.4 The performance of machine learning models and the explainability of those models.

the intricate algorithms employed in decision support systems (DSSs) are comprehensible not only to data scientists and engineers but also to medical practitioners, patients, and government agencies.

As shown in Figure 5.4, a model's interpretability changes depending on the stakeholders, the particular use case, and the decision-making context. Interpretability is not a universally applicable notion. Interpretability can take many forms, such as indicating the significance of a feature, producing decision rules, or presenting visuals that show how the model makes decisions.

5.3.2 Importance of Interpretability in Healthcare

Healthcare requires interpretability above [22,23] everything else for several important reasons, as shown in Figure 5.4. First and foremost, trust is necessary. Patient welfare is directly impacted by healthcare decisions, regardless of whether ML algorithms or human specialists make them.

The acceptability and use of these models will be hampered if patients and healthcare professionals cannot comprehend or trust their decisions. Second, ethical and regulatory compliance depends heavily on interpretability. Regulatory agencies like the Food and Drug Administration (FDA) stress how crucial it is for ML models used in healthcare to be transparent and comprehensible. Model [24] decisions must be explained in detail to comply with standards and laws. Healthcare practitioners need to comprehend and verify the suggestions provided by ML models in a clinical context. Interpretability guarantees that these experts can combine their clinical knowledge with algorithmic insights, resulting in better informed and cooperative decision-making. Interpretability also makes it easier to make improvements over time [25].

5.3.3 Challenges and Risks in Black-Box Models

The healthcare field faces certain risks because of black-box models. These are complex systems that are hard to understand. They use advanced methods like ensemble techniques and deep learning, and while they are good at predicting, they're not easy to see through. We know they're accurate, but we can't always follow their logic [26]. One big problem is that black-box models hide their reasoning. This is tricky for doctors. They might not trust or follow when they can't understand why a machine gives specific advice. They're worried about who is responsible if something goes wrong because of the model's advice. Another issue is when the models learn from biased data. If the information in the model is not fair, the outcomes will reflect that [27], which can worsen healthcare inequalities. It's essential to understand how these models think so we can spot and remove their biases. This makes sure the models are fair and valuable for everyone. Explaining what a model does is essential in healthcare, especially when new technology is involved. Making ML in healthcare clear and readable is key. It builds trust, ensures responsibility, and helps AI use the right way to care for patients.

5.4 INTERPRETABLE MACHINE LEARNING TECHNIQUES

5.4.1 Rule-Based Models

Rule-based models are ML that make decisions using definite rules. These modes are logical; they check specific conditions to determine what to do next. People understand the problem quite well. We often use these systems in areas like expert systems, finance, and medical care [28].

5.4.1.1 Rule-Based Algorithm for Disease Diagnosis

Step 1: Define Input Variables

Input variable, symptom, characteristics: It indicates as:

$$X = \{X_1, X_2, \ldots, X_n\}$$

Step 2: Formulate rules

Rule formulated based on medical knowledge are rule-based. Every rule consists of a variety of inputs and is associated with its outcome, and it is represented:

$$\text{Rule 1: If } X_1 > \theta_1 \text{ and } X_2 < \theta_2, \text{then Outcome} = A$$

$$\text{Rule 2: If } X_3 = \text{“Positive”}, \text{then Outcome} = B$$

Step 3: Evaluate conditions

Track and check the condition using the following:

$$\text{Condition } 1: X_1 > \theta_1$$

$$\text{Condition } 2: X_2 < \theta_2$$

$$\text{Condition } 3: X_3 = \text{“Positive”}$$

Step 4: Decision-making

Based on the criteria, it helps to decide based on rule-based knowledge and associated association rules.

$$\text{Decision : If Condition 1 and Condition 2, then Outcome} = A$$

$$\text{Decision : If Condition 3, then Outcome} = B$$

Step 5: Output

The output is shown as:

$$\text{Final\_Diagnosis} = \text{Outcome}$$

Example:

Let's consider a simple example for illustrative purposes:

$$\text{Rule } 1: \text{If } X_1 > 30 \text{ and } X_2 < 25, \text{ then Outcome} = \text{“High Risk”}$$

$$\text{Rule } 2: \text{If } X_3 = \text{“Positive”, then Outcome} = \text{“Positive Diagnosis”}$$

Given patient data:

$$X = \{X_1 = 35, X_2 = 20, X_3 = \text{“Positive”}\}$$

The algorithm evaluates the conditions:

$$\text{Condition } 1: 35 > 30(\text{True})$$

$$\text{Condition } 2: 20 < 25(\text{True})$$

$$\text{Condition } 3: \text{“Positive”} = \text{“Positive”}(\text{True})$$

The algorithm makes a decision based on the first satisfied rule:

$$\text{Decision : Outcome} = \text{“High Risk”}$$

The final diagnosis output is “High Risk.”

5.4.2 Surrogate Models

Surrogate models are like optimization. They copy the work of complex and heavy-duty models. People also call them meta models or even response-surface models. They're nifty because they quickly link what you put in and what you get out. Hence, these surrogate models help us guess outcomes or improve things much quicker. They're handy helpers in areas like ML and finding the best solutions [29].

5.4.2.1 Typical Methods of Surrogate Modeling

- **Gaussian Process Regression**: Kriging, or Gaussian process regression, is a Bayesian technique representing connections as spatial processes. In addition to forecasts, it offers estimations of uncertainty [30].
- **Radial Basis Function Interpolation**: This method interpolates between data points using radial basis functions (RBFs). It works well for high-dimensional spaces.

Neural networks can be trained to function as surrogate models using artificial neural networks (ANNs). They may not be interpretable, but they can capture intricate nonlinear interactions [31].

5.4.3 Explainable Neural Networks

Neural network topologies and approaches are referred to as explainable neural networks (XNNs) or interpretable neural networks (INDs) to improve the interpretability of their decision-making processes [32]. Because of their intricate designs, traditional neural networks, intense neural networks, are frequently referred to as "black-box" models since it can be challenging to comprehend how they make particular predictions, as shown in Figure 5.5. XNNs seek to improve the interpretability and accountability of neural networks by addressing this lack of transparency.

5.4.3.1 Relevance Propagation Layer-Wise

Layer-by-layer relevance (LRP): Using the propagation technique, each input feature is assigned a relevance score to determine how it affects the network's output. Although it is based on the concept of backpropagation, relevance scores are assigned to input features and neurons rather than gradients.

$$R_i = \frac{\sum_j a_{ij} \cdot R_j}{\sum_k a_{ik}}$$

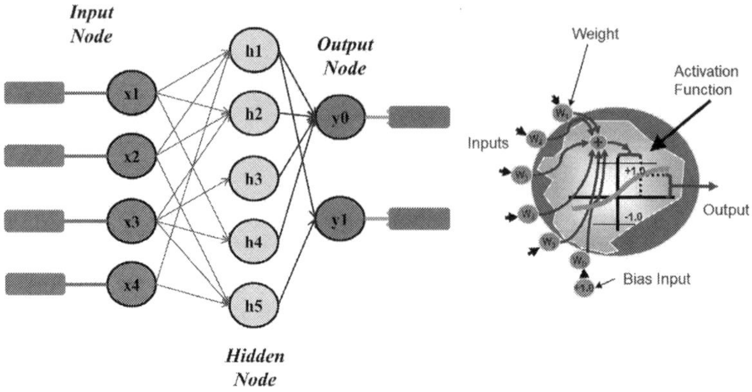

FIGURE 5.5 Representation of a black-box neural network.

5.4.3.2 Saliency Maps

Saliency maps draw attention to the key areas of the input image that support a particular hypothesis. The partial derivative of the output concerning the input is calculated using a gradient-based technique.

$$S_i = \frac{dy}{dx_i}$$

5.4.3.3 Interpretable Local Model-Independent Explanations

Any ML model, including neural networks, can have its predictions explained by local model-independent explanations (LIME), a model-agnostic technique. Around certain instances, it creates local surrogate models to simulate the behavior of the larger model.

$$\text{Minimize } L\left(f, g, \pi x\right) + \Omega\left(g\right)$$

5.4.3.4 Shapley Additive Explanations

According to the concepts of cooperative game theory, shapley additive explanations (SHAP) values assign the contributions of each feature to a prediction. It offers an equitable allocation of each feature's contribution to the forecast.

$$\phi_i(f) = \sum_{S \subseteq N \setminus \{i\}} \frac{S|!\left(|S|\,|N| - |S| - 1\right)!}{|N|!}\left[f\left(S \cup \{i\}\right) - f\left(S\right)\right]$$

5.4.3.5 Pruning Neural Networks

Some neurons or connections are pruned to simplify a neural network's structure. The network that has been pruned can reveal information about the significance of particular neurons or connections.

$$\text{Minimize } L(\theta) + \lambda \cdot \text{Pruning}_{\text{Cost}(\theta)}$$

5.5 USE CASES OF INTERPRETABLE MACHINE LEARNING IN HEALTHCARE

5.5.1 Systems for Clinical Decision Support

Overview: CDSS analyze patient data to guide medical professionals. These systems draw on strong evidence to provide advice. They make sure doctors understand their suggestions clearly, thanks to interpretable ML.

Advantages:

- Increased confidence between medical experts.
- Better communication and cooperation between ML models and physicians.

5.5.2 Diagnostic Predictive Modeling

Overview: Predictive modeling uses ML in healthcare to guess which diseases a person might have. To make these predictions, it looks at patient information, symptoms, and test results.

The Application of IML:

- Finding the most critical patient characteristics that affect the diagnosis and providing justifications for the decisions made is what feature importance analysis is all about.

Advantages:

- More certainty in the diagnosis's prognoses.
- The establishment of a channel of communication between medical professionals and AI systems.

5.5.3 Tailored Care Coordination

Overview: IML is essential in tailoring treatment plans to each patient by considering their unique characteristics and therapeutic responses.

The Application of IML:

- Rule-based models guarantee decision transparency by using understandable criteria for treatment decisions based on patient characteristics [33].
- What the model is predictions: Building rapport and comprehension by providing clear explanations for treatment plan suggestions.

Advantages:

- Individualized and patient-focused treatment plans.
- Improved patient acceptance and compliance with treatment regimens.
- Working together, ML models and healthcare providers can give individualized care.

5.5.4 Observation and Prompt Identification

Overview: Machine learning helps doctors catch health problems early. It constantly looks at patient data and spots small changes in health signs.

The Application of IML:

- Feature importance analysis is a method for identifying critical traits or biomarkers that suggest early warning signs.
- Reasons behind alerts: Helping medical professionals understand the reasoning behind notifications by providing understandable reasons for warnings generated by surveillance systems.

Advantages:

- Prompt action and averting situations from getting worse.
- Enhanced dialogue between healthcare providers and ML models.
- Systems of transparent decision-making that are reliable.

5.6 ADDRESSING ETHICAL AND REGULATORY CONSIDERATIONS

5.6.1 Ethical Implications of Healthcare AI

- Transparency is necessary for ethical AI in healthcare. Patients and healthcare professionals should know how AI models make judgments [34] to guarantee informed consent and promote trust.
- **Patient Autonomy**: It's critical to respect patients' right to autonomy. It should not be compromised for patients' autonomy to choose their healthcare providers by AI recommendations.
- **Accountability**: It's critical to set up distinct channels of accountability.

5.6.2 Regulatory Frameworks and Guidelines

- HIPAA Compliance, also known as the Health Insurance Portability and Accountability Act, sets forth regulations in the United States to safeguard confidential patient data. These directives are pertinent to every AI system within the healthcare sector.
- The European Union's General Data Protection Regulation (GDPR) provides a comprehensive structure for protecting personal data. Healthcare AI applications handling patient data must adhere to GDPR [35].
- The FDA holds regulatory authority over healthcare AI applications in the U.S., mainly if classified as medical devices.

New Developments in Regulations:

- The evolving landscape of healthcare indicates a growing need for specific regulations targeting AI. This underscores the potential emergence of novel frameworks tailored to address the unique challenges posed by AI technologies.

- The seamless integration of AI applications with existing healthcare systems may require regulations prioritizing the promotion of interoperability standards.

5.6.3 Privacy and Security Concerns

Data encryption is a crucial security measure that safeguards patient information during transmission and storage.

- Strict access controls must be implemented to limit who can access sensitive patient data. Only authorized personnel should be able to access patient data and AI models.
- To address privacy concerns, healthcare AI systems should incorporate methods for de-identifying and anonymizing patient data.
- Verifying the security of AI models before deploying them is of the utmost importance. Defensively protecting models against intrusions and hostile attacks is essential to safe deployment.

5.7 CASE STUDIES AND PRACTICAL IMPLEMENTATIONS

5.7.1 Real-World Examples of Interpretable Machine Learning in Healthcare

---

Case Study 1: Predicting the Risk of Readmission through the Use of Predictive Analytics

- **Goal**: Estimate the likelihood that patients with heart failure will return to the hospital.
- **Implementation**: A rule-based model with interpretable features, including medication. The model's clear risk scores allowed physicians to see what made each patient more likely to need to be readmitted.
- **Outcome**: Reduction in avoidable readmissions due to better patient management and resource allocation.

Case Study 2: Using Saliency Maps to Interpret Radiology Images

- **Goal**: Make AI in medicine more straightforward. This helps find odd patterns in medical scans.
- **Implementation**: We used "highlight maps" to show which parts of a scan matter. Doctors use these to see what guides the AI's choices.
- **Result**: Doctors gain trust in AI. They read scans faster and check if AI works right in real hospitals.

5.7.2 Lessons Learned and Best Practices

5.7.2.1 Lesson 1: Working with Domain Experts to Collaborate on Design

- **Lesson Learned**: Working with medical experts early ensures the model matches how clinics work. It also addresses real health concerns effectively.

5.7.3 Resolving Implementation Obstacles

First Challenge: Juggling interpretability and model complexity

- **Solution**: Make use of hybrid models, which incorporate interpretable elements.

Challenge 2: Ethical considerations and data quality

- Resolve biases in training data and prioritize data quality.

Challenge 3: Trust and acceptance by users

- User-friendly interfaces, conduct user-centric design and give concise justifications for model decisions. Promote a cooperative strategy between end users and ML developers.

5.8 CONCLUSION

ML and AI are transforming healthcare positively. These tools help us in predicting health occurrences, monitoring patients and supporting doctors. They could make healthcare work a whole new way. First, it must look hard at how the models do. Measures like recall and accuracy tell us if they work well. Doctors need to trust AI and understand how it makes choices. Things like saliency maps and rules help with this. Ethics in AI matter more as it grows in healthcare. Ideas like fairness and openness guide AI creation. To be fair to patients and earn their trust, we need to fix any bias in the AI. Makers of AI must be responsible for what it does.

GDPR and HIPAA are key, and new laws for AI in healthcare will come. We expect rules for sharing data safely and keeping patient details secret. AI privacy and safety are big deals. We keep data safe with encryption and by limiting who can see it. We also keep AI safe from attacks to keep diagnoses accurate. A new AI that's easier to understand looks promising. This transparent AI will ensure that it works right, is open, and is useful. We need more study and teamwork to handle AI's ethical and legal troubles. In short, blending ML with healthcare can make things way better. It calls for strong morals, obeying laws, and seeking safety and clarity. With the integration of AI in healthcare, we must carefully balance its advantages with caution toward its possible risks.

REFERENCES

1. Li, B.H.; Hou, B.C.; Yu, W.T.; Lu, X.B.; Yang, C.W. Applications of artificial intelligence in intelligent manufacturing: A review. *Front. Inf. Technol. Electron. Eng.* 2017, 18, 86–96.
2. Kaplan, A.; Haenlein, M. Rulers of the world, unite! The challenges and opportunities of artificial intelligence. *Bus. Horiz.* 2020, 63, 37–45.
3. Chien, C.F.; Dauzere-Peres, S.; Huh, W.T.; Jang, Y.J.; Morrison, J.R. Artificial intelligence in manufacturing and logistics systems: Algorithms, applications, and case studies. *Int. J. Prod. Res.* 2020, 58, 2730–2731.
4. Mittelstadt, B.; Russell, C.; Wachter, S. Explaining Explanations in AI. *Proceedings of ACM Conference on Fairness, Accountability, and Transparency (FAT* 2019)*, New York, USA, 2019; pp. 279–288.
5. Obermeyer, Z.; Powers, B.; Vogeli, C.; Mullainathan, S. Dissecting racial bias in an algorithm used to manage the health of populations. *Science.* 2019, 366(6464), 447–453.
6. Oh, J.; Makar, M.; Fusco, C.; McCaffrey, R.; Rao, K.; Ryan, E.E.; Washer, L.; West, L.R.; Young, V.B.; Guttag, J.; Hooper, D.C.; Shenoy, E.S.; Wiens, J. A generalizable, data-driven approach to predict daily risk of clostridium difficile infection at two large academic health centers. *Infect. Control Hosp. Epidemiol.* 2018, 39(04), 425–433.
7. Neff, G.; Tanweer, A.; Fiore-Gartland, B.; Osburn, L. Critique and contribute: A practice-based framework for improving critical data studies and data science. *Big Data.* 2017, 5(2), 85–97.
8. Kumar, P.; Sharma, S.K.; Dutot, V. Artificial intelligence (AI)-enabled CRM capability in healthcare: The impact on service innovation. *Int. J. Inf. Manag.* 2023, 69, 102598.
9. Aiken, R.M.; Epstein, R.G. Ethical guidelines for AI in education: Starting a conversation. *Int. J. Artif. Intell. Educ.* 2000, 11, 163–176.
10. Bansal, A.; Padappayil, R.P.; Garg, C.; Singal, A.; Gupta, M.; Klein, A. Utility of artificial intelligence amidst the COVID-19 pandemic: A review. *J. Med. Syst.* 2020, 44, 156.
11. Chee, M.L.; Ong, M.E.H.; Siddiqui, F.J.; Zhang, Z.; Lim, S.L.; Ho, A.F.W.; Liu, N. Artificial intelligence applications for COVID-19 in intensive care and emergency settings: A systematic review. *Int. J. Environ. Res. Public Health.* 2021, 18, 4749.
12. Minz, A.; Mahobiya, C. MR Image Classification Using Adaboost for Brain Tumor Type. In *Proceedings of the IEEE 7th International Advance Computing Conference*, Hyderabad, India, 5–7 January 2017; pp. 701–705.
13. Ribbens, A.; Hermans, J.; Maes, F.; Vandermeulen, D.; Suetens, P. Unsupervised segmentation, clustering, and group-wise registration of heterogeneous populations of brain MR images. *IEEE Trans. Med. Imaging.* 2014, 33, 201–224.
14. Strachan, O.; Asan, O. Reengineering Clinical Decision Support Systems for Artificial Intelligence. In *Proceedings of the IEEE International Conference on Healthcare Informatics*, Oldenburg, Germany, 30 November–3 December 2020; pp. 1–3.
15. Comito, C.; Falcone, D.; Forestiero, A. Current Trends and Practices. In *Smart Health Monitoring and Clinical Decision Support*. In *Proceedings of the IEEE International Conference on Bioinformatics and Biomedicine*, Seoul, Republic of Korea, 16–19 December 2020; pp. 2577–2584.
16. Bernardini, M.; Romeo, L.; Frontoni, E.; Amini, M.R. A semi-supervised multitask learning approach for predicting short-term kidney disease evolution. *IEEE J. Biomed. Health Inform.* 2021, 25, 3983–3994.
17. Yu, H.; Zhou, Z. Optimization of IoT-based artificial intelligence assisted telemedicine health analysis system. *IEEE Access.* 2021, 9, 85034–85048.
18. Chen, Z. An AI-based heart failure treatment adviser system. *IEEE J. Transl. Eng. Health Med.* 2018, 6, 1–10.

19. Dhieb, N.; Ghazzai, H.; Besbes, H.; Massoud, Y. A Secure AI-Driven architecture for automated insurance systems: Fraud detection and risk measurement. *IEEE Access*. 2020, 8, 58546–58558.
20. Merhi, M.I. An evaluation of the critical success factors impacting artificial intelligence implementation. *Int. J. Inf. Manag*. 2022, 69, 102545.
21. Sqalli, M.T.; Al-Thani, D. AI-Supported Health Coaching Model for Patients with Chronic Diseases. In *Proceedings of the 16th International Symposium on Wireless Communication Systems*, Oulu, Finland, 27–30 August 2019; pp. 452–456.
22. Zhou, L. A rapid, accurate and machine-agnostic segmentation and quantification method for CT-based COVID-19 diagnosis. *IEEE Trans. Med. Imaging*. 2020, 39, 2638–2652.
23. Tobore, I.; Li, J.; Yuhang, L.; Al-Handarish, Y.; Kandwal, A.; Nie, Z.; Wang, L. Deep learning intervention for health care challenges: Some biomedical domain considerations. *JMIR mHealth uHealth*. 2019, 7, e11966.
24. Kitsios, F.; Kamariotou, M. Information Systems Strategy and Strategy-as-Practice: Planning Evaluation in SMEs. In *Proceedings of the Americas Conference on Information Systems (AMCIS2019)*, Cancun, Mexico, 15–17 August 2019; pp. 1–10.
25. Wahl, B.; Cossy-Gantner, A.; Germann, S.; Schwalbe, N.R. Artificial intelligence (AI) and global health: How can AI contribute to health in resource-poor settings? *BMJ Glob. Health*. 2018, 3, e000798.
26. Kaur, A.; Garg, R.; Gupta, P. Challenges Facing AI and Big Data for Resource-Poor Healthcare System. In *Proceedings of the 2nd International Conference on Electronics and Sustainable Communication Systems*, Coimbatore, India, 4–6 August 2021; pp. 1426–1433.
27. Goodarzian, F.; Ghasemi, P.; Gunasekaren, A.; Taleizadeh, A.A.; Abraham, A. A sustainable-resilience healthcare network for handling the COVID-19 pandemic. *Ann. Oper. Res*. 2021, 312, 761–825.
28. Pee, L.G.; Pan, S.; Cui, L. Artificial intelligence in healthcare robots: A social informatics study of knowledge embodiment. *J. Assoc. Inf. Sci. Technol*. 2019, 70, 351–369.
29. Madurai, P.K.; Dewangan, Y.; Yadav, D.; Chauhan, S.; Singh, K. IoT Based Patient Health Monitoring Portable Kit. In *Proceedings of the 2nd International Conference on Advances in Computing, Communication Control and Networking*, Greater Noida, India, 18–19 December 2020; pp. 513–516.
30. Hossen, M.S.; Karmoker, D. Predicting the Probability of COVID-19 Recovered in South Asian Countries Based on Healthy Diet Pattern Using a Machine Learning Approach. In *Proceedings of the 2nd International Conference on Sustainable Technologies for Industry 4.0*, Dhaka, Bangladesh, 19–20 December 2020; pp. 1–6.
31. Xie, X.; Zang, Z.; Ponzoa, J.M. The information impact of network media, the psychological reaction to the COVID-19 pandemic, and online knowledge acquisition: Evidence from Chinese college students. *J. Innov. Knowl*. 2020, 5, 297–305.
32. Dharani, N.; Krishnan, G. ANN Based COVID-19 Prediction and Symptoms Relevance Survey and Analysis. In *Proceedings of the 5th International Conference on Computing Methodologies and Communication*, Erode, India, 8–10 April 2021; pp. 1805–1808.
33. Duan, L.; Street, W.N.; Xu, E. Healthcare information systems: Data mining methods in creating a clinical recommender system. *Enterp. Inf. Syst*. 2011, 5, 169–181.
34. Antoniou, Z.C.; Panayides, A.S.; Pantzaris, M.; Constantinides, A.G.; Pattichis, C.S.; Pattichis, M.S. Real-Time adaptation to time-varying constraints for medical video communications. *IEEE J. Biomed. Health Inform*. 2018, 22, 1177–1188.
35. Liu, J.; Ma, J.; Li, J.; Huang, M.; Sadiq, N.; Ai, Y. Robust watermarking algorithm for medical volume data in the internet of medical things. *IEEE Access*. 2020, 8, 93939–93966.

6 A Comprehensive Exploration of How Deep Learning Is Revolutionizing Patient Care in the Healthcare Landscape

Ali Mohammed Hendi,
Mohammad Alamgir Hossain,
Suresh Limkar, Naif Ali Majrashi,
and Mehebubar Rahman

6.1 INTRODUCTION

6.1.1 Background and Motivation

Precise diagnosis and individualized care have long posed challenges for the health systems. The review and assessment of medical data demand sophisticated tools due to its vast size and intricate nature. This study explores how advanced methods can better handle health care's modern complexities. As traditional approaches show declining effectiveness, the industry seeks solutions in deep learning [1] with its power to examine extensive data collections, uncover subtle connections, and provide essential understandings. Health care strives for more exact and streamlined delivery, making leveraging deep learning's promising abilities crucial.

This study comes from constantly trying to improve health outcomes using new ideas. Custom care plans, predicting trends, and exact diagnoses have all been hard on standard healthcare setups [2]. Deep learning's use is fair because it can review giant sets of facts, see hidden connections, and find practical knowledge. Healthcare information is getting harder to understand fast, and choices need to be quick and right, so we must use deep learning's powers to solve these problems.

6.1.2 Overview of Deep Learning in Health Care

Understanding how this technology works is key to understanding how learning helps health care fully. Deep learning, a part of artificial intelligence (AI), uses neural networks to try and mimic how humans make choices. Doctors and scientists are looking at medical information like scans and records with programs [3].

DOI: 10.1201/9781003479185-6

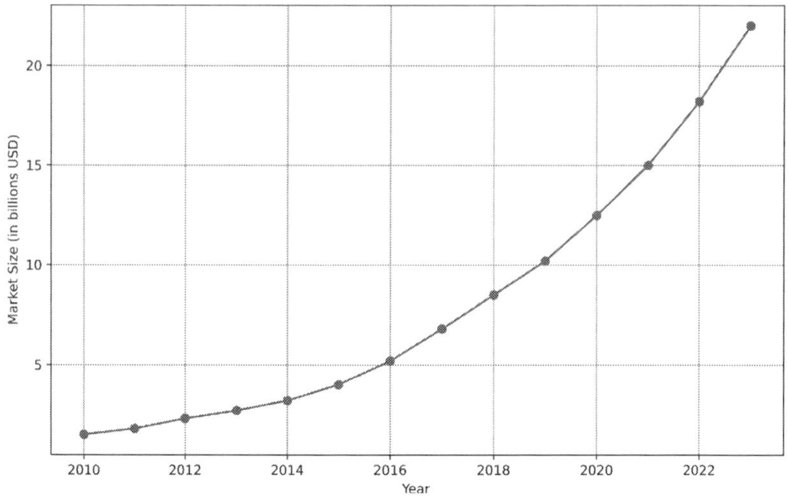

FIGURE 6.1 Deep learning in healthcare market size worldwide.

These programs use rules to see patterns. This beginning part discusses the basic idea of deep learning for all care. It can deal with many kinds of medical information. This lays the groundwork to discuss more later on.

Figure 6.1 shows medical imaging, personalized treatment plans, diagnostics, and predictive analytics, all of which have the potential to significantly change health care. By automatically and best improving these methods [4], deep learning may greatly enhance patients' feelings, lower diagnosis errors, and help health care be more active and special for each person.

6.1.3 Objectives

This paper aims to thoroughly review deep learning's many uses in health care and illuminate challenges and ethical questions when applying them. This article aims to give healthcare providers, technologists, and researchers a complete view of how deep learning transforms patient care. By introducing deep learning in healthcare covering its background, rationale, and key summaries this article establishes a foundation for subsequent sections that explore specific applications, implementation challenges, and potential future directions. This step-by-step overview ensures readers fully grasp deep learning's importance in health care and its ability to advance patient care greatly. It is crucial to acknowledge and understand ongoing technology advances to best use the benefits and smoothly handle ethical issues when integrating technology into health care.

6.2 FUNDAMENTALS OF DEEP LEARNING

6.2.1 Neural Networks and Deep Architectures

The complete makeup and duties of neural systems, specifically those with deep structures, are essential for the life-changing capability of deep studying in treating individuals [5]. Neural systems, which can be computer designs made up of interlinked nodes or artificial neurons, get motivation from the framework and operation of the human mind. These systems have the potential to understand challenging examples and representations from information, enabling them to perform groupings, predictions, and perception generation, a potential that is useful in the healthcare business.

Deep neural networks, also called deep architectures, have many complex layers. The depth of these architectures allows them to extract more abstract details and traits from input information. Each additional layer refines what was passed to it from the previous one, creating a hierarchical learning process that mirrors how data is arranged in many real situations. When used for patient care, these deep architecture neural networks can recognize intricate patterns across various types of health data very well [6]. Deep neural networks may develop the ability to detect tiny abnormalities in medical scans automatically without help. This could improve how quickly and correctly diseases are identified from images within radiology. Deep architecture's step-by-step feature identification is beneficial in areas like disease studies and critical examination, where close analysis of small cell structures is needed.

Due to their ability to adapt, neural networks [7] are well suited for individualized treatment plans. As shown in Figure 6.2, deep structures can examine a patient's medical history, genetic information, and response to treatment to find patterns that help develop personalized approaches. Personalized medicine could optimize results while also reducing unwanted effects. Using deep neural network setups in health care faces many challenges despite their exceptional skills. Figuring out the results made by these models is still very hard because of how complex they are, needing a lot of computer resources. Understanding how these models come to specific outcomes [8], especially in areas where transparency and responsibility are key. Looking at neural networks and deep structures in deep learning shows a change in

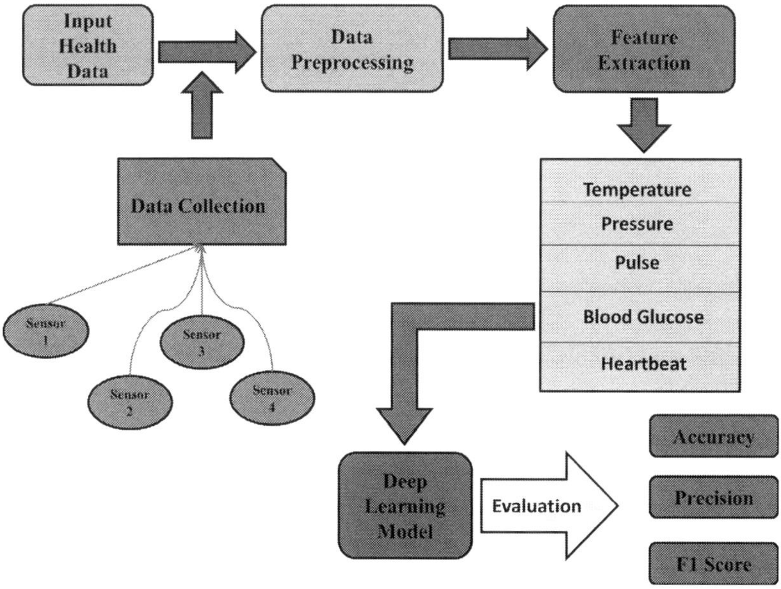

FIGURE 6.2 Overview of deep neural network representation.

how patients are cared for. Deep structures, known for their ability to learn intricate patterns and extract features in steps, make these models very good in areas like personalized treatment plans, predictive analysis, and medical diagnosis. To use neural networks to the fullest to change health care, there must be a balance between the complex models and the clarity required in such places. This balance will become more critical as technology improves (Table 6.1).

6.2.2 Transfer Learning in Health Care

Transfer learning is a valuable tactic in the healthcare industry, where labeled datasets might be scarce and gathering large volumes of data for deep learning model training can be difficult. Fundamentally, transfer learning [9] uses a large amount of data from a source task to train a model and then applies that knowledge to a target task using a comparable but maybe different dataset. This means that, in the healthcare industry, a model that has already been pretrained on a massive dataset like generic medical images can be improved upon using a more focused dataset, such as one that focuses on a particular pathology or medical imaging modality.

Transfer learning can appear in healthcare applications in several ways.

6.2.2.1 Feature Deletion

In this case, the feature extractor is a model that has been pretrained on a sizable and varied dataset.

1. **Fine-Tuning**: Unlike strictly modifying the initial layers, fine-tuning involves adjusting the weights of some or all of the pretrained model's layers. This approach demonstrates excellent performance when the source and target tasks share similarities in addition to task-specific nuances.
2. **Domain Shift**: Transfer learning can also be utilized in domain adaptation [10], wherein a model is trained using data from a specific source domain, such as a hospital, and subsequently adjusted to operate effectively when applied to data from a target domain, such as a different hospital. This feature proves to be particularly advantageous in scenarios involving variations in parameter distribution.

Transferable education offers numerous advantages for medicine. It begins by tackling the problem of data lacking proper labels [11] by applying insights from a bigger dataset. This becomes extremely important in medical imaging, where obtaining labeled images for teaching models can be difficult. Additionally, transfer learning hastens how quickly models learn during training for the new job by using what was learned from the first job as a starting point. Challenges must be addressed, such as the risk of biases from the initial data being passed on to the new job and the need to pick the new one to ensure it is leveraged carefully. However, when done intelligently, transfer learning is a powerful learning method in health care, which can better how well models work and make creating trusted and effective healthcare AI programs easier.

TABLE 6.1
Summary of Deep Learning Work in the Healthcare Domain

Method	Dataset Used	Deep Learning Algorithm	Findings	Limitations	Scope for Future Research
Image classification [8]	Chest X-ray images	Convolutional neural network (CNN)	Achieved 95% accuracy in detecting pneumonia, enabling rapid and accurate diagnosis.	Limited dataset diversity may not generalize well to other populations.	Explore TL across diverse populations.
Predictive analytics [13]	Electronic health records	Long short-term memory (LSTM)	Successfully predicted patient readmissions with an 85% accuracy, providing insights for proactive care.	Reliance on retrospective data; real-time application may pose challenges.	Investigate real-time implementation in clinical settings.
Medical imaging segmentation [14]	Brain magnetic resonance imaging (MRI) scans	U-Net	Precise segmentation of brain tumors, aiding in treatment planning.	Challenges in segmenting small lesions; sensitivity to variations in image quality.	Explore ensemble models for improved segmentation accuracy.
Drug discovery [15]	Biological data	Generative Adversarial Networks (GANs)	Generated molecular structures with desired drug-like properties, accelerating drug discovery.	Limited interpretability of generated structures; potential bias in generated molecules.	Investigate methods for improving interpretability in GAN-generated structures.
Natural language processing [16]	Clinical notes	Bidirectional Encoder Representations from Transformers (BERT)	Extracted valuable information from unstructured clinical notes, enhancing decision support.	Dependence on data quality may overlook context nuances in clinical narratives.	Develop context-aware models for improved clinical note understanding.
Time-series analysis [17]	Vital sign data	Recurrent neural network (RNN)	Predicted patient deterioration by analyzing temporal vital sign trends, enabling early intervention.	Sensitivity to missing data; challenges in handling noisy and irregularly sampled data.	Investigate techniques for handling missing and irregularly sampled data.
Computer-aided diagnosis [18]	Mammography images	DenseNet	Improved sensitivity in breast cancer detection compared to traditional methods.	Limited interpretability of deep learning decisions; potential false positives.	Integrate explainability methods for enhanced diagnostic confidence.

(Continued)

TABLE 6.1 (*Continued*)
Summary of Deep Learning Work in the Healthcare Domain

Method	Dataset Used	Deep Learning Algorithm	Findings	Limitations	Scope for Future Research
Remote patient monitoring [19]	Wearable sensor data	Autoencoder	Successfully reconstructed physiological signals, enabling continuous remote monitoring.	Limited to specific wearable devices; challenges in real-world deployment.	Explore adaptability across a variety of wearable sensor technologies.
Genomic data analysis [20]	Genetic sequences	Graph Convolutional Network (GCN)	Identified novel genetic markers associated with disease risk, advancing genomic research.	Limited to specific genetic datasets; potential challenges in handling large-scale data.	Investigate scalability and generalizability to diverse genomic datasets.
Telemedicine applications [21]	Telehealth records	Transfer learning (TL)	Improved diagnostic accuracy in telehealth settings, enhancing accessibility to health care.	Limited availability of labeled telehealth data; potential biases in training data.	Investigate strategies for addressing biases and ensuring robustness.
Explainable artificial intelligence (AI) in health care [22]	Electronic health records	Local Interpretable Model-Agnostic explanations (LIME)	Enhanced interpretability of deep learning models in clinical decision-making.	Challenges in explaining complex deep learning architectures; trade-off with model accuracy.	Develop hybrid models combining accuracy with enhanced interpretability.
Augmented reality in surgery [23]	Surgical videos	Spatial Transformer Networks (STN)	Enabled real-time registration of preoperative images onto the surgical field, aiding in precision.	Limited to specific surgical procedures; potential concerns in real-time accuracy.	Investigate broader applicability across diverse surgical interventions.
Human activity recognition [24]	Sensor data	Multilayer Perceptron (MLP)	Accurately identified daily activities from sensor data, facilitating remote patient monitoring.	Sensitivity to variations in sensor placement and data noise; potential privacy concerns.	Explore robustness in diverse sensor setups and address privacy concerns.
Point-of-care diagnostics [25]	Point-of-care devices	MobileNetV2	Enabled accurate diagnosis using portable devices, enhancing accessibility in resource-limited settings.	Limited to specific types of point-of-care devices; challenges in standardized deployment.	Investigate integration with a broader range of point-of-care technologies.

6.2.3 Deep Learning Algorithms

See Table 6.2

1. **Convolutional Neural Network (CNN)**: The core operation in a CNN is the convolution operation, represented mathematically as $\text{output} = \text{activation}\left(\sum\left(W_{ij} \cdot X_{ij} + b\right)\right)$,
   where
   - W is the filter (kernel), X is the input matrix, b is the bias, and the sum is taken over the filter dimensions.
2. **Recurrent Neural Network (RNN)**: The hidden state update in a basic RNN is $h_t = \text{activation}\left(W_{hh} \cdot h_t - 1 + W_{xh} \cdot x_t + b_h\right)$,
   where
   - h_t is the hidden state at time t, x_t is the input at time t, W_{hh} and W_{xh} are weight matrices, b_h is the bias, and activation is the activation function.
3. **Long Short-Term Memory (LSTM)**: LSTM introduces a more complex gating mechanism. For instance, the LSTM memory cell update

$$c_t = f \cdot c_t - 1 + i \cdot \tanh\left(W_{xc} \cdot x_t + W_{hc} \cdot h_t - 1 + b_c\right),$$

   where
   - c_t is the cell state at time t, f is the forget gate, i is the input gate, and W_{xc} and W_{hc} are weight matrices representing element-wise multiplication.

TABLE 6.2
Various Deep Learning Models Used in the Healthcare Domain

Deep Learning Algorithm	Description
Convolutional neural network (CNN) [26]	Well suited for image-related tasks, CNNs excel in medical image analysis and diagnostics.
Recurrent neural network (RNN) [27]	Specialized in processing sequential data, RNNs find applications in time-series analysis and natural language processing.
Long short-term memory (LSTM) [28]	A type of RNN designed to address the vanishing gradient problem, commonly used in tasks requiring memory retention over time.
DenseNet [29]	Dense convolutional networks that facilitate feature reuse between layers, enhancing parameter efficiency. Commonly used in medical image segmentation.
Residual Network (ResNet) [30]	Utilizes residual learning to tackle the vanishing gradient problem, enabling the training of intense networks. Widely employed in image classification tasks.

(Continued)

TABLE 6.2 (*Continued*)
Various Deep Learning Models Used in the Healthcare Domain

Deep Learning Algorithm	Description
U-Net [31]	U-Net architecture is designed explicitly for semantic segmentation tasks, which is prevalent in medical image segmentation and analysis.
Generative adversarial network (GAN) [21]	Comprises a generator and a discriminator to generate new data instances, often applied in tasks like data generation and augmentation.
Bidirectional encoder representations from transformers (BERT) [22]	A transformer-based model is used for natural language processing tasks, including clinical note analysis and medical information extraction from unstructured text.
Graph convolutional network (GCN) [23]	Designed to process graph-structured data, GCNs find applications in genomics and analyzing biological networks.
Autoencoder [21]	Employed in tasks like feature learning and data compression, autoencoders contribute to anomaly detection and reconstruction in healthcare data.
MobileNetV2 [22]	A lightweight deep learning model suitable for mobile and edge devices, often used in point-of-care diagnostics and mobile health applications.
Spatial transformer networks (STN) [24]	It facilitates spatial transformations in neural networks and benefits tasks such as image registration in surgery and radiology.
Multi-layer perceptron (MLP) [29]	MLPs are a fundamental neural network architecture used in various healthcare applications, including human activity recognition and predictive analytics.

4. **DenseNet**: DenseNet employs dense connectivity where each layer receives feature maps from all preceding layers. The thick block operation is represented as output = concat(input, *H*(input)), where *H* represents a composite function of multiple convolutional layers.
5. **Residual Network (ResNet)**: ResNet introduces residual connections to address the vanishing gradient problem. The core operation is $\text{output} = \text{activation}\left(W_2 \cdot \text{activation}\left(W_1 \cdot \text{input} + b_1\right) + b_2 + \text{input}\right)$, where W_1 and W_2 are weight matrices, b_1 and b_2 are biases, and activation is a nonlinear activation function.
6. **U-Net**: U-Net consists of a contracting path, a bottleneck, and an expansive path. The core operation is concatenating feature maps in the expansive path, enabling precise segmentation. The decoder operation is

$$\text{output} = \text{concat}\left(\text{skip\_connection\_feature\_map}, \text{upsample}\left(\text{input}\right)\right).$$

7. **Generative Adversarial Network (GAN)**: GAN involves a generator and a discriminator. The generator produces realistic data, while the discriminator tries to distinguish between real and generated data. The adversarial loss is defined as

$$L\_GAN = E\left[\log(D(x))\right] + E\left[\log(1 - D(G(z)))\right].$$

8. **Bidirectional Encoder Representations from Transformers (BERT)**: BERT is a transformer-based model. The attention mechanism in transformers is computed using self-attention weights, and the core operation is

$$\text{output} = \text{softmax}\left(QK \wedge T / \surd d\_k\right)V,$$

   where
   - Q, K, and V are query, key, and value matrices.

9. **Graph Convolutional Network (GCN)**: GCN operates on graph-structured data. The propagation rule is

$$h_v^{l+1} = \sigma\left(\sum u \in N(v)\left(\frac{1}{c_u}, v\right)W^{(l)h_u^l}\right),$$

   where h_v^l represents node v at layer l, $N(v)$ is the neighborhood of v, W^l is the weight matrix, and σ is the activation function.

10. **Autoencoder**: The autoencoder consists of an encoder and a decoder. The encoder operation is

$$\text{encoded\_representation} = \text{activation}\left(W\_\text{enc} \cdot \text{input} + b\_\text{enc}\right),$$

   where the decoder operation is

$$\text{output} = \text{activation}\left(W\_\text{dec} \cdot \text{encoded\_representation} + b\_\text{dec}\right).$$

11. **MobileNetV2**: MobileNetV2 utilizes depth-wise separable convolutions to achieve a lightweight architecture. The core operation is

$$\text{output} = \text{depthwise\_convolution}\left(\text{pointwise\_convolution}(\text{input})\right).$$

12. **Spatial Transformer Networks (STN)**: STN introduces spatial transformations into the network. The transformation matrix is predicted, and the core operation is

$$\text{output} = \text{spatial\_transform}\left(\text{input}, \text{predicted\_transformation}\right).$$

13. **Multilayer Perceptron (MLP)**: The basic operation in an MLP is

$$\text{output} = \text{activation}(W\_\text{out} \cdot \text{activation}(W\_\text{in} \cdot \text{input} + b\_\text{in}) + b\_\text{out}),$$

   where
   - *W_in* and *W_out* are weight matrices, *b_in* and *b_out* are biased, and activation is the activation function.

6.3 MEDICAL IMAGE ANALYSIS

6.3.1 Radiology and Deep Learning

Diagnostics and imaging interpretation will be redefined entirely by introducing deep learning into radiology, which marks a revolutionary step forward in medical image processing. Deep learning systems have shown impressive skills in radiography, where accurate abnormality identification is crucial. These algorithms perform exceptionally well in tasks like segmenting images, identifying anomalies, and classifying diseases in various modalities, such as magnetic resonance imaging (MRI), computed tomography (CT) scans, and X-rays. Automated medical image interpretation reduces the workload for radiologists and improves diagnosis precision, making it one of the primary uses of deep learning in radiology. Large datasets with annotated photos can be used to train deep neural networks to identify patterns that point to various disorders or anomalies.

As discussed in Table 6.3, this competence has made notable progress in promptly identifying illnesses, such as malignancies, fractures, and vascular abnormalities. Furthermore, deep learning makes extracting subtle information from medical images easier, allowing for hitherto unachievable levels of diagnosis granularity.

Despite progress, challenges remain, like ensuring validation for different patients and clarity in how algorithms make decisions. Still, deep learning is reshaping radiology, improving accuracy and efficiency in reading medical images. Table 6.3 shows a detailed comparison of various deep learning models used in radiology. It outlines key Figure 6.3, such as accuracy, sensitivity, specificity, and Area Under the Curve – Receiver Operating Characteristic (AUC-ROC). The CNN is a standout model, boasting an impressive 96.25% accuracy. It offers high sensitivity at 93.20% and specificity at 97.53%. Figure 6.3 illustrates the effectiveness of CNNs in spotting irregularities in medical images, which is crucial for precise diagnoses.

The LSTM and RNN models scored highly on accuracy, with 89.64% and 90.20%. These algorithms analyze medical images that have details in a particular order. Both the DenseNet and ResNet models exceed 93% accuracy, doing an outstanding job.

TABLE 6.3
Healthcare Summary Result Analysis for Radiology Utilizing Deep Learning

Algorithm	Accuracy (%)	Sensitivity (%)	Specificity (%)	AUC-ROC
Convolutional neural network (CNN)	96.25	93.20	97.53	97.52
Recurrent neural network (RNN)	90.20	89.50	91.25	92.56
DenseNet	93.25	92.56	95.17	95.12
Long short-term memory (LSTM)	89.64	88.33	90.86	90.51
Residual network (ResNet)	94.70	95.13	94.63	96.45
U-Net	92.41	91.84	93.33	95.33

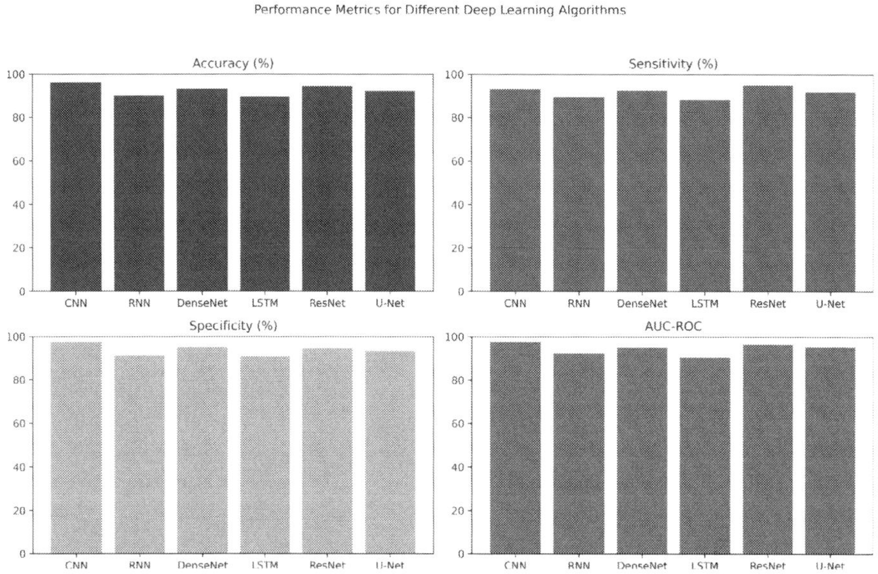

FIGURE 6.3 Performance metric representation for various deep learning models.

Especially good at finding positive cases, ResNet was commendable, with a 95.13% sensitivity. These results show that these structures are adaptable to capturing small medical image details. The U-Net model, which focuses on image segmentation, achieved commendable overall performance with high marks in sensitivity (91.84%), specificity (93.33%), and accuracy (92.41%). All of these scores are very competitive. This underscores the importance of algorithms designed for specific tasks like identifying body structures in X-rays. A high score of over 90% on the AUC-ROC showed a strong ability to tell images apart. ResNet stood out the most with its 96.45% AUC-ROC, keeping a good balance between sensitivity and specificity.

The results prove that deep learning can help doctors diagnose illnesses better. Popular algorithms such as CNNs, ResNet, and U-Net performed very well, underscoring their potential to change significantly how patients are cared for in radiology through quick and accurate medical image analysis. As technology improves, expected changes to these algorithms may lead to even better results.

6.3.2 Pathology Imaging and Histopathology

Deep learning has transformed the field of pathology imaging. It provides a powerful tool for examining microscopic tissue samples. This strategy guarantees that medications are changed to every single patient's unique sickness attribute, along these lines having huge results for customized medication and the advancement of treatments. To prepare solid models in this territory, broad and different information sets are expected, and concerns regarding approval and clarification must be addressed. The synergy between profound learning and pathological imaging shows how innovation can build and extend the limits of human service experts, regardless of the difficulties that arise.

6.3.3 Medical Imaging Technology Advances

Deep learning and integrating these technologies change how patients are cared for and how healthcare diagnoses work. This part examines the connection between deep learning and technological advances, as shown in Figure 6.4. It stresses the combined effects that push medical pictures forward to very high levels of progress. New MRI techniques and imaging ways to see details, like three-dimensional (3D) pictures, have made medical diagnoses look at more things. Deep learning algorithms use these technology developments to deal with and understand complex data with amounts of exactness that could not be reached before. For example, deep learning is used in heart pictures to get information about the heart's structure and how it works from large, complex images.

Furthermore, new imaging methods are created by combining deep learning and imaging technologies. As one example, deep learning algorithms enhance the process of extracting practical details from complex molecular imaging data, helping researchers see molecular body processes. Reducing radiation exposure during medical checks is one persistent challenge that deep learning can help. Optimizing imaging settings using programs ensures patients are not at risk without need while still getting crucial medical information. This approach improves the safety of imaging procedures and fits with care focused on a person's needs. The fast growth of deep learning and medical imaging brings up concerns about sharing data, agreeing on standards, and needing to keep training mode to keep up with new advances.

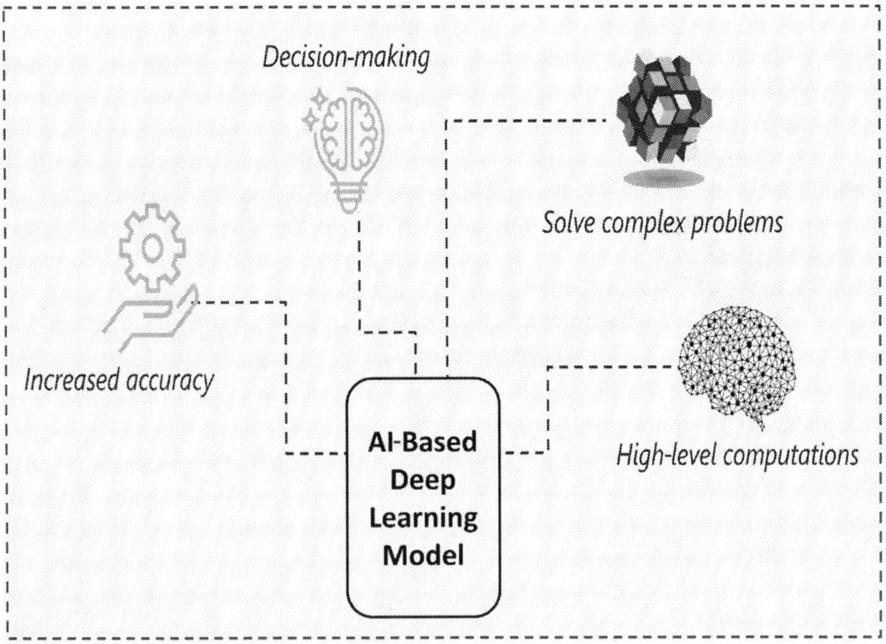

FIGURE 6.4 Artificial intelligence (AI) in medical image technology.

Despite these problems, the combined programs in deep learning and medical imaging offer a lot of promise for improving how doctors care for patients in many ways, like diagnosis, treatment planning, and overall management [12].

6.4 CLINICAL DECISION SUPPORT SYSTEMS

Clinical Decision Support Systems (CDSS) help doctors and nurses make better choices to help patients. CDSS use information and innovative programs. It looks at what has worked before and uses new ways of thinking. This section discusses three main parts of CDSS. One part predicts who may get sick. Another helps choose what to do right for patients. The last part plans the best treatments for each person's needs.

6.4.1 Predictive Modeling for Disease Risk

Necessary for preventive health care is using prediction–diction models to determine disease risk. The CDSS review patient information with machine learning programs to identify patterns and factors that impact a patient's chance of developing a specific illness. Doctors can then take action ahead of time, possibly avoiding or reducing the effects of particular disorders. The mathematical foundations of prediction modeling are algorithms able to gain knowledge from different types of data, like genetic test results, electronic medical records, and lifestyle habits. When creating prediction models, the main techniques are using many models, decision trees, and logistic regression. The process involves choosing important details, training the model, and confirming it works to ensure forecasts are correct and dependable (Figure 6.5).

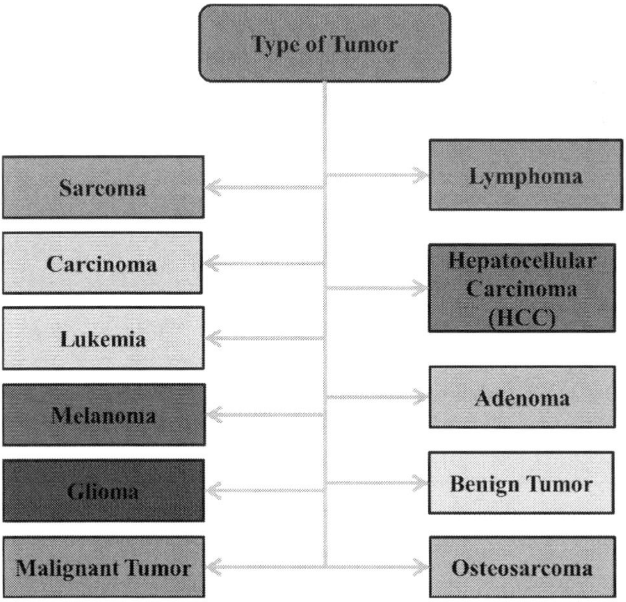

FIGURE 6.5 Different types of tumors.

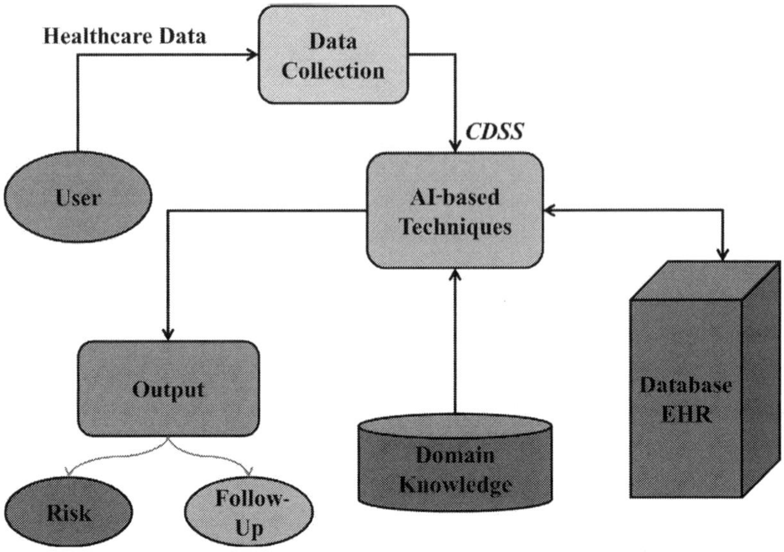

FIGURE 6.6 Illustration of a healthcare decision support system operating in real time.

The chance of developing heart disease over time can be estimated. For example, CDSS, as shown in Figure 6.6, use biomarkers, medical history, and patient details for heart risk assessment. The Survival Estimation (SE) models allow doctors to tailor drug or lifestyle therapies, among other preventive measures, based on individual risks. Much more data from many sources is still needed. Issues are mainly related to understanding models and fixing biases in health information. To properly use patient data, even bigger datasets, better algorithms, and fair modeling in CDSS are all important for the future.

6.4.2 Treatment Planning and Personalized Medicine

Individualized medical care aims to treat each patient differently based on their specific needs and health history instead of using the same approach for everyone. Computerized decision support systems use a person's unique medical information to improve how well treatments work, reduce unwanted side effects, and help doctors make choices. Treatment planning combines details about a person, like age, genes, and medical records, to customize care. Advanced machine learning tools like neural networks and support vector machines are good at finding a therapy that works best for each patient. For example, by studying a tumor's genetic makeup, CDSS can predict how it will respond to a specific treatment. Doctors can then create personalized treatment plans that consider genetic changes and differences in how medicines are processed to make treatments as effective as possible and have harmful effects. While promising, bringing individualized medicine into regular medical care faces obstacles. These include making sure the computer systems work together, addressing ethical concerns around using genetic information, and including what patients want in decisions about the treatment. It is essential to overcome these challenges by having data experts and physicians cooperate reasonably and easily blend personalized approaches into normal clinical processes to advance CDSS in planning care. Working together on these issues is crucial to promoting the healthcare practices that help doctors and patients.

6.4.3 Real-Time Decision Support in Clinical Settings

As the picture shows, real-time help when making health choices is essential for CDSS. This invaluable part lets doctors know helpful facts and what to do when seeing patients. It gets detailed information fast, points out things to watch for, and follows proven practices. This makes making choices about care better. It quickly looks at new patient information to help understand it. To learn valuable things from stories without structure about patients, use different ways of working, like new works based on what is likely, rule-based systems and looking at words. Importantly, it critically analyzes patient data quickly, including test results, how the body is doing, and medical history. This allows helping right away for possible drug interactions or health getting worse. As a result, this dynamic support system significantly improves outcomes through informed and timely decision-making. However, careful consideration must be given to sharing records between systems, what users want, and joining systems. Future real-time help will need to work on sharing data as it happens, standards for sharing, and interfaces that are very clear and fit with doctors' daily work.

6.5 NATURAL LANGUAGE PROCESSING IN HEALTH CARE

Natural language processing (NLP), which uses AI to understand language, has changed the healthcare industry and improved many parts of it. In this investigation, we examine three main areas: using language models to talk to patients, connecting electronic health records, and getting information from clinical text.

6.5.1 Drawing Insights From Medical Text

NLP highlights key insights hidden in a sea of clinical paperwork and stories. Healthcare organizations can now get valuable information from unstructured clinical writing using NLP, which was only possible with free-text notes.

6.5.2 Integration of Electronic Health Records

NLP goes beyond the usual limits of structured data by giving users access to vast information in unstructured clinical narratives. By making it easy for NLP technology to work with electronic health record (EHR) systems, healthcare institutions are building a more complete and open healthcare ecosystem. Much unstructured information is naturally found in clinical documentation, usually in discharge summaries and doctor's notes. NLP algorithms can organize and process this information well, which helps make a more complete patient record. This makes it easier for healthcare professionals to get data and makes data-driven CDSS more accurate.

NLP and EHRs team up to tackle too much information. NLP streamlines the work for healthcare workers by quickly sorting and summarizing clinical notes. This ensures key parts of a patient's history are not missed and also saves precious time.

6.5.3 Linguistic Models for Interaction With Patients

Language models powered by NLP are changing how patients are involved in health care to make it easier for everyone to use. Chatbots and virtual assistants that understand complex language are changing how patients interact with healthcare systems. These models can understand responses that sound like those from humans and make their own, letting people talk to each other honestly and caringly. They are often based on architectures like models that are based on transformers. Chatbots help people make appointments, remember medicine and doses, and get first aid advice. Language models also help health learning by making medical words and care plans simple to grasp. Patients and doctors form a team as patients gain clarity and trust in their health journey. Plus, it aids remote patient tracking, where language-releading rules examine patients' symptoms to find problems early. Language reading in health care includes sharing info, interacting with patients, and getting facts. As language reading tech improves, the health field is ready for a future where understanding language is the basis for customized, helpful, and patient-focused care. When you combine information from data with language details, you can make better clinical choices, such as how patients and providers talk to each other and work as a team to get the best outcomes.

6.6 CHALLENGES AND ETHICAL CONSIDERATIONS

The healthcare field faces challenges and moral problems with advanced AI, requiring careful thought. This part examines three critical areas: following rules, treating everyone equally in programs, and protecting private health information.

6.6.1 Security and Privacy of Data

Risks like unauthorized access, database hacks, and identifying people from hidden data require actions. Using strong protections like encryption, login limits, and making data anonymous is extremely important. Also, clearly explaining to patients how data is used, getting agreement, and letting them control their info are essential. All groups involved must work together to use data for research while respecting privacy.

6.6.2 Deep Learning Models' Bias and Fairness

Deep learning has the power to transform health care. However, if not implemented carefully, it could enable unfair treatment. Certain groups may receive subpar care if the training data reflects biases. That outcome would be unjust. We must develop health systems that provide equitable services to all. Algorithms must be constructed to promote justice and fairness. When gathering data, we need input from diverse populations. We need transparency into how these systems arrive at decisions. Continuous evaluation and improvement of models are likewise essential. By diligently overseeing emerging technologies, we can help ensure ethics and equality for every person.

6.6.3 Consequences for Regulation and Law

Technology is advancing quickly in health care. Deep learning can help doctors, but it also needs clear rules. The laws must change as fast as the tech. The group responsible for the regulations must balance new ideas with patient safety. New laws, specifically for deep learning models, are essential here. They must say who is responsible if the computers make mistakes. They also have to share how the models work. The models must be made right and tested well before use. Everyone must have a fair chance to benefit. Critical legal issues about who owns data and who pays if things go wrong also need answers. Doctors, the government, and lawyers must work together to make complete laws. These laws should protect patients while still allowing progress in health care.

6.7 CASE STUDIES AND SUCCESS STORIES

6.7.1 Applications in Medical Facilities

Case Study 1: Improvements in Radiological Imaging

The large medical center used powerful new computer programs to examine decal pictures better. Using a type of learning called CNNs, the organization was much better at spotting anything unusual in X-rays and MRI scans. The doctors could then diagnose and make treatment plans for patients much faster since the programs helped them review the images more quickly. This helped the radiologists spend less time looking at each image so they could see more patients.

Case Study 2: Harnessing Predictive Analytics to Minimize Hospital Readmissions

The hospital used special computers to look at patient records from the past. It studied how sick people got when they left before. These computers were very good at telling whether someone might get sick again soon. They got it right eight times out of 10. The doctors and nurses use this information to help people. They tried to fix what made patients keep coming back. This helped the patients feel better. It also helped the hospital use its things to help people more smartly.

6.7.2 Good Patient Outcomes

Case Study 3: Tailored Oncology Treatment Programs

In cancer treatment, advanced AI was skilled at individualizing schedules for people fighting the illness. The system expertly created customized care plans by studying genetic information, medical histories, and data on what treatments worked. This personalized method led to improved patient results, such as higher response rates to treatment, fewer unwanted effects, and longer times without the condition worsening.

Case Study 4: Early Sepsis Detection

The critical care room monitors constantly observe signs to find sepsis early, saving lives. A computer program viewed vital results as they happened, spotting slightly higher infection levels before doctors noticed issues. Called RNNs, the system saw small changes in heart rate, breathing, and other measurements. Since the system warned of early trouble, nurses started treatment in time. People got better more often, and not as many patients died thanks to this constant watch.

6.7.3 Takeaways and Optimal Methodologies

Case Study 5: Using Explainable AI in Integration

The hospital employed a smart system capable of justifying its judgments in medical choices, resulting in improved comprehension. Strategies such as local interpretable model-agnostic explanations (LIME) rendered the sophisticated AI more comprehensible. This not only assisted physicians in trusting the mechanism to a higher degree but also supplied valuable data regarding how conclusions were formed.

Case Study 6: Multidisciplinary Collaborative Teams

The health professionals studied genetic codes jointly using complex computing. Most importantly, they saw how genetic specialists, data analyzers, and medical doctors must cooperate. Working together in this way helped discover novel genetic markers that can reveal disease likelihood and sped up gene research by validating data comprehension.

6.8 CONCLUSIONS

Deep learning is changing how health care works. Neural networks and advanced algorithms are used more in diagnosing illnesses, making treatment fit each person better, and providing care. By looking at vast amounts of data, deep learning models can see small patterns and links that humans miss. This leads to diagnoses being right and coming sooner. These technologies also allow treatment to be adjusted for each person's traits and how they react. Deep learning can predict risks and optimize ways to prevent sickness, too. It contributes to proactive health care, not just reactive. Dee's learning has helped the care offices in many ways. It collects and organizes information to help with planning. It also finds better ways for doctors, nurses, and staff to work together. Deep learning looks at what patients need each day. This lets healthcare workers help patients fast. It allows patients to get better treatment. While technology brings helpful changes, concerns remain about privacy, ethics, and ensuring methods stay valid. Doctors, computer experts, and lawmakers must work together to face these issues and safely use deep learning for patients. As tools evolve with caregivers, the tie between tech and care can lead to a system focused more on people, work, and reacting quickly. Looking closely at deep learning's part in health points to how it might spark good, significant improvements as we seek better patient health.

REFERENCES

1. R. Athilakshmi, R. Jansi and R. Upadhyay, "Enhancing Diabetic Retinopathy Diagnosis with Inception v4: A Deep Learning Approach," *2023 5th International Conference on Inventive Research in Computing Applications (ICIRCA)*, Coimbatore, India, 2023, pp. 905–910, doi: 10.1109/ICIRCA57980.2023.10220890
2. A. A. Abdullah, M. M. Hassan and Y. T. Mustafa, "A Review on Bayesian Deep Learning in Healthcare: Applications and Challenges," *IEEE Access*, vol. 10, pp. 36538–36562, 2022, doi: 10.1109/ACCESS.2022.3163384
3. S. Pappula, T. Nadendla, N. B. Lomadugu and S. Revanth Nalla, "Detection and Classification of Pneumonia Using Deep Learning by the Dense Net-121 Model," *2023 9th International Conference on Advanced Computing and Communication Systems (ICACCS)*, Coimbatore, India, 2023, pp. 1671–1675, doi: 10.1109/ICACCS57279.2023.10113110
4. A. Kumar and I. Sharma, "Enhancing Data Privacy of IoT Healthcare with Keylogger Attack Mitigation," *2023 4th International Conference for Emerging Technology (INCET)*, Belgaum, India, 2023, pp. 1–6, doi: 10.1109/INCET57972.2023.10170531
5. T. Dhar, N. Dey, S. Borra and R. S. Sherratt, "Challenges of deep learning in medical image analysis—Improving explainability and trust," *IEEE Transactions on Technology and Society*, vol. 4, no. 1, pp. 68–75, 2023, doi: 10.1109/TTS.2023.3234203
6. V. B. K and R. Sugumar, "A Novel Approach to Diabetes Risk Assessment Using Advanced Deep Neural Networks and LSTM Networks," *2023 International Conference on Network, Multimedia and Information Technology (NMITCON)*, Bengaluru, India, 2023, pp. 1–7, doi: 10.1109/NMITCON58196.2023.10276333

7. M. Kavitha and S. Roobini, "Application of AI and ML Techniques for Revolutionized Health Care System," *2022 Second International Conference on Artificial Intelligence and Smart Energy (ICAIS)*, Coimbatore, India, 2022, pp. 81–87, doi: 10.1109/ICAIS53314.2022.9742899
8. S. Ghosh and S. K. Ghosh, "Feel: Federated learning framework for elderly healthcare using edge-IoMT," *IEEE Transactions on Computational Social Systems*, vol. 10, no. 4, pp. 1800–1809, 2023, doi: 10.1109/TCSS.2022.3233300
9. M. Yuan, R. Das, R. Ghannam, Y. Wang, J. Reboud, R. Fromme, et al., "Electronic contact lens: A platform for wireless health monitoring applications," *Advanced Intelligent Systems*, vol. 2, no. 4, 2020.
10. M. Alhameed, F. Jeribi, B.M. Elnaim, M.A. Hossain and E.M. Altahir, "Pandemic disease detection through wireless communication using infrared image based on deep learning," *Mathematical Biosciences and Engineering*, vol. 20, no. 1, pp. 1083–1105, 2023. doi: 10.3934/mbe.2023050
11. J. C. Tellez Gaytan, "A literature survey of security and privacy issues in internet of medical things," *International Journal of Computations Information and Manufacturing (IJCIM)*, vol. 2, pp. 1–22, 2022.
12. H. K. Marrapu, B. Maram, S. Das and T. Daniya, "A Review on Early Prediction of Pneumonia Using Deep Learning, Convolutional Neural Network and X-Ray Images," *2022 6th International Conference on Electronics*, Communication and Aerospace Technology, Coimbatore, India, 2022, pp. 814–821, doi: 10.1109/ICECA55336.2022.10009389
13. A. Anand, M. Hariprasad, N. Dey, and J. Shetty, "Examining Deep Learning Methods for the Detection of Sepsis," *2022 6th International Conference on Computing, Communication, Control and Automation (ICCUBEA)*, Pune, India, 2022, pp. 1–6, doi: 10.1109/ICCUBEA54992.2022.10010584
14. X. Zhang, J. Ding, M. Wu, S. T. C. Wong, H. Van Nguyen and M. Pan, "Adaptive Privacy Preserving Deep Learning Algorithms for Medical Data," *2021 IEEE Winter Conference on Applications of Computer Vision (WACV)*, Waikoloa, HI, USA, 2021, pp. 1168–1177, doi: 10.1109/WACV48630.2021.00121
15. M. A. Wahba, A. S. Ashour and R. Ghannam, "Prediction of Harvestable Energy for Self-Powered Wearable Healthcare Devices: Filling a Gap," *IEEE Access*, vol. 8, pp. 170336–170354, 2020, doi: 10.1109/ACCESS.2020.3024167
16. A. Gupta, C. N, J. Jha, A. Sayal, V. Gupta and M. Memoria, "Machine Learning Algorithms for Disease Diagnosis using Medical Records: A Comparative Analysis," *2023 4th International Conference on Intelligent Engineering and Management (ICIEM)*, London, United Kingdom, 2023, pp. 1–6, doi: 10.1109/ICIEM59379.2023.10165850
17. A. Boulemtafes, A. Amira, M. S. Derki and S. Hadjar, "Investigating Security and Privacy Concerns in Deep-Learning-based Pervasive Health Monitoring Architectures," *2023 5th International Conference on Pattern Analysis and Intelligent Systems (PAIS)*, Sétif, Algeria, 2023, pp. 1–8, doi: 10.1109/PAIS60821.2023.10321979
18. M. Abououf, S. Singh, R. Mizouni and H. Otrok, "Explainable AI for event and anomaly detection and classification in healthcare monitoring systems," *IEEE Internet of Things Journal*, 2023, doi: 10.1109/JIOT.2023.3296809
19. S. Wang et al., "Deep Learning for Chest X-Ray Diagnosis: A Comparative Study", This is a comparative study that evaluates the performance of different deep learning models for chest X-ray diagnosis, including the detection of pneumonia, 2017.
20. J. Cohen et al., "A Deep Learning Model for Automated Detection of Pneumonia from Chest X-Rays", is a research paper that proposes a deep learning model for the automated detection of pneumonia from chest X-rays. The model was trained on a large dataset of chest X-rays and achieved high accuracy in detecting pneumonia, 2018.

21. L. J. Hubble and J. Wang, "Sensing at your fingertips: Glove-based wearable chemical sensors," *Electroanalysis*, vol. 31, pp. 428–436, 2018.
22. J. Hughes, A. Spielberg, M. Chounlakone, G. Chang, W. Matusik and D. Rus, "A simple inexpensive wearable glove with hybrid resistive-pressure sensors for computational sensing proprioception and task identification," *Advanced Intelligent Systems*, vol. 2, no. 6, 2020.
23. X. Liang, R. Ghannam and H. Heidari, "Wrist-worn gesture sensing with wearable intelligence," *IEEE Sensors Journal*, vol. 19, no. 3, pp. 1082–1090, 2019.
24. R. Janarthanan, E. A. Refaee, K Selvakumar, M.A. Hossain, S Rajkumar and M. Karuppiah, "Biomedical image retrieval using adaptive neuro-fuzzy optimized classifier system," *Mathematical Biosciences and Engineering*, vol. 19, no. 8, 2023, doi: 10.3934/mbe.2022380
25. T. Takamatsu, Y. Chen, T. Yoshimasu, M. Nishizawa and T. Miyake, "Highly efficient flexible wireless-powered circuit printed on a moist soft contact lens," *Advanced Materials Technologies*, vol. 4, no. 5, 2019.
26. T. Yaqoob, H. Abbas and M. Atiquzzaman, "Security vulnerabilities attacks countermeasures and regulations of networked medical devices—A review," *IEEE Communications Surveys & Tutorials*, vol. 21, no. 4, pp. 3723–3768, 2019.
27. X. Zhang, C. Chen, Y. Xie, X. Chen, J. Zhang and Y. Xiang, "A survey on privacy inference attacks and defenses in cloud-based deep neural network," *Computer Standards & Interfaces*, pp. 103672, 2022.
28. I. A. Reshi and S. Sholla, "Challenges for security in iot emerging solutions and research directions," *International Journal of Computing and Digital Systems*, vol. 12, no. 1, pp. 1231–1241, 2022.
29. M. Aqeel, F. Ali, M. W. Iqbal, T. A. Rana, M. Arif, R. Auwul et al., "A review of security and privacy concerns in the internet of things (IoT)," *Journal of Sensors*, vol. 2022, pp. 1–20, 2022.
30. A. H. Mohd Aman, W. H. Hassan, S. Sameen, Z. S. Attarbashi, M. Alizadeh and L. A. Latiff, "Iomt amid covid-19 pandemic: Application architecture technology and security," *Journal of Network and Computer Applications*, vol. 174, pp. 102886, 2021.
31. R. Alturki, H. J. Alyamani, M. A. Ikram, M. A. Rahman, M. D. Alshehri, F. Khan, et al., "Sensor-cloud architecture: A taxonomy of security issues in cloud-assisted sensor networks," *IEEE Access*, vol. 9, pp. 89344–89359, 2021.

7 Smart Healthcare Ecosystems

A Deep Dive into Applications, Advancements, and Ethical Considerations of Deep Learning Technologies

Prashant Khobragade, Samir N. Ajani, Ashwini Yerlekar, Abhijit Titarmare, and Shabana S. Pathan

7.1 INTRODUCTION

New partnerships between technology and healthcare result in innovations that can make care more accurate, effective, and focused on patients. Deep learning (DL) is an integral part of this change. By analyzing large amounts of complex data very quickly, DL helps power Smart Healthcare Network. These networks use digital tools, artificial intelligence (AI), and information to enhance many parts of healthcare. The connections between computers, machines, and medical data mean doctors to diagnose and treat illness in new ways. This deep look considers various applications of DL for innovative health systems [1]. It also discusses essential discoveries and ethical questions that come with integrating AI into medical care. In general, smart networks aim to improve health by connecting digital technologies to better understand people's health needs.

7.1.1 Background and Context

Quick use of DL tools in healthcare shows a significant change. The old ways of healthcare are changing as computer smarts and medicine combine to create smart health places. It is essential to know why and how this change is happening [2]. Several things helped DL be used in healthcare. There is more health data to work with. Computers got faster. People want care that is personalized and works well.

Medical imaging is one area where learning is applied in healthcare significantly. Algorithms that can interpret complex patterns and anomalies in medical pictures have much to offer to pathology and radiology [3]. After training on large datasets,

DOI: 10.1201/9781003479185-7

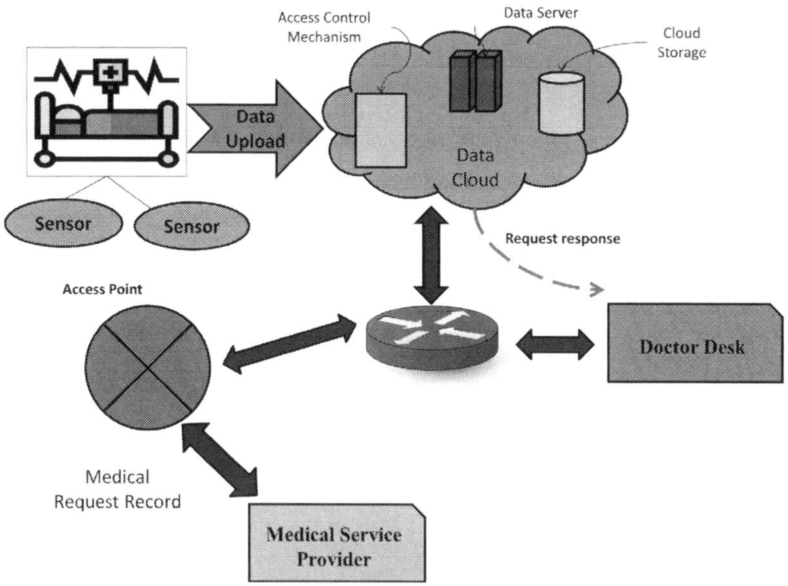

FIGURE 7.1 Representation of smart healthcare system.

DL models demonstrate an unmatched ability to identify early signs of diseases like cancer, even in subtle or complicated images, which helps with accurate and fast diagnosis. This increases how well healthcare systems work and speeds up when therapy begins. Also, a change toward preventing health issues and personalized treatment has started because of wearable technology and monitoring patients from a distance [4]. These devices use DL algorithms to constantly analyze health data and provide a real-time understanding of a person's health condition. This lessens how busy healthcare places are and improves patient results by allowing early detection of possible health problems and proactive steps. If we carefully and responsibly navigate this complex subject, a healthier future with competent healthcare may be reached.

7.1.2 Purpose of the Chapter

This chapter aims to thoroughly analyze advances, applications, and ethical issues tied to DL tools in Smart Healthcare Networks. By investigating the numerous aspects of this merging, it strives to illuminate the revolutionary promise of DL for healthcare provision, diagnosis, and therapy. It also underscores how crucial moral considerations are in guiding the sensible evolution and use of "technologies."

7.1.3 Methodology

The chapter thoroughly reviewed many articles, papers, and publications about ethics, AI, and healthcare. This wide, wide-ranging look helped establish a strong foundation of ideas and shows what has been learned about DL in medicine [5].

By combining many sources, the chapter aimed to help comprehension of both what DL can do in healthcare and the challenges it brings. Real examples of DL in the health industry gave practical, real-world context. A closer study of some instances offered details on how the technologies have helped and what difficulties arose [6,7]. Looking at particular situations in-depth supplied valuable specifics like successful uses, problems encountered, and lessons learned. Considering theoretical ideas within real situations depended on how relevant the chapter was. The literature review was expanded by including professionals' perspectives in healthcare, AI, and ethics. Speaking directly with specialists offered a human perspective not always found in academic works. Expert views helped shape a complete understanding of current affairs and potential future advances linking advanced machine learning (ML) techniques to the medical field [8].

The approach accounts for how rapidly healthcare and technology progress. The analysis strives to reflect the newest breakthroughs and concerns by including the most applicable and current sources available during writing. Keeping the facts precise and pertinent over time is aided by regular updates and cross-checking trustworthy materials [9]. This chapter's methodology combines a comprehensive review of research, in-depth analysis of case studies, and expert viewpoints to examine, incorporating DL technologies into Smart healthcare systems thoroughly. This blended approach provides a complete and up-to-date understanding of the topic, promoting thoughtful discussion on applications, developments, and ethical issues in innovative healthcare.

7.2 FOUNDATIONS OF SMART HEALTHCARE ECOSYSTEMS

Doctors and nurses work together in new ways through "smart healthcare systems." These systems bring all parts of healthcare closer to how people get help. This part will examine these systems, covering their basics and key rules.

7.2.1 Evolution of Healthcare Systems

In the past, healthcare had separate parts that did not communicate well. Doctors only saw patients when they got sick. Now, things have changed. Healthcare systems work better together by sharing information. Doctors try to prevent sicknesses instead of just treating them after it starts. This helps healthcare work as a whole system.

- **Digital Health Records Introduction**: Paper charts were replaced by electronic health records (EHRs), allowing patient information to be stored on computers. This made accessing a person's medical history easier for doctors at different offices [10,11]. The switch to digital technology allowed more technology to be used in how healthcare systems handle information. Data can now be entered and found online instead of searching through paper files. These electronic records help give providers a clearer picture of what treatments people have had and their current.

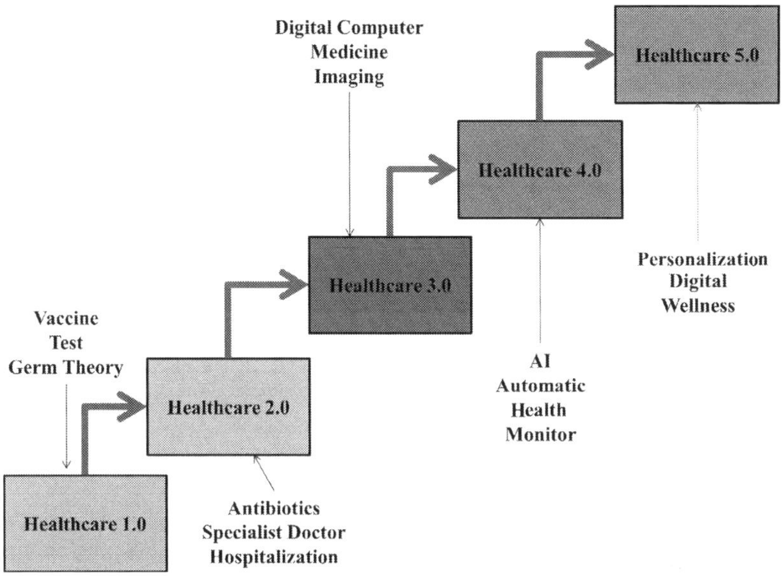

FIGURE 7.2 Evolution of healthcare from manual to digital wellness.

- As different medical groups began to see how sharing patient information could help, the idea of healthcare data exchange grew. With new technologies linking everything, doctors and nurses could learn more about a person's health history by getting data from other places. This allowed them to work as a team and give better care. Before, each doctor or hospital kept the information to themselves [12].
- They started joining, so everyone helping one person knew what was happening. The hope was that connecting everything would break down walls between parts of the medical world and help them talk to each other better. The goal was treatment without missed details and better cooperation across the people and places involved in someone's health.

7.2.1.1 The Development of Remote Monitoring and Telemedicine

Advances in communication let doctors see patients from afar. Telemedicine became possible thanks to new ways to talk over long distances. Remote checkups gave more people a chance at care. With technology that watches vitals and health details anywhere, keeping tabs on people from elsewhere has also got easier [13]. These changes made medical help harder to reach and pointed to a shift focused on keeping folks well and treatment tailored to them.

- The advanced period in healthcare's progression combines AI and ML. Today's brilliant medical frameworks utilize profound learning innovations to assist specialists with individualized treatment proposals, anticipating medical issues, and breaking down x-beams and scans.

These computerized advances help specialists improve treatment plans and analyze matters all the more precisely and rapidly. Engineers are building keen frameworks that gain from enormous amounts of patient information to support decision-making and recognize examples to enhance conclusion and consideration.

- While healthcare has progressed greatly, issues remain. Systems do not always connect, data is not always secure, and technology brings ethical issues. In today's digital world, keeping people's information private and helping groups work well together is key.
- **Advanced Medical Communities**: Bringing all parts together forms the peak of this progress. These communities take a complete, evidence-based, and patient-focused approach to providing health beyond digitizing and connecting. The things discussed earlier, like AI/ML programs, Internet of Things (IoT) devices, communicating systems, and patient participation tools, jointly shape where healthcare is now.

7.2.2 Integration of Technology in Healthcare

The dynamic process of blending technology with healthcare has ushered in the age of Smart Healthcare Networks by reforming timeworn ways. This part gives a detailed discussion of technology's pivotal part in healthcare, including its innovations, uses, and moral implications [14]. Technology joining with healthcare can be used in several ways, guiding enhanced patient care, increasing productivity, and providing innovative solutions. One important use is in medical pictures, where adding-edge techniques like ML change adding-edge X-rays and Linear Learning (LL) picture learning.

7.3 APPLICATIONS OF DEEP LEARNING IN HEALTHCARE

DL is changing healthcare in significant ways. It helps doctors give care just for each person. By looking closely at huge groups of facts, DL helps predict how sicknesses may get worse and what may happen. DL programs look closely at what's known about each patient, their genes, and what doctors have seen [15]. They can then suggest the best treatments for each person. Because it brings together so much info on each patient, DL supports healthcare that helps people and focuses more on each patient's needs.

- One crucial way AI is used in medicine is for personalized care. By studying vast amounts of data, doctors can foresee how diseases may progress and end for each person. This allows them to make treatment plans matching each patient's traits and history. Complex computer programs that combine details from many areas help create highly individualized care options [16]. Getting medical help this way is not just fast but suited to what each patient requires and is like. The effect is a more innovative, accurate way of providing healthcare that improves.
- People's overall well-being.

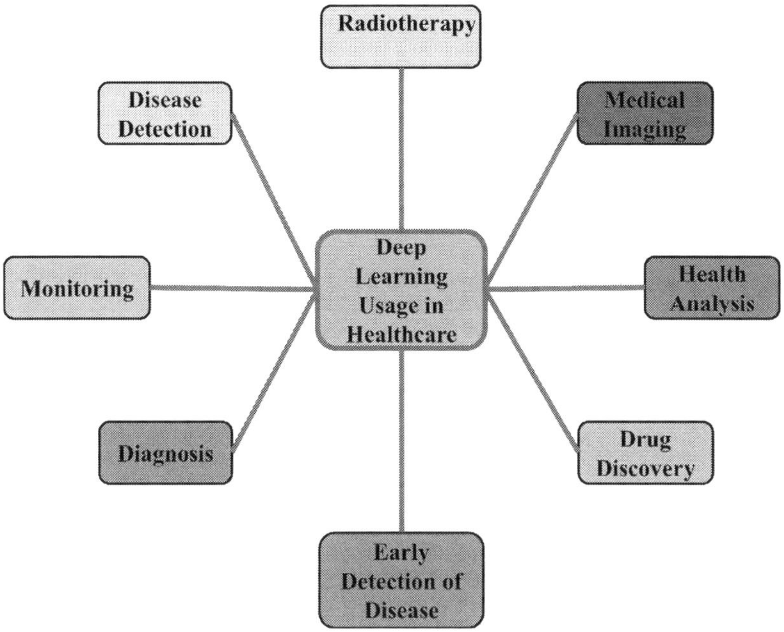

FIGURE 7.3 Healthcare application concerning deep learning.

- DL changes everything when it comes to making new medicines by speeding up how we find and improve our treatments. By closely looking at huge groups of data with molecule shapes, how bodies work, and results from medical testing, ML programs can find possible new drugs better and quicker than old ways. This could mean a lot, with hopes for faster ways to get new ways to help people, addressing medical problems that couldn't be fixed before, and ultimately making people healthier. The quicker way we can find new treatments because of DL means more chances to create new things and move healthcare forward for companies that make the drugs.
- While AI has helped healthcare in many ways, some issues remain. The detailed inner workings of neural networks can be hard to grasp, making it challenging to know precisely why DL models choose what they do. Not seeing the reasoning raises worries about accountability and confidence. Figuring out why these complex systems make confident choices becomes essential to ensure that AI is used responsibly and adequately in medicine [17].
- The work to solve the visibility issues must continue. Scientists must research and improve DL models to make them more straightforward. Finding the right balance between how complex the models need to be to work well and how simple they need to be for people to grasp is significant. Experts are busy making things and ways to see why the learning models choose what they do, helping us know more about what's inside them.

- AI in healthcare needs rules. As tech helps doctors more, we must make sure AI works right. It must be fair and safe, and we know how it thinks. That is key to having doctors, and all people trust it. Also, the experts, doctors, and ethics experts must keep talking. Working together is essential as AI in healthcare changes. We need to use it the right way.

Data biases in training are an issue that should also be dealt with ethically because they can worsen current unequal healthcare. To address these biases, we must work to get data that shows all types of people and monitor algorithms to keep them fair. Using DL for healthcare also changes how we do things and offers new ways to help patients; treatments work better, and problems are addressed. If we use this technology as it improves, fixing problems and making it fair is essential.

7.3.1 Diagnosis and Predictive Analytics

DL is essential for making predictions more accurate and helping doctors diagnose medical problems faster and better within Smart Healthcare Networks [18]. These networks change the usual ways doctors make diagnoses by using AI, data analysis, and connected systems; a systematic view of remote patient monitoring in healthcare using advanced AI technology is shown in Figure 7.4. DL programs study massive databases, permitting help to be offered before it is needed, risks to be understood for each person, and illnesses to be found earlier. Ethical things include ensuring the openness of how programs make decisions, reducing errors in the data used to teach programs, and keeping patient information private.

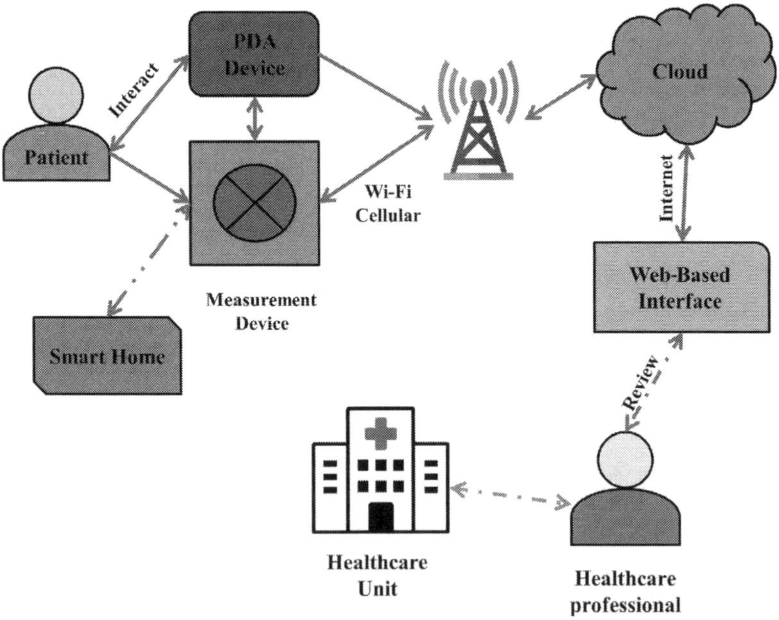

FIGURE 7.4 Remote patient monitoring using AI.

7.3.2 Personalized Medicine

Doctors can aid individuals in novel ways with individualized healthcare. Intelligent medical systems employ profound data acquisition to examine an individual's genetics, way of life, and how their body responds to therapy. If doctors formulate a blueprint precisely for each patient, it performs better and has fewer unwanted side effects. When medications suit a person's circumstances, anticipatory screenings can assist healthcare in transitioning from correcting issues to preempting them.

7.4 ADVANCEMENT IN DEEP LEARNING TECHNOLOGIES

DL helps doctors find illness, check people faster, and find new ways to help people. This part looks at how DL in healthcare is changing, focusing on neural networks and how they are made, the use of talking to computers, and the use of computers close to patients to help healthcare systems [19].

7.4.1 Neural Networks and Architectures

Changes to how neural networks are built and designed have been very crucial for improving how DL can help with healthcare. Convolutional neural networks (CNNs), a neural network, have significantly changed how doctors view medical pictures. CNNs are better at finding small details in X-rays, MRIs, and CT scans. This helps doctors diagnose illnesses faster and more correctly. Using CNNs to study mathematical pictures has made it much quicker. It gives doctors a critical way to see inside the body [20].

Doctors have better tools now for learning from medical records over time. Networks that remember past details can follow how patients' health changes. These help look at a person's whole medical story. Details from long ago add to what doctors see today. Together, all the information gives caregivers a fuller picture [21]. They can use that complete data to make smarter choices about the best treatments. Neural systems now focus better on what matters most, thanks to attention guides. Transformers use these to help the models comprehend more. They let networks spotlight essential details. This expands on how these systems can assist healthcare. Developers keep improving how neural layers are arranged. These tweaks show the promise of networks tackling challenging medical puzzles. Progress here marks a key step where technology and treatment team up.

7.4.2 Natural Language Processing in Healthcare

Natural language processing (NLP) [22] lets computers work with human language in new ways. It helps machines read, understand, and create text like doctors' notes, research papers, and patient histories. This new technology helps uncover essential facts hidden in words and sentences. It shows promise for learning from all the information doctors and scientists write down daily to give people better care. Doctors are learning a lot from computers about reading health papers and reports. Programs that summarize long medical documents and find essential facts from research articles

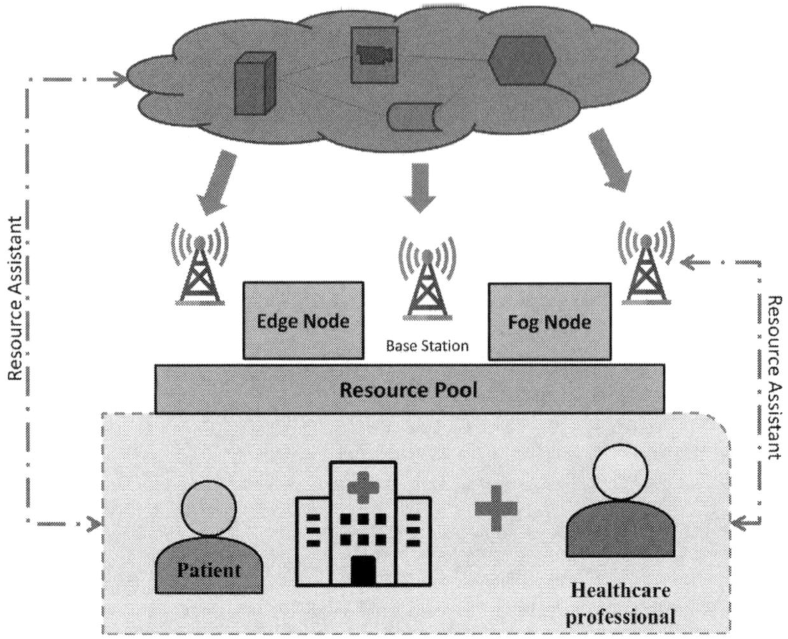

FIGURE 7.5 AI-based edged-based healthcare system.

are also helping doctors. Programs also look at what people say about their health online to see how they feel. By having computers do some reading and writing tasks, doctors have more time to help people. They can learn from many papers, studies, and posts without reading them all day. This helps doctors make good choices to keep people healthy. Doctors and researchers can learn more from words with new language tools. These tools can look at words, not in a special way [23]. They can find facts hidden in reports and papers. This new way of understanding words changes how doctors learn from the past and make choices to help people feel better. Words and healthcare are working together in new ways. This allows doctors to take better care of patients.

7.4.3 Edge Computing for Healthcare Applications

Wearable technology and sensors today create a lot of information. Edge computing helps by processing some of this data on the devices before sending everything to large computer systems. This edge computing is essential for healthcare. It can efficiently deal with the vast amounts of data from things like fitness trackers and heart monitors. Small machines with smart StePS can look at details immediately, finding what they need without sending everything to the big servers so fast. This does not just cut down on the servers but ensures people get what they need on time. The fast steps of small machines help make choices quicker, improving how folks are helped when fast work counts. Bringing edge computing to healthcare changes how systems work, and many small computers are used to help doctors help people better. This works with the big focus now on caring for each person and being there when they need it. It shows that technology will be essential in how we care for people in the future.

7.4.4 Integration of Internet of Things

The linking of systems, machines, and detectors through new networks has drastically changed healthcare with the IoT allowing smooth information sharing. IoT is key for deep studying since it gives ongoing, real-world information for inspection. Clever wearables, associated medical tools, and tracking sensors add to massive information sets that different types utilize for personalized treatment options, future investigation, and analysis. Integrating IoT assists the shift toward proactive and stoppable healthcare and better ring choices dependent on information.

Wearable devices provide constant health information for each person. Some parables use DL to study exercise levels, body features, and other medical details. Doctors can check patients remotely using this data, find issues early, and offer help quickly. The details that wearables collect help create custom care plans for each patient. So wearables also aid personalized medicine. DL and parables work together to give our patients more control over their health. Doctors get helpful facts, too. Advances in DL have changed healthcare in many ways. A more intelligent, more responsive system is the result. Changes include complex neural networks, NLP, and edge computing. Also, things connected to the internet to share information well. Wearables add to these benefits by allowing health tracking anywhere. The future of healthcare looks very promising because these technologies work well together. They encourage new ideas, better patient results, and a more efficient, personalized healthcare system.

7.5 ETHICAL CONSIDERATIONS IN SMART HEALTHCARE

New ideas like DL make healthcare systems smarter and change how care is given. However, this change has moral problems that must be fixed to be fair, safe, and focused on patients. Important moral points are looked at here, like privacy and security worries, who owns data and needs Oks, unfairness in DL rules, and the importance of laws and following rules.

7.5.1 Security and Privacy Issues

While security and confidentiality are essential to properly introducing intelligent healthcare networks, patient details must transfer seamlessly. Since these systems rely on private medical records, strong protections are crucial.

7.5.2 Ownership of Data and Consent

It is essential to get informed permission before any data collection, sharing, or examination to protect individuals' freedom over using health facts. Trust between patients, doctors, and the bigger system is made by openly talking about the aims and possible results of data use.

7.5.3 Deep Learning Algorithms' Bias and Fairness

The use of DL algorithms in healthcare raises moral issues regarding fairness and prejudice, mainly when they are used to make choices about diagnosis and care. Since the algorithms are taught using past information, models that contain biased data risk worsening existing healthcare wrongs. It is essential to fix biases in the training information and continuously check that the results of algorithms are fair. Also important is making sure the info used for teaching is presentative of and different to avoid algorithmic bias, which may unjustly harm certain groups of people. Transparency in telling patients and medical workers about possible biases and limits of DL models is needed to make ethical progress.

7.5.4 Compliance and Regulatory Frameworks

Regulations play an essential role in healthcare technologies. Strict rules ensure new ideas follow the laws and moral rules we agree on. Groups are responsible for setting rules and policies for patient privacy and data safety, and doing the right thing with new tools. Following standards like the General Data Protection Regulation (GDPR) in Europe and the Health Insurance Portability and Accountability Act (HIPAA) in America is key. As tech changes, so should the rules to address new moral issues. The guidelines must adapt to join ethics and progress as friends.

Thoughtful and patient-focused healthcare settings largely depend on moral problems in innovative healthcare environments. To ensure the prospective benefits of leading technologies are shared fairly and patient trust remains at the core of healthcare practice, progress must be balanced with privacy, safety, fairness, and obeying rules. As these environments keep changing, a forward-thinking and adaptable moral structure is essential to handle the intricate connections between technology, patient care, and societal hopes. Innovation and ethics working together will play a key part in making a future in healthcare that takes advantage of technology but also adheres to the strictest moral standards.

7.6 CASE STUDIES AND SUCCESS STORIES

New tools are helping hospitals work better together. Some places are using computers and phones to take care of people. They are trying different ways to help patients feel better faster at a lower cost. This part will look at real examples and good things that happened.

7.6.1 Smart Healthcare Implementations in the Real World

7.6.1.1 AI's Effect on Diagnostic Imaging

The hospital uses innovative computer programs to help with medical pictures. Doctors could focus on complex cases and talking to people because it took less time to look at the pictures. The programs were very good at finding problems and helping doctors name faster what was wrong. This story showed how clever technology could help doctors do their jobs, making diagnoses more exact and working better.

Case Study 1: Remote Monitoring of Patients with Chronic Illnesses

The doctors use watches and internet-connected things in a program to check patients from far away with prolonged illnesses like diabetes and hypertension. Helpers in healthcare now can see how patients are feeling and act fast if something is wrong because of putting together the real information from the things into an innovative system for healthcare. The patients improved in the end, and a few returned to the hospital because they were using the things. This case shows how watching before problems and quick action can well take care of long-time illness through competent healthcare.

7.6.2 Effect on Results for Patients

7.6.2.1 Tailored Cancer Patients' Treatment Programs

The doctors at a famous hospital that treats cancer use a computer program to help plan each patient's care. The program looked at DNA tests and what happened to other people before getting different treatments. It helped the doctors make better treatment plans for each person. The results showed that patients were treated better and had fewer problems. This showed that using computer programs in healthcare can improve treatments and have fewer side effects. The program helped because it used what it learned from each patient to pick treatments that fit each person's needs.

7.6.2.2 Wearable Technology Improving Heart Health

The research thoroughly investigated how wearable devices could assist with heart health. Patients with cardiovascular issues are tested with smartwatches and trackers designed to consistently track activity levels and significant body signals. The constant sharing of this information with doctors through technology allows problems to be spotted earlier. Fewer health issues occurred because of the system, demonstrating how wearable technology incorporated into intelligent health networks can enhance what doctors can do for people. By continuously collecting and sending data, we helped providers monitoring patients closer and react quicker when signs of trouble started to show.

7.6.3 Efficiency and Cost-Effectiveness Gains

Case Study 1: Enhancing Resource Allocation through the Application of Predictive Analytics

The hospital group uses predictive analytics to help with resource planning. DL models predicted when more patients would need care and when things would be quieter. This helped the staffing schedule match the patient workload better. They could avoid having too many workers when few patients needed help or too few workers when lots of patients came in. By forecasting demand, they optimize staff numbers. Matching resources to the patient load improved how they worked. It saved the hospital network a lot of money.

Case Study 2: Using NLP to Simplify Administrative Procedures

The hospital developed new computer programs to help schedule appointments and write medical records. The programs used NLP to understand written words like a person. In a case study, the programs helped lower the workload for the staff. Workers had more time for patients because the computer took over some paper tasks. It costs less to run the hospital with few staff spent on paperwork. The changes showed that the new system saved money and worked well.

The stories and examples demonstrate how smart healthcare environments truly impact people's feelings, how money matters, and how work gets done. Innovative technologies in healthcare can change how care is provided in real-life situations, like making sure the right things are where needed, watching patients from afar, and individualizing care plans. These examples light the path as these environments keep changing, showing direction for healthcare as technological improvements will help people and make systems work better and stronger.

7.7 FUTURE DIRECTIONS AND EMERGING TRENDS

Advances in DL and AI will help improve smart healthcare systems over the next decade. This section discusses what may happen in healthcare over the coming ten years, new ways DL can help with medicine, and how intelligence is altering smart healthcare communities.

7.7.1 Forecasts for the Future

1. **Patient-Centered, Holistic Care**: Over the next ten years, innovative healthcare systems aim to focus more on overall patient care. Bringing together different types of information, such as lifestyle, social factors, and genetic details, would give doctors a clearer picture of each person's situation. This complete view may enable customization and preemptive strategies. The goal is to identify issues early and act fast to help patients stay healthy. Doctors could use this comprehensive approach to identify risks and find better ways to prevent or delay diseases.
2. **Improved Data Exchange and Interoperability**: Healthcare organizations will work together better in the future. Groups will agree on the same ways to share facts between them. This will let details move smoothly between different programs and machines. People making choices about treatment will have more to go by because of the connection between groups. Doctors and nurses will be able to work together better to help people. They will not repeat the steps or papers. Everyone will see the same notes on how a person is doing with their health.
3. **Decentralized Models of Healthcare**: Doctors may share health information in new ways using edge computing and blockchain. These technologies could spread healthcare to more places by letting data be stored on

many different computers. Patients could have more say over where the information goes. They might take charge of their health records instead of leaving them with one group. This would help people play a bigger role in staying healthy.

7.7.2 Advances in Healthcare Using Deep Learning

7.7.2.1 Clinical Decision Support with Explainable AI

Explainable AI will be the primary focus of the upcoming wave of DL advances in the medical field. Some models will give clear reasons for their choices, as not knowing why a model decides something can cause problems for doctors using it. Making algorithms easier to grasp will boost how much doctors trust and accept them in hospitals and clinics.

7.7.2.2 Federated Learning for Analytics that Preserve Privacy

Federated learning, a technique that keeps personal information private, may become more common in healthcare. This discovery allows doctors to work together to improve AI models used for patients. The models learn from many different hospitals and clinics without sharing actual records. Patient privacy is protected because the tails remain in their device or place. This makes it very relevant for innovative health systems connecting doctors, hospitals, and patients. In those networks, a person's privacy and data security matter greatly.

7.7.2.3 Combining Multiple Modes of Data for Detailed Examination

Dee's learning advancements will help combine different types of health information for improved medical understanding. In addition to routine scans, these models should also be capable of analyzing genetic information, data from medical devices, and doctors' clinical notes. Considering all this information together can help doctors gain a deeper understanding of a patient's condition and develop treatments tailored specifically to them.

7.7.3 Artificial Intelligence's Impact on Healthcare

7.7.3.1 Strengthening Medical Experts

While AI can help doctors and patients in the future, machines will not replace human doctors. AI programs may take over simple routine tasks to give doctors more time to think hard about complex cases and focus on helping patients feel better. These computer helpers could find patterns in medical information to help with diagnoses. They may also automate boring, repetitive jobs, and plan treatment options. This would allow doctors to spend their time on the vital work of caring for people who need medical care. AI assistants will support doctors in many ways, such as analyzing test results, prescribing appropriate therapies, monitoring patient progress, predicting potential complications, and providing decision support for personalized treatment plans.

7.7.3.2 Predictive Analytics and Population Health Management

Population health will change a lot with AI helping. AI can find groups who may get disease soon using past health details. It looks at big databases with all our health info. The AI programs try to see what diseases may happen and where. This helps send help to the right places. It aims to keep people from getting ill in the first place or stop the disease from spreading to others. Resources can be used in the best way. People may get care early before issues grow worse.

7.7.3.3 Democratizing Healthcare Access

AI can help more people get medical care no matter where they live or their access to doctors. Telemedicine and AI tools may diagnose illnesses and check on patients from far away. This could help communities without many clinics and hospitals. It fits with a bigger goal of making healthcare smart. The goal is for everyone to be able to get healthcare when they need it, no matter what. The possibilities for intelligent healthcare networks are vast, pushed forward by constant improvements in DL and artificial thinking. Predictions for the following ten years show a change toward decentralized healthcare models, better ability of different systems to work together, and complete patient-focused care all about one person. Explaining results, keeping private information private during the analysis, and bringing together different types of information for complete health checks will be the main areas of advancement in DL. Artificial thinking will play a revolutionary role in managing the health of whole populations, making healthcare services available to more people and helping those who care for people's health. The joining of technological advances and careful thinking about ethics will be necessary in deciding how these technological changes happen and how intelligent healthcare networks will reshape how healthcare is provided worldwide.

7.8 CONCLUSION

Innovative healthcare systems combine late technologies with focusing on patients. This thorough look covers how DL is used, what's being made, and essential questions. DL helps medical tests a lot. It leads to better medical pictures and finding illnesses earlier. Preventing illness is helped by parables and internet devices. They let doctors watch patients from anywhere. Personalized medicine uses DL to make treatments fit each person. Telemedicine made healthcare easier to get. Neural networks, talking to computers, and edge computing are essential for advances in innovative healthcare systems. They make accurate diagnoses, let doctors look at data immediately, and improve healthcare steps. Also, we interpret many kinds of data together to understand patients' health better. Innovation and privacy must be balanced carefully thinking about ethics. Strong security and privacy rules are needed to protect private information. The good use of AI depends on fixing unfair thinking and being open about computer choices. New laws must change to ensure new technologies are used well and safely. DL healthcare systems with smarts hold the hope of a medical field that is good and right for people both now and in the future. A significant change in healthcare starts with all the new things, discoveries, and important questions. This time promises better patient care and a healthcare system focused more on each person.

REFERENCES

1. S. Das, T. K. Samal, B. K. Mohanta and A. Nayak, "Emerging Cyber Threats in Healthcare: A Study of Attacks in IoMT Ecosystems," *2023 7th International Conference on I-SMAC (IoT in Social, Mobile, Analytics and Cloud) (I-SMAC)*, Kirtipur, Nepal, 2023, pp. 77–82, doi: 10.1109/I-SMAC58438.2023.10290147
2. V. Puri, A. Kataria, S. Rani and P. K. Pareek, "DLT Based Smart Medical Ecosystem," *2023 International Conference on Network, Multimedia and Information Technology (NMITCON)*, Bengaluru, India, 2023, pp. 1–6, doi: 10.1109/NMITCON58196.2023.10276204
3. M. Wazid, J. Singh, A. K. Das and J. J. P. C. Rodrigues, "An ensemble-based machine learning-envisioned intrusion detection in Industry 5.0-driven healthcare applications," *IEEE Transactions on Consumer Electronics*, doi: 10.1109/TCE.2023.3318850
4. V. Sharma, P. Saxena, S. K. Yadav, D. Singh, S. Ranka and R. Dhabliya, "Smart Contract Based Sensitive Data Hashing for Security in Healthcare Environment," *2023 International Conference on Data Science and Network Security (ICDSNS)*, Tiptur, India, 2023, pp. 1–7, doi: 10.1109/ICDSNS58469.2023.10245390
5. N. Chakraborty, S. Iqbal and M. Zulkernine, "Risk Assessment in Smart Aging Care Systems: An Elderly-Centered Perspective," *2023 IEEE International Conference on Digital Health (ICDH)*, Chicago, IL, USA, 2023, pp. 1–12, doi: 10.1109/ICDH60066.2023.00012
6. N. R. Rajeswari, G. Arunkumar, M. S. Vadivu, M. Gupta, R. Sethuraman and M. Rajkumar, "Development of Healthcare Monitoring System with Pollution Control in Industrial Sectors Using the Internet of Things," *2023 5th International Conference on Inventive Research in Computing Applications (ICIRCA)*, Coimbatore, India, 2023, pp. 1392–1397, doi: 10.1109/ICIRCA57980.2023.10220589
7. A. Abugabah and N. Nizamuddin, "Smart Healthcare Ecosystem for Elderly Patient Care," *2020 43rd International Convention on Information, Communication and Electronic Technology (MIPRO)*, Opatija, Croatia, 2020, pp. 365–370, doi: 10.23919/MIPRO48935.2020.9245404
8. V. Bhatt and S. Chakraborty, "Real-Time Healthcare Monitoring Using Smart Systems: A Step towards Healthcare Service Orchestration Smart Systems for Futuristic Healthcare," *2021 International Conference on Artificial Intelligence and Smart Systems (ICAIS)*, Coimbatore, India, 2021, pp. 772–777, doi: 10.1109/ICAIS50930.2021.9396029
9. R. Lebre, M. Pedrosa, M. G. Pose and C. Costa, "A Safe Architecture for Authorization Grant in Healthcare Ecosystems," *2020 IEEE International Conference on Healthcare Informatics (ICHI)*, Oldenburg, Germany, 2020, pp. 1–5, doi: 10.1109/ICHI48887.2020.9374380
10. F. F. Alruwaili, B. Alabduallah, H. Alqahtani, A. S. Salama, G. P. Mohammed and A. A. Alneil, "Blockchain enabled smart healthcare system using jellyfish search optimization with dual-pathway deep convolutional neural network," *IEEE Access*, vol. 11, pp. 87583–87591, 2023, doi: 10.1109/ACCESS.2023.3304269
11. E. Kim, "Smart City Service Platform Associated with Smart Home," *2017 International Conference on Information Networking (ICOIN)*, Da Nang, Vietnam, 2017, pp. 608–610, doi: 10.1109/ICOIN.2017.7899557
12. A. Abugabah, N. Nizamuddin and A. A. Alzubi, "Decentralized telemedicine framework for a smart healthcare ecosystem," *IEEE Access*, vol. 8, pp. 166575–166588, 2020, doi: 10.1109/ACCESS.2020.3021823
13. H. Xie, X. Zhang, N. I. Xuefeng, H. Jiang and L.I. Dongjing, "Application of telemedicine in the elderly population," *Chinese Journal of General Practitioners*, vol. 15, no. 10, pp. 805–808, 2016.

14. J. Boudy, J. L. Baldinger, F. Delavault, M. Muller, I. Farin, R. V. Andreao, et al., "Telemedicine for an Elderly Patient at Home. In Smart Homes and Beyond," *4th International Conference on Smart Homes and Health Telematics (ICOST 2006)*, vol. 19, pp. 74–81, Belfast, Northern Ireland, 2006, June.
15. P. P. Ray, "Home Health Hub Internet of Things (H 3 IoT): An architectural Framework for Monitoring the Health of Elderly People," *2014 International Conference on Science Engineering and Management Research (ICSEMR)*, pp. 1–3, Chennai, India, 2014, November.
16. S. J. Park, M. Subramaniyam, S. E. Kim, S. Hong, J. H. Lee, C. M. Jo, et al., "Development of the elderly healthcare monitoring system with IoT," In *Advances in Human Factors and Ergonomics in Healthcare*, vol. 482, pp. 309–315, Springer, Cham, 2017.
17. N. Sultan, "Making use of cloud computing for healthcare provision: Opportunities and challenges," *International Journal of Information Management*, vol. 34, no. 2, pp. 177–184, 2014.
18. S. P. Ahuja, S. Mani and J. Zambrano, "A survey of the state of cloud computing in healthcare," *Network and Communication Technologies*, vol. 1, no. 2, pp. 12, 2012.
19. B. C. Drolet, J. S. Marwaha, B. Hyatt, P. E. Blazar and S. D. Lifchez, "Electronic communication of protected health information: privacy security and HIPAA compliance," *The Journal of Hand Surgery*, vol. 42, no. 6, pp. 411–416, 2017.
20. G. C. Doolittle and R. J. Spaulding, "Defining the needs of a telemedicine service," In *Introduction to Telemedicine*, Second edition. CRC Press, pp. 79–92, 2017.
21. M. Sajid and Z. Raza, "Cloud Computing: Issues & Challenges," *International Conference on Cloud Big Data and Trust*, vol. 20, no. 13, pp. 13–15, 2013, December.
22. M. P. Mcbee and C. Wilcox, "Blockchain technology: Principles and applications in medical imaging," *Journal of Digital Imaging*, vol. 33, no. 3, pp. 726–734, January 2020.
23. Y. Chen, S. Ding, Z. Xu, H. Zheng and S. Yang, "Blockchain-based medical records secure storage and medical service framework," *Journal of Medical Systems*, vol. 43, no. 1, pp. 1–9, 2019.

8 Healing Intelligence

A Deep Dive into the Cognitive Revolution of Health care through Advanced Deep Learning Technologies

Nilesh P. Sable, Vijay U. Rathod, Pallavi K. Parlewar, Masira S. Kulkarni, and Sheetal Dhande

8.1 INTRODUCTION

Deep learning is a branch of artificial intelligence (AI) that learns from data and finds helpful answers by mimicking the way our brains work [1]. The start of healing wisdom can be found in deep learning. It offers a new approach to understanding, diagnosing, and addressing health issues.

8.2 BACKGROUND

In the first section of our investigation, we explore the fundamentals of [2] deep learning in health care. We dissect the complexities of this groundbreaking technology and look at how it powers healing intelligence. By breaking down the fundamentals of deep learning and charting its development within the framework of medical data analytics, we create the foundation for comprehending the revolutionary potential that lies ahead. The story then moves past the theoretical underpinnings and explores the real-world uses of deep learning in diagnostics.

A deep learning and healing intelligence-based system for recommending medical medications is shown in Figure 8.1. This sophisticated model represents a paradigm shift in healthcare decision-making by combining patient data, medical history, and state-of-the-art algorithms to offer individualized prescription recommendations. Healing intelligence transforms medical imaging, a vital component of contemporary health care, improving its accuracy and efficacy. With [3] the help of sophisticated algorithms, diagnostic decision support systems become indispensable resources that give medical personnel unmatched precision and insights when recognizing and analyzing patient conditions. Our exploration into intelligence and

DOI: 10.1201/9781003479185-8

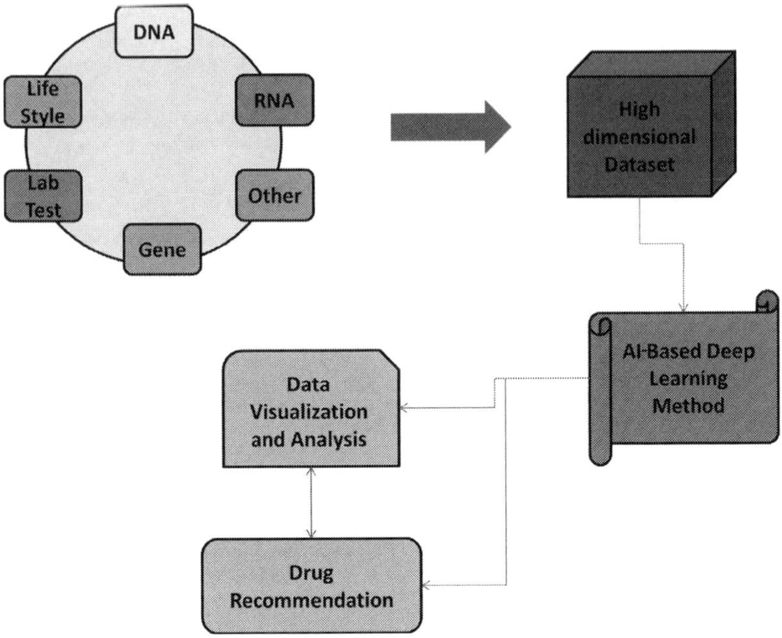

FIGURE 8.1 Healthcare medicine recommendation using deep learning with healing intelligence.

its impact on how treatments are planned continues. The new approach personalizes treatment on a person's genes and molecules, moving past therapy that sees all patients as alike.

8.3 OBJECTIVES

The work checks out how deep learning analyzes vast datasets, such as gene sequences and body chemistry, to tailor plans for each individual. Compared to the old standard-size-for-all therapies, personalized medicine could mean therapies targeting people are better with fewer steps.

This study aims to clarify how AI can change how we care for patients. It focuses on virtual assistants with advanced AI skills. These virtual assistants can provide patients with individualized advice, assistance, and relevant information. The study also examines how deep learning and prediction analysis can expand patient care beyond normal hospitals. This includes monitoring people remotely. These technology tools may help create a more dynamic and adaptable healthcare system. The system could better serve people before problems become severe.

This article thoughtfully examines important questions about using smart tech in medical care. It discusses issues like programs mistreating some groups and keeping people's information private and safe. The writer also shares ideas on how to fix problems [4]. Furthermore, it helps us think about what could happen next as tech gets more intelligent and wiser. This will help learners, doctors, and teachers understand the right and wrong of these significant changes.

This section offers a complete and thoughtful examination of the study's effect on health care sparked by superior cognitive technologies. We aim to clarify how these technologies may change matters and offer insight into the moral problems surrounding such an essential switch by analyzing the levels of therapeutic knowledge. We stand where invention and duty meet as we delve deeply into healthcare's long run, led by therapeutic knowledge. We are mapping a path toward a healthcare system that is smarter, more reactive, and kinder.

8.4 FOUNDATIONS OF DEEP LEARNING IN HEALTH CARE

Advanced learning methods help doctors care for people, plan treatments, and detect sicknesses in a new way during changes in thinking about health care. This chapter examines how the best deep learning methods improve healing intelligence in healthcare today.

8.4.1 Overview of Deep Learning

Looking back over deep learning's basics is key before advancing to more intricate methods. Neural stems act as the foundation for deep learning since they emulate the intricate structure of the human thought process. Convolutional neural networks (CNNs) and recurrent neural networks (RNNs)—with ground-laying structures—are helpful in healthcare use [5]. While RNs work well for handling data that changes through time, like inpatient tracking, CNNs excel at recognizing pictures, rendering them invaluable for medical photo analysis.

8.4.2 Integration Challenges

While advancements have been made with deep learning techniques in medicine, issues remain. Researchers must strike a balance between innovation and ethics, privacy, and the production of interpretable results. Approaches that combine deep learning with technologies such as rating and blockchain show promise. Federated deep learning decentralizes model training while blockchain enables safe data sharing [6]. Quantum computing coupled with deep learning may vastly increase processing power for complete health analysis. Quantum EEP learning could harness quantum computers' unique abilities. This is quantum and deep learnings strengths to further medical research. Faster drug discovery and optimized treatment optimization may occur with unprecedented efficiency [7,8].

The field of medical advancement [9] is evolving due to deep learning techniques being added to changes in how health care uses knowledge. Different methods, like AI that can be explained, attention processes, and copying learning from other tasks or GANs to learning through trial and error or learning that can be explained, not only improve how well EP learning models work but also deal with essential problems like not having enough data and being able to explain the reasoning. The [10] joining of cutting-edge methods points us toward a future where medical advancement is powered by technology but also does what is right, is open about how it works, strongly helps patients get better, and changes how healthcare is given as we deal with change brought about by new ideas and health care.

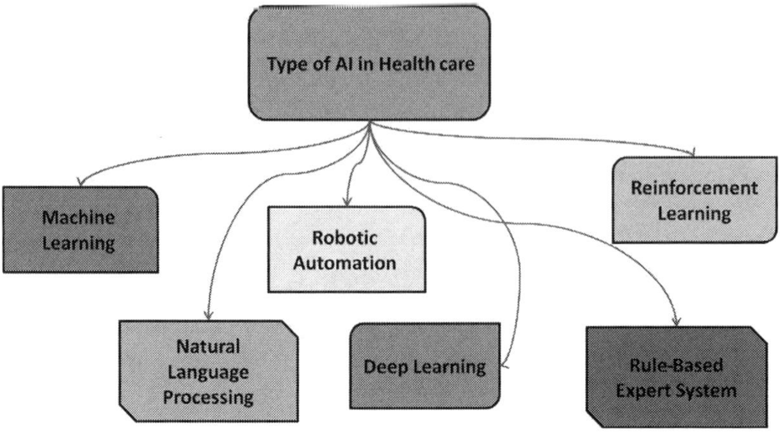

FIGURE 8.2 Types of AI in health care.

8.4.3 Advanced Deep Learning Techniques

Doctors are learning new ways to help people by using deep learning. Deep learning uses computers to find patterns in large amounts of data. Doctors study these patterns to better understand diseases and discover new treatments. Deep learning also helps doctors diagnose illnesses. It looks for clues in scans, tests, and medical histories. This lets doctors know what's wrong with a patient and make a treatment plan. Deep learning is transforming what doctors thought they knew about healthcare. It is like doctors helping people in new ways. This chapter tells more about how deep learning and health care work together (Figure 8.2).

8.4.4 Convolutional Neural Networks (CNNs)

CNNs are at the forefront of deep learning approaches in the medical field. This [11] particular class of neural networks is beneficial in medical imaging because of its superior ability to interpret and extract hierarchical characteristics from organized grid data. CNNs have a significant role in improving the accuracy of diagnosis in the context of healing intelligence. In radiology, for example, CNNs can identify minute patterns in medical images, which help diagnose and identify anomalies early. As CNNs, the architecture shown in Figure 8.3, have developed, attention mechanisms have been included, which allows the networks to concentrate on important characteristics and improves their diagnostic performance.

8.4.4.1 CNN Algorithm

Step 1: Convolution Operation

$$(I * K)(i,j) = \sum D_m \sum I_n \; I(i+m, j+n) \cdot K(m,n)$$

Step 2: Activation Function

$$f(x) = \max(0, x)$$

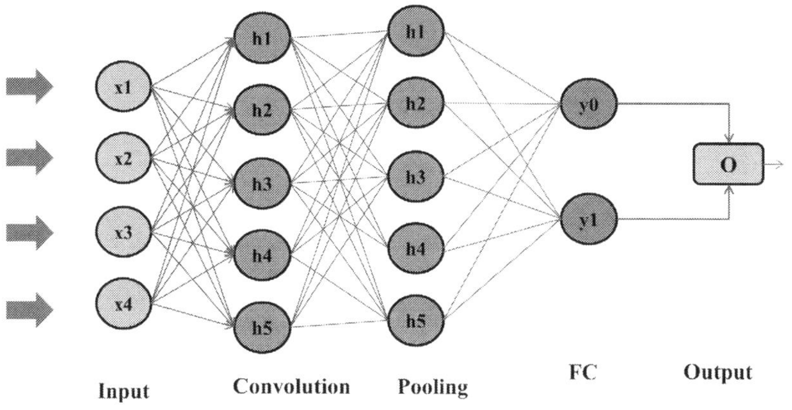

FIGURE 8.3 Systematic architecture of CNN.

Step 3: Pooling (Subsampling)

$$\text{MaxPooling}(x) = \max(xi,\ j)$$

Step 4: Flattening

$$\text{Flatten}(\text{Pooling})$$

Step 5: Fully Connected Layer
Step 6: Output Layer
Step 7: Loss Function and Backpropagation

$$\text{MSE} = \frac{1}{N}\sum_{i=1}^{N}(y_i - \hat{y}_i)^2$$

8.4.5 Temporal Data Analysis with Recurrent Neural Networks (RNNs)

Healthcare data, such as patient records and continuous monitoring data, are temporally structured; hence, methods that can capture [12] sequential dependencies are required. RNNs are a cutting-edge deep learning technique well-suited for temporal data analysis. RNNs are proving to be extremely useful in the cognitive revolution of health care as they can anticipate patient outcomes, spot trends, and tailor treatment regimens to each patient's changing health state. Patient care can be provided more dynamically and responsively thanks to RNNs' capacity to remember previous states.

8.4.6 Using Generative Adversarial Networks (GANs) to Generate Synthetic Data

A paradigm shift is introduced [13] by the incorporation of GANs, which enable the synthesis of synthetic medical data. GANs provide a novel option when obtaining large and diverse datasets for deep learning model training is difficult because of data shortages or privacy concerns, as shown in Figure 8.4. GANs enable training deep

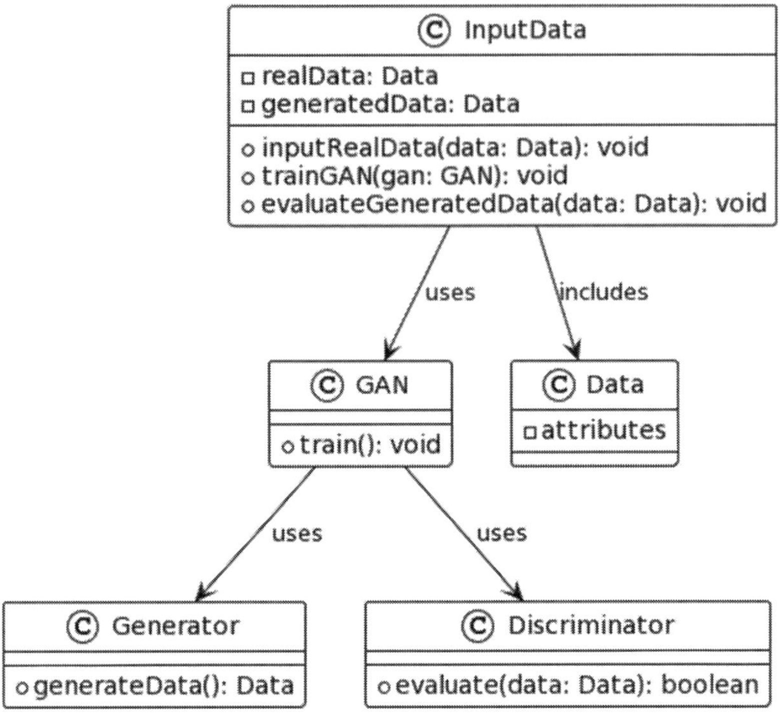

FIGURE 8.4 Workflow of GANs to generate synthetic data.

learning models without jeopardizing patient privacy by producing realistic synthetic data. This app approach has become essential in fields such as medical imaging, where robust model performance requires access to a broad range of images.

8.4.7 Transfer Learning for Knowledge Transfer across Domains

In the cognitive revolution of health care, transfer learning appears as a powerful tool to address the persistent problem of scarce labeled data in some medical regions. Transfer learning facilitates knowledge transfer to the target healthcare domain by utilizing pre-trained models on big datasets from similar domains [14]. As a result, much less labeled data is required, which speeds up the creation of reliable and accurate deep learning models.

8.4.8 Reasonable Artificial Intelligence (XAI) for Open Decision-Making

Transparency and understanding complex healthcare programs are becoming more necessary as deep learning models evolve. Explainable AI technique gives insights into involved models' thinking. In health care, where choices matter, grasping why a model's diagnosis or plan is essential. Doctors can trust each other more when using XAI techniques, like paying attention to things and ways that work with any model, which helps develop learning models clearer and ensures that AI is used correctly to help people.

In short, changes in how health care uses thinking are mainly due to cutting-edge deep learning techniques being added. CNNs help doctors with diagnosis, and RNNs help with info over time [15]. This all was AI to handle the medical facts well. Transfer learning speed using deep learning models for specific medical areas. GANs help when there isn't much data. Explainable AI techniques ensure models' choices are clear, and people trust the m. The store has more than just technology as we learn more. We see the effects of what's right and their important part in making health care that responds well, is smart, and works well [16].

8.5 HEALING INTELLIGENCE AND DECISION SYSTEM IN HEALTH CARE

Doctors now use computers to help with medical decisions. Machines that find problems and pictures that show inside the body are changing how doctors decide what's wrong with patients. This part talks about how computers help doctors check sick people and make choices about their care. It shows how technology in health care is causing big changes in finding illnesses and deciding what to do.

8.5.1 Medical Imaging Advancements

Medical imaging has dramatically improved thanks to deep learning. While old ways of medical imaging sometimes have problems, deep learning helps. CNNs are a type of deep learning commonly used now. CNNs help medical imaging be more accurate and fast. CNNs are excellent at recognizing images, which is useful when analyzing medical imaging. Healing intelligence improves diagnosis accuracy in various fields, including radiology and pathology. It does this by painstakingly deciphering minute details in images and assisting in detecting anomalies, lesions, and subtle patterns that the human eye might miss. Furthermore, by including transfer learning, these models can take advantage of the knowledge gathered from various datasets, which improves their capacity to adjust to particular medical imaging domains [17]. Healing intelligence improves diagnostic precision in medical imaging while simultaneously speeding up the procedure.

Deep learning has helped doctors make quicker choices, which can save lives. It looks at medical pictures better and faster than people. This part talks about real examples of smart machines helping sick people. The machines found problems in pictures before doctors could, allowing doctors to help patients sooner with the right treatment.

8.5.2 Systems for Diagnostic Decision Support

Diagnostic decision support systems [18] are a key part of the smart revolution in health care, supporting advances in medical imaging. These technologies, made stronger by cutting-edge deep learning methods, signal a new time when medical staff have access to thoughtful, information-driven information to guide their clinical decisions. Diagnostic decision support systems are collaborative technologies that improve rather than replace healthcare providers' knowledge. This chapter dives into the complexities of these systems in this part, clarifying how they use deep

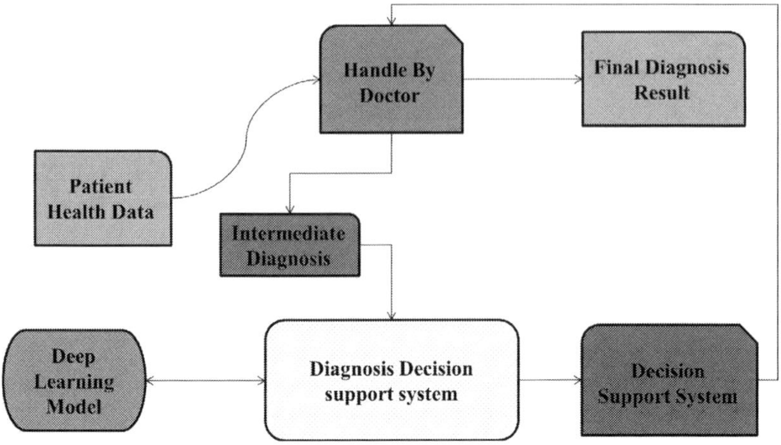

FIGURE 8.5 Representation of systems for diagnostic decision support.

learning algorithms to handle large sets of data that include patient histories, medical imaging outcomes, and a variety of other clinical data points. A detailed and delicate picture of a patient's condition is ensured for doctors by the teamwork of decision support systems and healing intelligence [19].

When these systems join together, how well do doctors diagnose illness, and how quickly are they improved? Doctors' ideas are meant just for that patient based on what they know about the patient before and what doctors learn now. This chapter also talks about the part these systems have in care, not just for each person. That kind of care makes suggestions for treatment based on understanding each patient's health situation. Even though GH help systems for diagnosis have come a long way, this chapter addresses the hard questions that come up when they are a part of how doctors work. Talks about using machines to help diagnose need to deal with privacy, needing to explain what the machines say, and balancing what machines think with what doctors think are all important subjects (Figure 8.5).

8.5.3 Prospective Pathways and Obstacles

Better conclusions may result from combining details about patients from various areas, which brings together data regarding a person from multiple origins for a complete picture. Additionally, explainable AI strategies address the issue of interpretation by analyzing how intelligent healing systems make choices that [20] are clear and comprehensible to medical experts. The section notes that problems remain, such as biased algorithms, private health information, and the smooth integration of supportive systems into precise medical care. By thinking about what may happen next, the section guides searchers, leaders, and doctors to navigate where wise choices and diligent healing meet. It encourages us to move toward a future where innovative tech works with human knowledge to reshape healthcare choices.

8.6 TREATMENT PLANNING AND PERSONALIZED MEDICINE

The way doctors make treatment plans is changing in the time of Smart Health. Instead of treating everyone the same way, care becomes more tailored just for you. This part discusses how looking at a person's genes and molecules and powerful computer learning changes treatment planning. It leads to the most accurate and customized care possible.

8.6.1 Tailoring Treatments with AI

Doctors can now customize care for each person using AI. AI helps doctors learn from large amounts of patient data in new ways. Deep learning programs in computers can help make treatment plans. These pans are tailored to each person's specific needs. The programs examine many details about lifestyle, genes, and health [21]. They help make sure care works well and is customized for each person. This chapter also talks about how AI helped plan care for cancer. Cancer research needs to consider many genetic and treatment factors. AI can do this better than old ways. As AI is more with care, ethical issues are more critical. Doctors and patients must work together to make decisions.

8.6.2 Molecular and Genetic Profiling

The groundbreaking advances in genetic and molecular testing go hand in hand with breakthroughs in AI-guided rapid planning. This section explains how high-throughput sequencing technologies and mapping the human genome weave a unique pattern of customized medicine, serving as the foundation of healing wisdom in treatment methods. Doctors have profound insights into hereditary causes of sicknesses and responses to treatments when someone's genetic code is solved [22]. This chapter delves into the complicated nature of genetic profiling by exploring deep learning algorithms' analysis of massive genomic data sets and tiny variations and mutations that may impact disease susceptibility and development. Also, rapid planning that includes genetic information ensures that actions target the exact biological mechanisms that cause a patient's disease [23].

Molecular profiling allows doctors to examine proteins, metabolites, and other biomolecules in a patient's body, helping them understand illnesses in more detail. This chapter discusses how mass spectrometry and other laboratory tests can find molecular signatures that signal health problems. Including these molecular profiles in treatment planning gives doctors a clearer picture of disease pathways.

8.7 HEALING INTELLIGENCE IN PATIENT CARE

Adding healing intelligence into patient care is a significant step forward for health care, profoundly changing how people see and interact with the system. This considerable change joins advanced AI learning with healthcare services to boost personal support, effectiveness, and fast responses. A key part of this change is the important job done by virtual health friends, which have become essential because of healing intelligence. These helpers go beyond just providing info and offer patients real answers right away using what they know about each situation and their ability to understand language. Reminders about my medicines, help manage a lifestyle, and quick replies to questions all contribute to patients feeling more involved and able to make better choices. Furthermore, the range of patient care goes beyond normal doctor's offices by improving monitoring from far away with the help of predicting what will happen. Healing intelligence lets healthcare providers constantly study a considerable amount of patient data, including behavior patterns and signs of health. By planning the ad, possible problems can be seen coming and dealt with before they get worse. This leads to better results for patients and less strain on healthcare systems by stopping issues that could have been avoided and people having to return to the hospital.

The joining of healing knowledge also involves the change toward knowing future health issues and preventing sickness before it starts. Advanced formulas, powered by past patient information, foresee dangerous signs and possible medical problems. This power to events that may come enables the doing of a plan to treat issues early, focusing on early help and encouraging overall health. Healing knowledge makes it easier for doctors to use care before sickness happens by looking at past patients. This helps healthcare providers shift from treating after sickness to preventing illness, improving how people feel. While health care is changing, some significant issues need focus. Keeping patient info safe and private and fixing problems in AI is extremely important. To gain trust and show what's done, a careful balance between new tech and ethics must stay. Using healing intelligence for care uses the best tech but also changes how people deal with doctors. Health care is moving toward the LP made for each person, works well, and follows the rules of right and wrong. This helps with virtual helpers and data number work to make sure that everyone's health and happiness are looked after in today's digital world.

8.7.1 Virtual Health Assistants

Virtual health assistants, or VHAs, are emerging tools changing health care. These co-op programs use advanced language understanding and context knowledge to improve how patients get at. They start a new time of personalized interaction, support, and sharing information. They show that VHAs help in their ability to connect patients to the complex healthcare system as middlemen. VHAs have extensive collections of medical facts. It quickly handles patient questions about symptoms, prescriptions, and other treatment options. Immediate access to information gives patients power and helps them feel in control of managing their health. What makes virtual health assistants unique is their ability to comprehend discussion topics. This all was for them to meet the specific needs of each individual and have difficult yet important conversations. For instance, a virtual helper can provide customized guidance by considering a person's medical background and personal choices. These automated assistants decrease the likelihood that treatment will end and help ensure medication is taken as intended. In doing so, virtual health assistants enhance patients' feelings and optimize how health care operates.

8.7.2 Remote Monitoring and Predictive Analytics

8.7.2.1 Remote Monitoring

Recently, technology has changed the way doctors help people stay healthy. New machines let doctors see how the body is doing from far away. This lets doctors take care of patients outside of clinics and hospitals. Devices constantly watch numbers about a person's body. They tell doctors lots of details about how organs work. Doctors understand a person's health very well by looking at patterns in signs and actions. This lets them find minor problems before they get big. Finding issues early helps people and makes health care easier. Remote monitoring especially helps those with long-term sickness. It makes sure treatment changes as needed without always needing to visit the doctor's office. The speed and effectiveness of AI remote monitoring change how health care is provided. It allows care that is prepared for each person and improves their feelings. It also introduces stress on regular healthcare buildings.

8.7.2.2 Predictive Analytics

Healing intelligence uses predicting patterns from past patient records to help health care. By finding problems before they start, this new way uses big math from lots of health data. It looks at all the info to see what might get sick later. This helps doctors start treatments and fixes before symptoms, changing how care works from reacting to acting first. Using healing intelligence not only makes people healthier but also cuts costs for medical care. Since it stops people from returning to hospitals or dealing with more issues, this change also helps save money and helps people do more with less. The star of healing intelligence marks a vital step, signaling a move from usual care methods to a future where figuring out patterns is key to shaping a more innovative, patient-centered, and long-term healthcare system.

8.7.2.3 Ethical Considerations and Integration

In healthcare technology, protecting patient privacy and remaining free of bias is extremely important, as are transparency and security. Developing new tools requires careful consideration of both benefits and ethics. Finding the right path between progress and principles is key. Being honest, trustworthy, and responsible with information is crucial to show technology respects people. Making these a top focus shields what is private and creates trust in the advance. By putting light and safety first, healthcare technology can work well within guidelines, proving to those that it helps that their good health comes before all else. This was all about people and progress to work together well for better care.

8.7.2.4 Prospective Courses

In coming years, adding the agency to remote remodeling and predictive analysis may assist health care in novel ways. Computer programs and AI are becoming more proficient at formulating highly accurate predictions and targeted assistance. It will be crucial for medical practitioners, designers, and ethics experts to collaborate effectively as changes occur. They could learn computer regulations more intelligently, examine new data types for improved forecasts, and establish equitable rules upon which all concur. To allow intelligence to aid individuals and the entire healthcare system most beneficially, medical professionals must continue their education regarding novel tech and perform what is just.

8.8 CHALLENGES AND ETHICAL CONSIDERATIONS

8.8.1 Security and Privacy

During Smart Care, advanced tech is blended smoothly with how people get help when sick or hurt. Keeping things safe and private for those using services is essential. With how much personal health info is made and worked with, strong steps must be taken to stop bad access, leaks, and possible misuse of data. There are many sides to security in health care. Protecting electronic health records, patient information, and how people talk to each other is very important. Encryption, secure login methods, and regular checks help keep information safe. We must also make the devices and systems that store or send health data safe from themselves or those not allowed to see it. Respect for patient privacy is a key part of doing right by people; it means guarding their health information and ensuring they agree and know how their information will be used. Having clear privacy rules, getting permission first, and letting patients control their own information helps individuals and builds trust in the healthcare system.

8.8.2 AI Algorithm Bias

Addressing bias in how AI systems make decisions involves acknowledging and trying to lessen biases from the data used to teach the systems, the algorithms that guide the m, and how they are made. If the data does not represent different types of people, biases can be learned and spread. It is essential to gather data from many kinds of groups to try to avoid unfair outcomes. Understanding exactly how a system decides things lets biases be found and fixed. Also, continuously checking AI systems over time can notice and correct biases that develop late or change with the data. However, dealing with biases in AI isn't one-size-fits-all. There must be room for new ideas in AI and a responsibility to ensure that all kinds of people share benefits fairly.

8.8.3 Juggling Creativity and Accountability

Creating AI that helps people while avoiding unnecessary problems takes care of work. Developers must encourage new ideas to advance technology. However, they must also ensure that their programs treat all groups equally and fairly. Balancing these goals is challenging. Developers need room to explore different solutions. Yet accountability is also essential. They must check their work does not accidentally spread or strengthen unfair biases against any members of society.

Creating a fair system requires careful planning from the start. It is important to get views from different people when developing and improving AI. Data scientists, ethics experts, doctors, and community members should work together.

Their perspectives can spot unfair treatment early and fix problems. It is also key for people to understand how decisions are made. Developers must show what information is used and how bias is stopped. This helps make sure the system is fair and earns trust. Learning does not end after making the AI. Healthcare workers and developers must keep learning new ideas about fairness and ways to stop bias. Regular training can help the teams working on projects stay ready to deal with challenging ethical issues when using AI to help people.

8.9 FUTURE TRENDS AND POSSIBILITIES

8.9.1 Integration of Healing Intelligence

Combining all intelligence also allows for new types of teamwork between groups with different areas of knowledge. Doctors, data scientists, morality experts, and technology makers working together can improve things. They can work as a team to solve complex problems and best use AI in health care. Schools, companies, and hospitals that partner up may make significant progress in creating algorithms, protecting information, and establishing fair rules. This could help AI in health care grow in a way that takes care of people.

Nevertheless, incorporating healing intelligence into the future will not be devoid of obstacles. Key areas of focus will continue to be ethical considerations, concerns regarding data privacy, and the necessity for regulatory frameworks to keep up with technological advancements. Establishing a harmonious equilibrium between innovation and moral responsibility will be crucial to constructing and sustaining public confidence in these revolutionary technologies.

8.9.2 Emerging Technologies

With its unmatched processing capacity, quantum computing holds the potential to transform the way complicated healthcare datasets are analyzed thoroughly. The new features of quantum computers can be utilized by quantum deep learning algorithms, which could open up new avenues for medication development, therapy optimization, and medical research. The chapter imagines a time when healing intelligence strengthened by quantum mechanics will happen more quickly in the future.

Blockchain technology appears to be a game-changer for handling and protecting health data. Blockchain's decentralized and impenetrable structure guarantees patient data integrity and privacy. This chapter examines how blockchain enables safe data exchange between healthcare practitioners, promoting more data-driven and cooperative methods of research, treatment planning, and diagnosis.

Data privacy issues are addressed via federated learning, a decentralized method of training models. Federate learning improves the creation of reliable and broadly applicable AI models by enabling machine learning models to be trained across numerous local datasets without centralizing sensitive data. In the future, this chapter sees federated learning helping to securely and morally deploy healing intelligence in various healthcare contexts.

8.10 CONCLUSION

The investigation into healing intelligence's principles, practices, and uses demonstrated how complex medical imaging insights, individualized treatment plans based on genetic and molecular profiling, and the use of virtual health assistants to redefine patient involvement could transform diagnostics. This chapter also covered the ethical issues of algorithmic bias, privacy, security, and predictive analytics in the proactive sphere of remote surveillance. The future confluence of developing technologies and the incorporation of healing intelligence into standard clinical operations presents a vision of intelligent, networked healthcare systems. To advance healing intelligence into a future where accuracy, safety, and patient-centeredness come together, quantum computing, blockchain, and federated learning emerge as friends. The conclusion challenges researchers, policymakers, and healthcare professionals to forge ahead with a resolute dedication to innovation, accountability, and a common goal of a thoughtful, adaptable, and caring future for health care as we stand on the brink of this cognitive revolution.

REFERENCES

1. M. H. Abidi, U. Umer, S. H. Mian, and A. Al-Ahmari, "Big data-based smart health monitoring system: Using deep ensemble learning," *IEEE Access*, vol. 11, pp. 114880–114903, 2023, doi: 10.1109/ACCESS.2023.3325323
2. K. Muhammad, S. Khan, J. D. Ser, and V. H. C. d. Albuquerque, "Deep learning for multigrade brain tumor classification in smart healthcare systems: A prospective survey," *IEEE Transactions on Neural Networks and Learning Systems*, vol. 32, no. 2, pp. 507–522, Feb. 2021, doi: 10.1109/TNNLS.2020.2995800
3. K. Mehta, Aayushi, C. Singh, H. Chugh and M. Kumar, "Revolutionizing healthcare by accessing the opportunities for virtual and augmented reality," *2023 7th International Conference on Intelligent Computing and Control Systems (ICICCS)*, Madurai, India, 2023, pp. 836–841, doi: 10.1109/ICICCS56967.2023.10142447
4. H. Elayan, M. Aloqaily, and M. Guizani, "Sustainability of healthcare data analysis IoT-based systems using deep federated learning," *IEEE Internet of Things Journal*, vol. 9, no. 10, pp. 7338–7346, 2021, doi: 10.1109/JIOT.2021.3103635
5. Á. Garai, A. Adamkó, and I. Péntek, "Reflective bio-sensory signal-processing: implementing personal assisted e-Health," *2018 9th IEEE International Conference on Cognitive Infocommunications (CogInfoCom)*, Budapest, Hungary, 2018, pp. 000185–000190, doi: 10.1109/CogInfoCom.2018.8639701
6. M. Saleemi, M. Anjum and M. Rehman, "The ubiquitous healthcare facility framework: A proposed system for managing rural antenatal care," *IEEE Access*, vol. 7, pp. 161264–161282, 2019, doi: 10.1109/ACCESS.2019.2951739
7. A. Kapoor and R. Mishra, "Genetic algorithm optimized gain augmented dual band printed antenna for cognitive eHealth Care (IoMT) applications," *2022 IEEE 11th International Conference on Communication Systems and Network Technologies (CSNT)*, Indore, India, 2022, pp. 6–11, doi: 10.1109/CSNT54456.2022.9787572
8. A. Buzachis, G. M. Bernava, M. Busa, G. Pioggia, and M. Villari, "Towards the basic principles of osmotic computing: A closed-loop gamified cognitive rehabilitation flow model," *2018 IEEE 4th International Conference on Collaboration and Internet Computing (CIC)*, Philadelphia, PA, USA, 2018, pp. 446–452, doi: 10.1109/CIC.2018.00067
9. M. Chen, J. Yang, Y. Hao, S. Mao, and K. Hwang, "A 5G cognitive system for healthcare," *Big Data and Cognitive Computing*, vol. 1, no. 1, pp. 2, 2017.

10. M. N. Ahmed, A. S. Toor, K. O'Neil, and D. Friedland, "Cognitive computing and the future of health care cognitive computing and the future of healthcare: The cognitive power of IBM Watson has the potential to transform global personalized medicine," *IEEE Pulse*, vol. 8, no. 3, pp. 4–9, 2017.
11. M. Simsek, A. Aijaz, M. Dohler, J. Sachs and G. Fettweis, "5G-enabled tactile internet," *IEEE Journal on Selected Areas in Communications*, vol. 34, no. 3, pp. 460–473, 2016.
12. Y. Siriwardhana, G. Gur, M. Ylianttila and M. Liyanage, "The role of 5G for digital healthcare against COVID-19 pandemic: Opportunities and challenges," *ICT Express*, vol. 7, no. 2, pp. 244–252, 2021.
13. L. Mishra, Vikash, and S. Varma, "Seamless health monitoring using 5G NR for the internet of medical things," *Wireless Personal Communications*, vol. 120, pp. 2259–2289, 2021.
14. S. Manna, T. Bose, and R. Bera, "Wearable antennas for medical application: A review," In: Kalam, A., Das, S., Sharma, K. (eds) *Advances in Electronics, Communication and Computing. Lecture Notes in Electrical Engineering*, vol 443, 115–130, Springer, Singapore, 2018.
15. P. Babbar, S. Mishra, A. Rajawat, and S. Saxena, "Design and analysis of a 5G wide band antenna for future mobile applications," *International Conference on Advances in Electrical Computing Communication and Sustainable Technologies (ICAECT)*, Bhilai. India, pp. 1–4, 2021.
16. R. Mishra, R. Dandotiya, A. Kapoor and P. Kumar, "Compact high gain multiband antenna based on split ring resonator and inverted F slots for 5G industry applications," *ACES Journal*, vol. 36, no. 8, pp. 999–1007, 2021.
17. R. Mishra, "An overview of microstrip antenna," *HCTL Open International Journal of Technology Innovations and Research (IJTIR)*, vol. 21, no. 2, pp. 39–55, 2016.
18. A. Kapoor, R. Mishra and P. Kumar, "Compact wideband-printed antenna for sub-6GHz fifth-generation applications," *International Journal on Smart Sensing and Intelligent Systems*, vol. 13, no. 1, pp. 1–10, 2020.
19. A. Kapoor, R. Mishra, and P. Kumar, "Frequency selective surfaces as spatial filters: Fundamentals analysis and applications," *Alexandria Engineering Journal*, vol. 61, no. 6, pp. 4263–4293, 2022.
20. S. Panda, A. Gupta, and B. Acharya, "Wearable microstrip patch antennas with different flexible substrates for health monitoring system," *Materials Today: Proceedings*, vol. 45, no. 4, pp. 4002–4007, 2021.
21. A. Kapoor, R. Mishra and P. Kumar, "Wideband miniaturized patch radiator for Sub-6GHz 5G devices," *Heliyon*, vol. 7, no. 9, pp. 1–10, 2021.
22. R. S. Uqaili, J. A. Uqaili, S. Zahra, F. B. Soomro, and A. Akbar, "A study on dual-band microstrip rectangular patch antenna for Wi-Fi," *Proceedings of Engineering and Technology Innovation*, vol. 16, pp. 1–12, 2020.
23. M. Salimitorkamani, H. Odabasi, and A. Najafi, "A dual-band microstrip patch antenna for brain machine interface applications," *15th European Conference on Antennas and Propagation (EuCAP)*, Dusseldorf, Germany, pp. 1–5, 2021.

9 Innovating at the Nexus

Unraveling the Impact of Deep Learning on Healthcare and Its Transformative Effect on Patient-Centric Solutions and Clinical Decision Support

Nilesh P. Sable, Vijay U. Rathod, Pramod Dhamdhere, Shinde Babaso, and Vishal Shankarrao Rakh

9.1 INTRODUCTION

New ideas have come from connecting deep learning and healthcare, as in medicine. This brought new ways to help people. Deep learning is a type of artificial intelligence (AI) that learns from lots of data [1]. It has become beneficial for healthcare. It can look at large, complex medical facts better than anyone. Using this technology focuses on each patient. It makes their unique traits the primary focus for diagnoses and treatment. Cutting-edge computer programs look beyond normal ways to see patterns in genes, medical histories, and what the body is doing now. As a result, patients can get care that meets their needs and gives them confidence in their health. Deep learning also changes systems that help doctors. Strengthened by advanced programs, these systems aid medical workers through complex patient information. They provide insights that improve the chosen treatment and the accuracy of the diagnosis [2].

Deep learning programs are great at finding patterns and giving helpful information. This makes clinical decision-making work better. This is clear in their ability to handle large amounts of electronic medical records and examine medical scans for minor problems. There are obstacles like needing good rules, privacy concerns, and ethical issues. This highlights how important it is to use this technology carefully. Deep learning can change clinical decision support and patient-focused care as we learn more. This will help make healthcare not just reactionary but also predictive and customized [3]. That will improve outcomes and create a more caring and effective healthcare system.

DOI: 10.1201/9781003479185-9

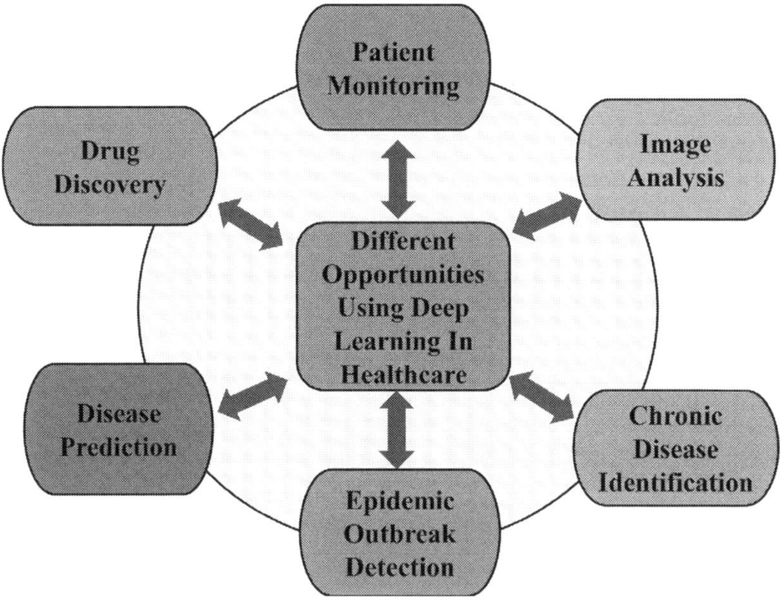

FIGURE 9.1 Deep learning for healthcare.

As our exploration advances, it becomes clear that a universal solution for integrating deep learning into healthcare does not exist. Instead, the synergy of advanced technology and empathetic patient care creates a dynamic and evolving environment, promising a more efficient, accurate, and personalized healthcare ecosystem. The foundation has been established for unraveling the intricate network of innovation where deep learning intersects with healthcare [2], providing a comprehensive understanding of its implications and groundbreaking potentials, as illustrated in Figure 9.1. This underscores the importance of recognizing the nuanced and ever-changing landscape where these two domains intersect, emphasizing the need for adaptable and patient-centric approaches to harness the transformative power of deep learning in healthcare fully [4].

9.1.1 Background

Doctors and scientists are always looking for better ways to help patients. They want treatments to work well and not miss essential details. A big step forward is using deep learning for health care. Much patient information is complex, and there is much of it daily. Traditional ways of understanding this data may not find everything helpful [5]. This challenge led to trying new advanced tools like deep learning. It can help experts navigate the large amounts of complex medical facts. One of the earliest applications of deep learning was in medical imaging analysis. There was a strong desire for quicker and more precise diagnoses, leading deep learning and healthcare to intersect initially. Mode is that automatically identifying patterns in medical images has revolutionized radiology and pathology. These models are built upon early computer-assisted diagnosis attempts. Deep learning algorithms have shown the ability to recognize minute image details that are sometimes invisible to the human eye. This enables earlier and more accurate identification of illnesses such as certain cancers. In addition, collecting patient information electronically through digital health records helped develop learning for healthcare. Models that learn in an advanced way are beneficial for assisting clinicians since they can study large sets of data containing patient backgrounds, exam results, and how the treatment worked out. Studying all this available information with models can provide an understanding of the best ways to treat people, possible dangers, and personalized care plans for each unique person [6].

Foundational research involves worldwide collaboration between scientists, doctors, and engineers. Complex AI has been applied in many medical areas, like predicting disease progression and improving treatment plans. By delving deeper into these problems, the background research acknowledges them as key parts of today's discussion about properly and ethically applying deep learning in healthcare [7]. To summarize, the context and associated research presented here demonstrate the origins of the deep learning-healthcare relationship, which is based on the demand for creative approaches to address the complexity of healthcare data [5]. As the layers of this convergence are unwrapped, we see that in addition to its potential to transform decision support and diagnostics, an ethical landscape must be navigated to ensure that the transformative impact is responsibly harnessed for the benefit of patients and the larger healthcare ecosystem [8].

9.1.2 Objectives

- **Examine the Development of Deep Learning in Healthcare**: This course will help you gain a thorough grasp of technological evolution by examining the historical development and significant turning points in integrating deep learning techniques within the healthcare industry [8].
- Examine how deep learning aids in creating patient-centered medical solutions, emphasizing telehealth, remote monitoring, and personalized medicine. Analyze how these applications affect patients' general experiences and results [9].

9.2 FUNDAMENTALS OF DEEP LEARNING IN HEALTHCARE

9.2.1 Overview of Deep Learning

Deep learning uses layers of linked nodes to examine and comprehend enormous datasets, fundamentally copying how neural systems in the human brain work [10]. This new way of processing and grasping complex data has developed in AI [11]. By analyzing intricate examples within vast amounts of information, deep learning can vary how medical analysis, finding issues, and therapy planning are done in doctor care settings [12].

Deep learning can automatically learn complex data relationships. This allows it to identify essential features from large datasets. In healthcare, deep learning can

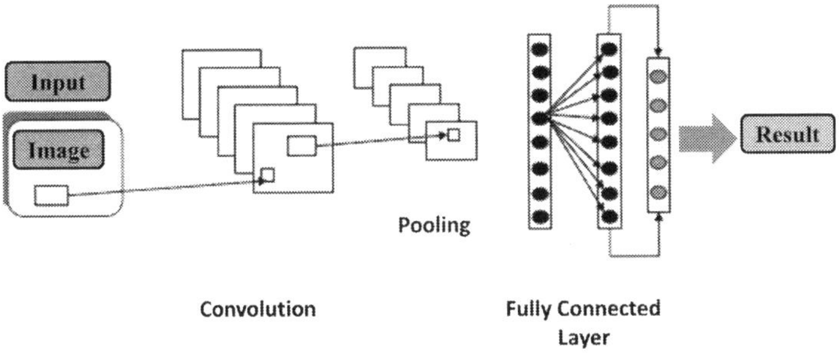

FIGURE 9.2 Overview of CNN architecture.

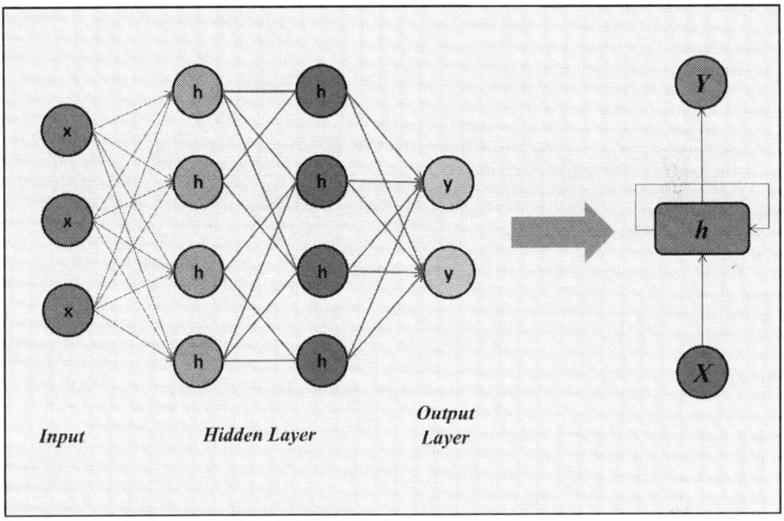

FIGURE 9.3 Overview of RNN architecture.

analyze many types of information such as genes, medical records, and medical images [13]. Convolutional Neural Networks and Recurrent Neural Networks are commonly used in deep learning models. They have proven very effective for tasks like analyzing sequences of data and recognizing images. Deep learning in healthcare includes identifying small patterns in data more accurately than older methods [14].

This permits earlier and more precise disease detection. As shown in Figures 9.2 and 9.3, doctors can better foresee potential health risks and consequences using deep learning models. The SE models enhance predictions by understanding intricate links within data. Researchers continue making deep learning algorithms better medical applications as they push the boundaries of what is possible [15].

9.2.2 Adoption in Healthcare

Deep learning in healthcare signals a significant switch in how medical professionals leverage technology to aid their essential choices. This groundbreaking change can be seen in several areas of healthcare, such as how treatment is planned, finding medical issues, and medical pictures [16]. Deep learning programs have proven extremely good at looking at medical pictures to spot unusual things in lab slides and X-rays. Getting diagnoses faster and more accurately results from these programs' ability to handle massive data sets and teach them to learn. Furthermore, deep learning is used in finding medical issues by reviewing many patient records to find tiny patterns that point to sicknesses. Deep learning programs help healthcare become more active and customized by helping to find illnesses sooner and predict how diseases will progress [17].

While deep learning adoption offers promising opportunities, several complex challenges must first be addressed. Healthcare systems must ensure patient privacy and allow different medical data sources to be shared and used. Deep learning models also need rigorous testing to prove their accuracy in various healthcare scenarios. However, once these complex issues are solved, the broader medical industry will recognize deep learning's ability to completely change how patients receive care by improving accuracy, personalizing treatments, and increasing effectiveness. The foundation of deep learning in healthcare combines cutting-edge computation with medical expertise. Studies show that deep learning excels at analyzing complicated data structures. Its applications in real-world healthcare are transforming patient outcomes and evolving medical practices. Continued research could lead deep learning and medicine to open new doors for customized care, diagnosis, and treatment centered around each patient [18].

9.2.3 Patients-Centric Solutions and Clinical Decision Support Using Deep Learning

Deep learning can help make healthcare more focused on each person and assist doctors. It is important for tools that customize care for each patient and for systems that give doctors better advice. Patient-centered care aims to treat people as individuals instead of treating everyone the same way. Clinical decision support uses the latest methods to help workers make more right and thoughtful choices. Deep learning can achieve these goals by studying large and different data sets to find patterns [19].

Tools using deep learning and large datasets can help doctors help patients. Learning is part of AI and uses computers to learn from patterns. It can spot diseases sooner and find the best care for each person. This puts patients first. It gives doctors ideas to help patients in new ways. It allows doctors to make choices faster with fewer mistakes. All of this means better help for people. But computers must keep info private and explain why they think what they think. Overall, these tools let doctors focus more on each patient's needs. They help change how healthcare works to make it more for people [20].

9.2.3.1 Recurrent Neural Networks (RNNs) for Clinical Decision Support

Connecting medical records to computer systems is essential for today's healthcare, trying to help people, make work easier, and increase how well things run. Electronic health records are digital paper charts saved on computers containing a person's medical past, diagnoses, medicines, treatment plans, vaccine dates, allergies, X-ray photos, and lab test results. Adding these records to healthcare computer systems provides advantages and difficulties—health info changes over time. Models are used to spot patterns in information from different times. RNNs can do this well since they are made to learn from information that happens at various points. RNNs' ability to remember past states through a hidden part makes them unique. This lets the network hold onto context and memory across the whole information series, an essential skill for dealing with changing medical situations. For example, RNNs can skillfully notice and locate signs of worsening well-being, sending essential warnings in the ongoing tracking of long-term illnesses. This proactive method allows for quick actions, possibly decreasing the need for repetitive trips to the hospital and lessening the load on patients and medical care systems [21].

In addition, RNNs' ability to change is invaluable for healthcare. RNNs can adjust treatments based on how people react and changing health issues. This allows doctors to change plans to make them work better. RNNs let doctors update what they do to help people feel better and avoid problems. Using neural networks repeatedly helps doctors with tools that spot how health details change over time. This allows care for each patient to change based on their needs. It improves healthcare and puts patients in the middle of the system. As repeating neural networks improve at learning, they may change how healthcare and choices are made. They focus on acting quickly, providing treatments for each person, and always making things better to give patients the best results [22].

9.2.3.1.1 Clinical Decision Support Using Recurrent Neural Networks (RNNs)

1. Initialization:

   Set the initial to Zero as given below:

$$h_0 = 0$$

2. Input Processing at Time Step t:

$$h_t = \text{ReLU}\left(W_{\{hx\}} * X_t + W_{\{hh\}} * h_{\{t-1\}} + b_h\right)$$

   where X_t represents the information present at time t, W represents how much that information influences late r calculations, H represents the current understanding, and b_h adds flexibility. The hidden state H from the previous time step is combined with the new input and weights, and the rectified linear unit activation function ReLU ensures only positive values progress to the next step, step-by-step building understanding over time.

3. Output Prediction at Time Step t:

$$Y_t = \text{softmax}\left(W_{\{yh\}} * h_t + b_y\right)$$

   where

   $W_{\{yh\}}$ is the weight matrix connecting the hidden state to the output, b_y is the bias term, and softmax is the softmax activation function.

4. Loss Calculation:

$$\text{Loss}_t = -\sum_{N=t-i}^{n} N * \log\left(\breve{I}_{\{t,i\}}\right)$$

The loss at time step t is computed using the predicted probabilities ($\breve{I}_{\{t,\, i\}}$) and the true labels ($y_{\{t,\, i\}}$).

5. Backpropagation Through Time (BPTT):

$$\frac{\partial \text{Loss}_t}{\partial W_{\{hx\}}}, \frac{\partial \text{Loss}_t}{\partial W_{\{hh\}}}, \frac{\partial \text{Loss}_t}{\partial W_{\{yh\}}}, \frac{\partial \text{Loss}_t}{\partial b_h}, \frac{\partial \text{Loss}_t}{\partial b_y}$$

Compute the gradients of the loss concerning the model parameters using backpropagation through time.

6. Parameter Update (Gradient Descent):

$$\theta_{\{\text{new}\}} = \theta_{\{\text{old}\}} - \alpha * \nabla_\theta \text{Loss}_t$$

Update the parameters (θ) of the model using gradient descent, where α is the learning rate.

7. Repeat Steps 2–6 for Each Time Step:
   - Repeat for $t = 1, 2, \ldots, T$
   - Iterate through the time steps, processing inputs, making predictions, calculating loss, and updating parameters.

9.2.3.2 ResNet50 for Clinical Decision Support

In clinical decision support (CDS), ResNet50, a deep learning model using a multilayered design with over 50 layers, has proven to successfully assist doctors by analyzing medical scan results. This neural network architecture addresses training difficulties by connecting layers so information can readily move between them. Clinicians can apply what ResNet50 learns from numerous photos to assist with complicated cases [23].

ResNet50 can spot minimal differences and problems in medical pictures because it is very good at using the number layers it has to look closely. The early parts find features, but the later parts help it understand important things for doctors even better. A path-driven method enhances the model's capacity to spot tumors, section organs, and recognize anomalies by boosting its awareness of minor visual clues that may point to many health issues. ResNet50's employment of residual blocks is fundamental for maintaining and using past knowledge, allowing the model to grasp complicated connections in the clinical material [19,21].

9.3.2.2 ResNet50 for Clinical Decision Support Algorithm

1. Input Image and Preprocessing:

   The input image is (X, O) for reprocessing and resizing it

2. Convolutional Block 1:

   The input used for convolution is represented as:

$$X_1 = \text{Conv}(X_0, W_1) + b_1$$

$$X_2 = \text{ReLU}(X_1)$$

3. Residual Blocks 2–5:

$$X_i = \text{ResidualBlock}\left(X_{\{i-1\}}, W_i\right)$$

where $i=2, 3, 4, 5$

Residual blocks repeat, introducing skip connections and additional convolutions, enhancing the network's representational capacity.

4. Global Average Pooling:

$$X_{\text{pool}} = \text{GlobalAveragePooling}(X_5)$$

Global Average Pooling reduces the spatial dimensions of the feature maps to a fixed size.

5. Fully Connected Layer and Softmax Activation:

$$Y = \text{Softmax}\left(\text{FC}\left(X_{\text{pool}}, W_{\text{fc}}, b_{\text{fc}}\right)\right)$$

The global features are connected to a fully connected layer (FC), and the softmax activation produces class probabilities.

6. Loss Calculation:

$$\text{Loss}_t = -\sum_{N=t-i}^{n} N \,\text{Loss}\, n * \log\left(\breve{I}_{\{t,i\}}\right)$$

Compute the categorical cross-entropy loss using predicted probabilities ($\breve{I}_i$) and accurate labels (y_i).

7. Backpropagation and Gradient Descent:

$$\frac{\partial \text{Loss}}{\partial W_i}, \frac{\partial \text{Loss}}{\partial b_i}$$

Calculate gradients of the loss concerning the model parameters for backpropagation and update using gradient descent.

8. Repeat Training Iterations:
   - Mathematical Equation:

     Repeat for multiple training iterations

   Iterate through the training dataset, adjusting weights to minimize the loss and enhance the model's ability to make clinical predictions.

9. Model Deployment:
   - Mathematical Equation:

     Deploy trained ResNet50 model for CDS

   The trained ResNet50 model can be deployed to predict clinical outcomes based on new data.

9.3 PATIENT-CENTRIC SOLUTIONS

9.3.1 Personalized Medicine

Deep learning's introduction into the medical field has accelerated the development of personalized medicine, which is a radical departure from conventional one-size-fits-all methods. Personalized medicine aims to customize care for each person using deep learning models that analyze genetics, genomics, and clinical records. These complex algorithms find patterns across massive datasets that were once impossible to see. They have given doctors new insights into how genes, biomarkers, and treatments affect people. Healthcare providers can now create exact plans for each patient using this focused approach. This minimizes unwanted reactions and maximizes healing results. Deep learning is key for studying personalized medicine through genetics because it spots gene variants and mutations linked to certain diseases. The data helps find diseases early and determines which drugs are most likely to work. Combining medical and "omics" information gives a complete picture of health. It also makes it easier to see individual risks and ways to prevent illness. Personalized care leads the changing of healthcare. In the future, treatments may be tailored precisely to each person's unique biology as learning technology improves [24].

9.3.2 Remote Patient Monitoring

New learning methods have made it possible for watching sick people from far away (RPM) to become a brand new way to help patients. RPM gets health facts from patients as things happen while they do what they do each day by using things worn, tools that sense, and other linked stuff. For dealing with long-term sicknesses, especially, smoothly adding deep learning rules to watching sick people from far away (RPM) is a significant change in healthcare. Deep learning adds a fluid and ready-to-act part of caring for patients by dealing with and knowing the meaning of steady flows of body function facts. More than usual health checks now and then; this changing ability lets you watch vital signs, follow the medical schedule, and make life choices.

AI and algorithms are crucial for managing long-term sickness, where monitoring is necessary. Through cautiously examining ongoing statistics streams, these algorithms are extremely good at spotting minute variations in health measures. Spotting alterations early is critical because it allows speedy movements that prevent problems and worsening signs and symptoms. Deep gaining knowledge of faraway affected person tracking is proactive in a way that goes beyond basic monitoring; it offers a scientific body of workers the potential to look at health developments in advance and increase tailored, preventive movements that can enhance affected person outcomes, additionally, including deep gaining knowledge of faraway affected person tracking facilitates an ongoing comments loop between scientific pros and sufferers. This offers sufferers a feeling of manipulation and involvement at the same time, additionally improving the effectiveness of the healthcare supply. The non-stop verbal exchange that was far away affected the person's tracking, and deep knowledge

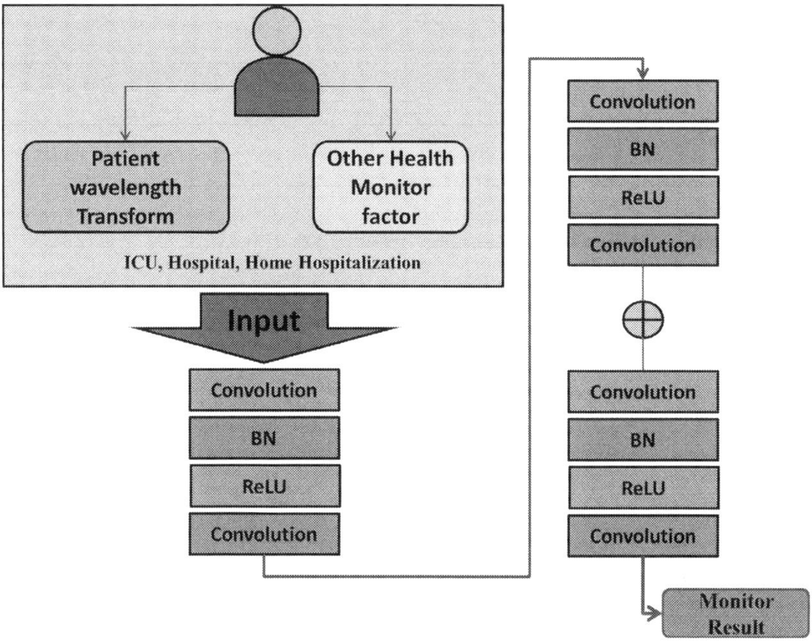

FIGURE 9.4 Systematic overview of the remote patient monitoring system.

of insights permitted the affected person's care to turn into a creative endeavor. With admission to real-time records, sufferers take an active role in their health and are empowered to make informed decisions about their care. The decrease in health facility admission prices is among the notable effects of this integration. Healthcare executives can lessen the desire for emergency interventions by addressing emerging issues before they worsen by acting early in response to insights gained through steady tracking (Figure 9.4).

9.3.3 Patient Engagement and Empowerment

Computer programs that learn from large amounts of data can help people better care for their health. These "deep learning" programs can suggest when to take medicine and give advice on healthy living. They adjust the information based on what interests each person and how well they understand medical topics. Deep learning makes complete medical info easier to grasp. This empowers patients to make health choices, work with doctors as equal partners, and follow treatment plans. Doctors now know that involving patients fully in their care leads to better results. Deep learning ensures solutions spot problems, check them, and let people actively look after themselves. Programs that learn from data are changing healthcare. Patients will play a bigger role in decisions about their care, get treatments tailored to them, and have their health monitored closely. Closely following each person's unique needs and giving more control and customized care make healthcare work better for each individual.

9.4 CLINICAL DECISION SUPPORT SYSTEMS

9.4.1 Enhancing Diagnostic Accuracy

Deep learning technologies have helped CDS systems become essential tools for making diagnoses more accurate in healthcare. CDSS can improve how health workers make choices by using advanced formulas to assist them in examining clinical information, medical images, and patient backgrounds. When checking for intricate patterns and unusual things in medical photos, deep learning does very well and helps find illnesses earlier. Deep learning algorithms excel at tasks involving feature extraction, segmentation, and picture identification for diagnostics. In radiology, for example, deep learning CDS systems may spot tiny anomalies in MRIs, CT scans, and X-rays that human eyes could miss. Seeking similarities between different medical records helps lead to more precise diagnoses and earlier care, which could help patients. Using deep learning in programs that assist doctors makes diagnoses more correct while allowing flexibility in choices. With time, how well these programs work gets better because they keep learning, learning, and changing to new facts. Repeated learning helps make better diagnostic rules and grows knowledge of many health issues. Clinical decision programs play a larger part in the proper diagnosis as learning technology improves and is used more in current medicine.

9.4.2 Treatment Optimization

Treatment optimization is one area where deep learning can influence clinical decision-making beyond diagnosis. This [24] ensures therapies are effective while tailored to limit unwanted effects. Including deep learning in therapy selections also addresses issues of unpredictability in clinical settings.

9.4.3 Integration with Electronic Health Records

The connection between clinical decision-making support systems and electronic health records significantly improves the management of healthcare information. Some records are easier to use and connect, providing thoughtful analysis within clinical workflows, while others require deep analysis. This link simplifies accessing essential data, assisting in diagnosis and treatment planning, and promoting more effective and knowledgeable care and delivery.

Bringing together medical records and healthcare systems is essential, with goals to better help people, make work easier, and improve how things run. Electronic health records are digital patient files containing a person's health history, diagnoses, medicines, treatment plans, immunization dates, allergies, X-ray photos, and lab test results. Merging these records into medical systems provides advantages and difficulties.

9.4.3.1 Benefits of EHR Integration

- **Efficient Information Access**:
  - Patient data is digitally stored, allowing doctors fast and protected access to essential health details. This electronic system saves time otherwise used for finding and handling physical documents.

- **Interoperability**:
  - Healthcare integration enables different medical systems and doctors to work together, allowing easy sharing of patient information between various programs.
- **Support**:
  - Electronic health records have the potential to include helpful clinical programs. These systems can offer doctors and nurses evidence-based recommendations, important notices, and reminder messages. The goal is to help providers make smart choices and avoid patient treatment mistakes.
- **Data Accuracy and Legibility**:
  - Electronic records eliminate issues associated with handwriting legibility and reduce the risk of errors due to misinterpretation, enhancing the accuracy and reliability of patient data.

9.5 ETHICAL CONSIDERATIONS AND CHALLENGES

9.5.1 Privacy and Security

Keeping patient data safe is key when using deep learning in healthcare. Looking at complex health info needs strong, easy-to-use systems focusing on privacy. It's vital to follow encryption rules and handle data well. We must know privacy issues, discuss patient fears, and show how to protect data to build trust. Putting patient privacy first makes the use of deep learning in healthcare better. It helps doctors, patients, and stakeholders work well together. Keeping things private is essential for the ethical and practical use of learning in healthcare.

9.5.2 Bias and Fairness

AI can greatly help doctors, but some parts of school information may cause problems. The numbers could treat some people unfairly without meaning to. This is a big problem that needs fast, complete answers. We must ensure that all sick people get the same quality of care when using computer programs for medicine. That way, nobody gets hurt by mistakes in the math. Creating fair machine learning requires constant examination and fixing of algorithms to remove unfair judgments. We must always look again at and improve these models so everyone has the same chance to succeed, no matter who they are or where they come from. To deal with this problem will require work from many sides.

It's essential to first find and fix biases in the information used to teach. Since past wrongs may have slipped into what the systems learned from, people must look closely for and eliminate them. Also, using different kinds of information during training can lead to more wide-ranging patterns and show more people. Including details from many sources and types of people ensures the systems can understand how patients can be different, helping treat everyone fairly and correctly.

Understanding how algorithms arrive at conclusions and being open about the process are essential for creating reliability and enabling further examination.

People should comprehend how the math works out choices, encouraging visibility that helps medical professionals and their clients grasp what's evaluated in their treatment blueprints. This visibility not only sets responsibility for utilizing these algorithms but also advances faith in how choices are made. Always pay close attention, be willing to change, and accept different ideas to reduce unfair treatment. Using computers to help with health care means checking on how things are going often. Doctors must be ready to fix problems when they come up and make sure machine learning fairly helps all types of patients. By watching algorithms and changing them when needed, healthcare providers can lower bias and make sure everyone gets help. The blending of machine learning in healing is a thoughtful tactic to handle likely unfairness and biases. By taking complete tactics, like improving coaching information, diversifying information categories, guaranteeing openness, and promoting watchfulness, the healthcare field can use the power of machine learning while keeping the rules of equal treatment and fairness for every patient.

9.5.3 Regulatory Environment

To keep morals strong and patients safe, we need smart rules. Setting standards for checking algorithms is a big challenge. So, it talks about how a computer makes decisions and works according to different laws worldwide. To use learning in healthcare well, we need to work. Regulators, tech people, and healthcare workers have to work together. They must apply rules based on good values and the patient's well-being. The only way to safely and responsibly use deep learning in healthcare is to work together. This will help create a good balance and connection between rule makers, tech creators, and healthcare workers. The goal is to get the most out of this progress.

9.6 CASE STUDIES

9.6.1 Effective Applications

Deep learning shows real effectiveness in health care by helping analyze X-rays. For example, a medical imaging center used deep learning to examine chest X-rays. This system was able to spot early signs of lung cancer with amazing accuracy. This means doctors could find cancer quickly and give more exact diagnoses. Deep learning is changing how doctors can see and treat illness. It makes diagnostic tests more accurate. These changes also improve the way care is given and boost patient outcomes. Thanks to deep learning, treatment can start earlier, patients have a better chance of getting better, and it shows a new way of standard diagnostic procedures. Science is helping to make health care more personalized. A respected correctional hospital used advanced computer software to examine patients' genes. This data lets them create unique treatment plans for each patient based on their cellular responses and DNA differences. This shows how computers can adjust treatment to fit a person's characteristics. This improvement in precise medicine also changes how therapies specifically target cancer. Deep learning is also helpful for watching patients remotely and managing long-term sicknesses. The healthcare system uses arable technology with learning to monitor patients with chronic illnesses like heart failure.

The system can always analyze the patients' physical data to spot warning signs early. The doctors can step in and help at the right time. This technology lets patients be active in their care, reduces the number of hospital readmissions, and highlights a care-driven and patient-focused way of health care.

9.6.2 Failure-Related Lessons

Deep learning in healthcare has faced challenges; though some results were promising, case studies give helpful lessons from errors. Doctors at hospitals have tried using computer programs to help diagnose serious illnesses in patients. The program was supposed to learn from examples to spot patterns. It worked well at first. However, doctors soon found problems when using the program on different kinds of sick people in the real world. It didn't help as much with some groups. This shows that testing computer programs on many patients is very important before using them for genuine medical care. Programs also need careful thought about how well the therapy might work for all patients.

In one example, a hospital started a small test using a computer program that understands language through learning from large amounts of data within their electronic patient records system. The goal was to find practical details from doctors' notes, but significant problems came up as the program had trouble changing to different ways doctors share information. The language program made wrong ideas because it struggled to understand and pull out information from text without a clear form. This shows it is essential to know the small details of medical writing and continually improve the learning models to get the best results. Doctors must carefully check computer programs used for healthcare. Tests can find problems, so the programs help all types of patients. The programs must learn the words doctors use every day. Healthcare information has changed a lot. The computer models need to change, too. This ensures that the programs work well and that people get better medical care.

Another case study on treatment optimization illustrated the downside of relying heavily on past information. A provider extensively utilized retrospective data, hoping to personalize the recommendations using deep learning. However, some historical data became outdated due to rapid medical knowledge and treatment advances, resulting in less helpful suggestions. The scenario highlights the need for regularly updating training datasets and dynamic models that can adjust to changing medical practices.

9.7 FUTURE DIRECTIONS AND RECOMMENDATIONS

9.7.1 Advancements in Deep Learning

Deep learning in healthcare is expected to bring many new ways to help people that will significantly change how doctors research sickness, find what's wrong with people, and treat them. The best way healthcare helps people and how it could be improved is by continuing to enhance deep learning programs, especially those that teach themselves and those that learn as they go. To be sure, deep learning models are easy for doctors to understand, gain trust in, and use widely, work making AI more straightforward to understand will also be the key. Also, new ideas for understanding hard-to-figure-out sicknesses will come from combining different data types, like test pictures, gene facts, and personal medical records. Pushing to do as much as possible where deep learning and healthcare meet will need people from different groups working together, like engineers, doctors, and researchers.

9.7.2 Overarching Guidelines for Ethical Application

It is necessary to be transparent about how algorithms make decisions so patients and healthcare providers understand why specific suggestions are made. To keep things fair and equal requires following standard testing steps, upgrading information, and always watching for bias. It is also essential to work together across countries to build excellent ethical rules. These rules should deal with private information, ensure patient information is used correctly, and skillfully handle the challenges of different rules in different places. Involving many affected people, like patients, in talks about using deep learning for health would help develop moral guidelines that prioritize people's well-being and trust in the healthcare system.

9.8 CONCLUSION

Dee's learning and healthcare coming together is a game-changer. This union opens new doors for better patient care and decisions in the clinic. Thanks to advancements in deep learning tech, we're seeing exciting changes. These changes can lead to better results for patients. Cutting-edge algorithms and neural networks have the power to change the way we diagnose and treat patients. Advanced machine learning strengthens personalized healthcare. It offers customized solutions tailored to each patient's unique needs. Deep learning models can analyze large amounts of data like medical records, scans, and genetic information. Understanding conditions allows them to detect illnesses early and pinpoint exact treatments.

REFERENCES

1. J. N. Odhiambo and N. Muganda Ochara, "Precision Health Care for Sustainable Patient Centric Solutions," *2018 Open Innovations Conference (OI)*, Johannesburg, South Africa, 2018, pp. 194–197, doi: 10.1109/OI.2018.8535905
2. D. Saraswat, P. Bhattacharya, A. Verma, V. K. Prasad, S. Tanwar, G. Sharma, P. N. Bokoro and R. Sharma, "Explainable AI for Healthcare 5.0: Opportunities and Challenges," *IEEE Access*, vol. 10, pp. 84486–84517, 2022.
3. R. Gupta, A. Shukla, and S. Tanwar, "AaYusH: A Smart Contract-Based Telesurgery System for Healthcare 4.0," *Proceedings of IEEE International Conference on Communications Workshops (ICC Workshops)*, pp. 1–6, Dublin, Ireland, 2020.
4. E. Mbunge, B. Muchemwa, S. Jiyane, and J. Batani, "Sensors and Healthcare 5.0: Transformative Shift in Virtual Care through Emerging Digital Health Technologies," *Global Health Journal*, vol. 5, no. 4, pp. 169–177, 2021.
5. C. F. Pasluosta, H. Gassner, J. Winkler, J. Klucken and B. M. Eskofier, "An Emerging Era in the Management of Parkinson's Disease: Wearable Technologies and the Internet of Things," *IEEE Journal of Biomedical and Health Informatics*, vol. 19, no. 6, pp. 1873–1881, 2015.

6. P. A. Laplante and N. Laplante, "The Internet of Things in Healthcare: Potential Applications and Challenges," *IT Professional*, vol. 18, no. 3, pp. 2–4, 2016.
7. B. Mohanta, P. Das and S. Patnaik, "Healthcare 5.0: A Paradigm Shift in Digital Healthcare System Using Artificial Intelligence IoT and 5G Communication," *Proceedings of International Conference on Applied Machine Learning*. (ICAML), pp. 191–196, Dalian, China, 2019.
8. U. Pawar, D. O'Shea, S. Rea and R. O'Reilly, "Incorporating Explainable Artificial Intelligence (XAI) to Aid the Understanding of Machine Learning in the Healthcare Domain," *Proceedings of Irish Conference on Artificial Intelligence and Cognitive Science*, pp. 1–12, Dublin, Ireland, 2020.
9. A. Verma, P. Bhattacharya, M. Zuhair, S. Tanwar and N. Kumar, "VaCoChain: Blockchain-Based 5G-Assisted UAV Vaccine Distribution Scheme for Future Pandemics," *IEEE Journal of Biomedical and Health Informatics*, vol. 26, no. 5, pp. 1997–2007, 2022.
10. A. N. Navaz, M. A. Serhani, H. T. El Kassabi, N. Al-Qirim and H. Ismail, "Trends, Technologies, and Key Challenges in Smart and Connected Healthcare," *IEEE Access*, vol. 9, pp. 74044–74067, 2021, doi: 10.1109/ACCESS.2021.3079217
11. J. Amann, A. Blasimme, E. Vayena, D. Frey and V. I. Madai, "Explainability for Artificial Intelligence in Healthcare: A Multidisciplinary Perspective," *BMC Medical Informatics and Decision Making*, vol. 20, no. 1, pp. 310, 2020.
12. M. H. Abidi, U. Umer, S. H. Mian and A. Al-Ahmari, "Big Data-Based Smart Health Monitoring System: Using Deep Ensemble Learning," *IEEE Access*, vol. 11, pp. 114880–114903, 2023, doi: 10.1109/ACCESS.2023.3325323
13. M. Kumar, W. Zhang, M. Weippert and B. Freudenthaler, "An Explainable Fuzzy Theoretic Nonparametric Deep Model for Stress Assessment Using Heartbeat Intervals Analysis," *IEEE Transactions on Fuzzy Systems*, vol. 29, no. 12, pp. 3873–3886, 2021, doi: 10.1109/TFUZZ.2020.3029284
14. K. Muhammad, S. Khan, J. D. Ser and V. H. C. d. Albuquerque, "Deep Learning for Multigrade Brain Tumor Classification in Smart Healthcare Systems: A Prospective Survey," *IEEE Transactions on Neural Networks and Learning Systems*, vol. 32, no. 2, pp. 507–522, 2021, doi: 10.1109/TNNLS.2020.2995800
15. H. Elayan, M. Aloqaily and M. Guizani, "Sustainability of Healthcare Data Analysis IoT-Based Systems Using Deep Federated Learning," *IEEE Internet of Things Journal*, vol. 9, no. 10, pp. 7338–7346, 2022, doi: 10.1109/JIOT.2021.3103635
16. A. A. Abdullah, M. M. Hassan and Y. T. Mustafa, "A Review on Bayesian Deep Learning in Healthcare: Applications and Challenges," *IEEE Access*, vol. 10, pp. 36538–36562, 2022, doi: 10.1109/ACCESS.2022.3163384
17. T. Mahara, V. L. H. Josephine, R. Srinivasan, P. Prakash, A. D. Algarni and O. P. Verma, "Deep vs. Shallow: A Comparative Study of Machine Learning and Deep Learning Approaches for Fake Health News Detection," *IEEE Access*, vol. 11, pp. 79330–79340, 2023, doi: 10.1109/ACCESS.2023.3298441
18. S. Chi, Y. Tian, F. Wang, Y. Wang, M. Chen and J. Li, "Deep Semisupervised Multitask Learning Model and Its Interpretability for Survival Analysis," *IEEE Journal of Biomedical and Health Informatics*, vol. 25, no. 8, pp. 3185–3196, 2021, doi: 10.1109/JBHI.2021.3064696
19. X. Chen, X. Lin, Q. Shen and X. Qian, "Combined Spiral Transformation and Model-Driven Multi-Modal Deep Learning Scheme for Automatic Prediction of TP53 Mutation in Pancreatic Cancer," *IEEE Transactions on Medical Imaging*, vol. 40, no. 2, pp. 735–747, 2021, doi: 10.1109/TMI.2020.3035789
20. X. Zeng, S. Lin and C. Liu, "Multi-View Deep Learning Framework for Predicting Patient Expenditure in Healthcare," *IEEE Open Journal of the Computer Society*, vol. 2, pp. 62–71, 2021, doi: 10.1109/OJCS.2021.3052518

21. F. C. Ghesu, E. Krubasik, B. Georgescu, V. Singh, Y. Zheng, J. Hornegger and Comaniciu, D, "Marginal Space Deep Learning: Efficient Architecture for Volumetric Image Parsing," *IEEE Transactions on Medical Imaging*, vol. 35, no. 5, pp. 1217–1228, 2016, doi: 10.1109/TMI.2016.2538802
22. B. Wu, Z. Cai, W. Wu, and X. Yin, "AoI-Aware Resource Management for Smart Health Via Deep Reinforcement Learning," *IEEE Access*, vol. 11, pp. 81180–81195, 2023, doi: 10.1109/ACCESS.2023.3299340
23. X. Zhou, W. Liang, K. I. -K. Wang, H. Wang, L. T. Yang and Q. Jin, "Deep-Learning-Enhanced Human Activity Recognition for Internet of Healthcare Things," *IEEE Internet of Things Journal*, vol. 7, no. 7, pp. 6429–6438, 2020, doi: 10.1109/JIOT.2020.2985082
24. F. Hajjej, M. Javeed, A. Ksibi, M. Alarfaj, K. Alnowaiser, A. Jalal, N. Alsufyani, M. Shorfuzzaman and J. Park, "Deep Human Motion Detection and Multi-Features Analysis for Smart Healthcare Learning Tools," *IEEE Access*, vol. 10, pp. 116527–116539, 2022, doi: 10.1109/ACCESS.2022.3214986

10 Enhancing Healthcare Data Governance and Security

The Role of Adaptive Data Management Middleware in Federated Cloud Environments

Vikas K. Kolekar and Sachin R. Sakhare

10.1 INTRODUCTION

10.1.1 Background and Context

Integrating security protocols, interconnected cloud systems, and flexible Middleware can revolutionize the dynamic domain of healthcare data management. Imagine a healthcare system with interconnected federated clouds, enabling the smooth and dynamic flow of patient data. Imagine a future where patient-centric care is not just a concept but a data-based reality. The rapid and exponential increase of healthcare data, along with the complex network of interconnected cloud systems, necessitates the implementation of an advanced adaptive Middleware layer. It will be interesting to learn about various difficulties and opportunities related to the interdependent relationship between adaptive Middleware and the governance and security of healthcare data in a federated cloud environment. Adaptive Middleware will be crucial in seamlessly integrating technological expertise and responsible data management.

10.1.1.1 Objectives of This Chapter

This chapter explores the complex domain of healthcare data governance and security in a federated cloud environment, with the aim of achieving many objectives. The main objectives are to analyze and understand how adaptive data management Middleware and federated cloud infrastructures interact and affect the healthcare sector.

- **Illuminate the Domain**: The aim is to clarify the complex structure of federated cloud architecture and its essential components, providing a clear understanding of the multifaceted terrain that serves as the foundation for

DOI: 10.1201/9781003479185-10

the exploration. This exposure acts as the initial stroke, establishing the context for a thorough comprehension of the difficulties and possibilities present in the federated cloud environment.

- **Extract the Essence of Adaptive Middleware**: This chapter explores the core of adaptive data management Middleware, uncovering its complicated functioning and crucial role in improving data governance. The goal is to find the fundamental nature of adaptive Middleware, highlighting its ability to bring about significant changes in healthcare systems and its smooth integration with federated cloud infrastructure.
- **Navigate the Regulatory Horizon**: To navigate the intricate regulatory domain that governs healthcare data, the objective is to create a thorough map of the regulatory frameworks and requirements for compliance. This purpose entails deciphering the current rules and predicting the future development of the regulatory domain, ensuring a proactive viewpoint.
- **Showcase Security as an Adaptive Art**: Within federated cloud environments, security is not a fixed condition but a flexible skill. Exploring the specific security issues that arise in federated cloud systems, emphasizing the role of adaptive Middleware in strengthening the security measures. Encryption, access control, and authentication are key components of this security masterpiece.
- **Illuminate Practical Insights with Case Studies**: In addition to theoretical exploration, the objectives encompass practical insights from real-world case studies. The aim is to highlight instances where adaptive Middleware has been efficiently implemented in the healthcare sector and present examples of federated cloud environments that have successfully overcome hurdles. These case studies function as dynamic narratives, connecting theoretical concepts with practical applications.
- **Peer into the Future**: Concluding the chapter by examining the future of adaptive Middleware, federated cloud environments, and their impact on healthcare data governance and security. Expecting the advancement of technologies and the emergence of new trends and how they may affect the healthcare sector. This will provide a forward-thinking viewpoint for scholars, practitioners, and stakeholders.

10.1.1.2 Significance of Healthcare Data Governance and Security in Federated Cloud Environments

In the complex domain of contemporary healthcare, where patient data is transmitted effortlessly across interconnected networks, maintenance and security are crucial priorities. In navigating the domain of federated cloud environments, the management and protection of healthcare data are usable to an intermediary, leading an orchestra toward seamless collaboration.

- **Harbinger of Precision Medicine**: In the current age of personalized healthcare, when treatment approaches are customized to individual characteristics, the importance of healthcare data governance becomes a guiding principle that leads to precision medicine. Federated cloud environments are utilized as the platform where various medical datasets are integrated. Efficient administration guarantees this combination's honesty, availability, and ethical utilization, promoting advancements in diagnostics, therapies, and preventive care.

- **Guardians of Patient Trust**: In the healthcare sector, where trust is of the utmost importance, ensuring strong data security in federated clouds protects patient confidentiality. A breach not only endangers personal privacy but also undermines patients' essential confidence in the healthcare system. With this in mind, the chapter explores the complex interaction between adaptive Middleware, protecting sensitive information, and the extensive scope of the federated cloud.
- **Resilience amid Digital Transformation**: The healthcare industry is experiencing a transformation, shifting toward a digital environment where information surpasses geographical limitations. The orchestration of adaptive Middleware plays a crucial role in federated cloud environments, providing resilience against ever-changing cyber threats. This adaptable architecture protects against criminal attacks and guarantees continuous access to vital healthcare data, even in the presence of technological setbacks.
- **Navigating Regulatory Currents**: Complying with rules in federated cloud settings is challenging within a complex healthcare system. The chapter examines the role of adaptive Middleware as a guiding tool for navigating the intricate realm of healthcare data governance. This sheds light on the mutually beneficial relationship between the ability of Middleware to adapt and the constantly changing landscape of regulatory frameworks.

Examining healthcare data governance and security in federated cloud environments involves more than a technical explanation. It is a process that involves the complex interaction of technological advancement, patient confidence, compliance with regulations, and the unwavering commitment to accuracy in healthcare provision. Beginning this journey, the reader is encouraged to explore the intricate layers of meaning included in the adaptive Middleware that coordinates managing and protecting healthcare data in federated clouds.

10.2 FOUNDATIONS OF FEDERATED CLOUD ENVIRONMENTS

10.2.1 Understanding Federated Cloud Architecture

The federated approach in current cloud computing is a revolutionary paradigm change. Imagine a synchronized ensemble of interconnected clouds, each utilizing its distinct capabilities to form a balanced ecosystem collaboratively [1].

- **Symphony of Clouds**: In the conventional cloud approach, a sole supplier coordinates the whole infrastructure. Nevertheless, inside the federated cloud architecture, numerous cloud providers cooperate in a unified manner. Consider this scenario as a symphony, wherein each cloud provider functions as an instrumental section, collaborating to produce a cohesive and robust composition.

- **Interconnected Nodes of Innovation**: Federated clouds are not simply isolated entities but function as nodes within an extensive innovation network. Every node contributes distinct skills, such as increased computational capacity, specialized services, or regional experience. The interlinked nodes create a collaboration network, optimizing efficiency and broadening the technical environment.
- **Dynamic Resource Allocation**: Resource allocation in a federated cloud is characterized by dynamic and flexible processes rather than following a fixed and preset routine. Envision an astute ballet in which resources effortlessly migrate between clouds according to demand, availability, and performance criteria. Dynamic allocation guarantees the most efficient use of resources, quick response times, and the ability to scale up as needed.
- **Resilience through Diversity**: Diverse elements inside federated cloud architecture enhance its strength. A federated cloud, characterized by its multitude of providers, services, and locations, possesses intrinsic robustness against disruptions, similar to how a diversified ecosystem exhibits resilience to environmental changes. The system is robust and benefits from diversity, making it resistant to individual sources of failure.
- **Empowering Innovation and Customization**: Federated clouds enable enterprises to customize their cloud experience. Consider it a selection of cloud services, resembling a buffet, from which enterprises can selectively choose the offerings that most closely match their specific requirements. This customization promotes creativity, enabling firms to experiment, develop, and explore the limits of what can be achieved in the cloud.
- **The Intelligent Intermediator**: Middleware's Role—The core of this symphony is adaptive Middleware, which acts as an intelligent conductor coordinating the collaboration. Middleware enables efficient communication among various cloud providers while optimizing resource allocation, ensuring robust security measures, and improving overall system performance. The maestro guarantees the synchronized performance of the federated cloud orchestra.

Figure 10.1 shows that system users can be patients, doctors, practitioners, nurses, and private clouds. Based on the requirements of respective users, adaptive Middleware will act as an intermediator to facilitate services between users and cloud service providers (CSPs). Federation of CSPs is a win-win situation for the users and CSPs. To grasp the concept of federated cloud architecture is comparable to comprehending a magnificent orchestral performance—intricate, ever-changing, and surpassing its components' combined value. A harmonious blend of innovation, collaboration, and adaptability characterizes the future aspect of cloud computing.

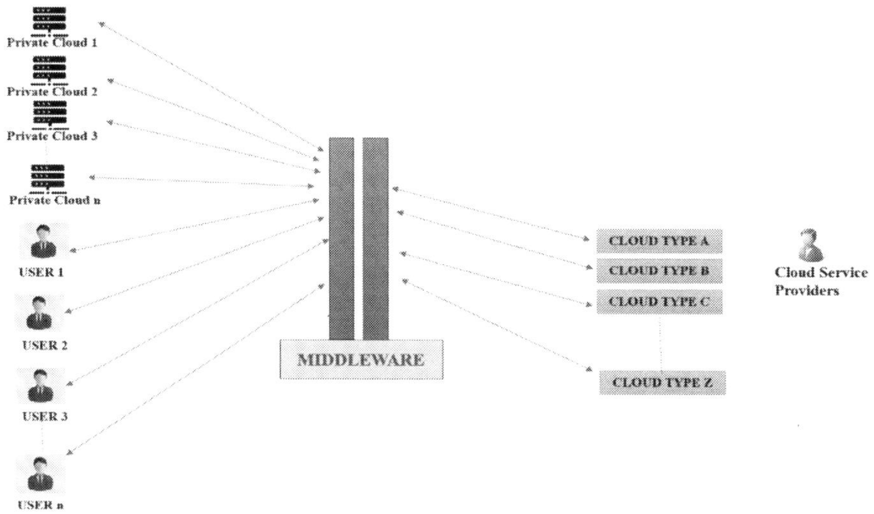

FIGURE 10.1 Proposed overview of cloud users, Middleware, and federated cloud service providers [2].

10.2.2 Key Components and Technologies

Federated cloud environments signify a fundamental change in the understanding and utilization of distributed computing. This section explores the complexities of the essential components that constitute the core of these ever-changing ecosystems.

Intelligent Orchestration Frameworks: Discover the underlying principles of intelligent orchestration frameworks that efficiently manage and optimize the allocation of resources across many cloud nodes. Examine how these frameworks adjust instantaneously to different workloads, guaranteeing the best possible performance and usage of resources.

Decentralized Identity Management: Explore the domain of decentralized identity management solutions that redefine security in federated clouds. Observe the transition from old authentication methods to advanced decentralized alternatives, which provide a strong and user-focused system for verifying identity while reducing security vulnerabilities.

Distributed Data Storage Architectures: Explore the cutting-edge methods of distributed data storage that form the foundation of federated cloud environments. Discover how different designs, ranging from sharding approaches to blockchain-based data integrity, transform data storage, retrieval, and resilience in response to the changing demands of healthcare data.

Adaptive Networking Protocols: Explore the array of adaptive networking protocols specifically developed to optimize communication efficiency across interconnected cloud nodes inside a federation. Analyze the ability of these protocols to adapt to changes in network conditions, guaranteeing fast response times and efficient data transfer for healthcare applications with strict data management regulations.

Edge Computing Integration: Observe the incorporation of edge computing as a crucial element in federated clouds. Examine the impact of edge nodes in healthcare as they bring computing capacity closer to the endpoints of healthcare systems. This reduces the delay in data processing and allows for real-time analysis while adhering to strict data governance regulations.

Machine Learning in Resource Allocation: Enter the domain of artificial intelligence (AI) and machine learning algorithms that dynamically coordinate the distribution of resources. Discover how these sophisticated systems assess past consumption patterns, forecast future demands, and independently optimize the allocation of resources, guaranteeing efficiency and cost-efficiency.

Optimal resource management in a federated cloud environment is a crucial aspect that will signify the system's effectiveness and performance. The ultimate goal should be to enhance user experience and maximize resource utilization [3]. Examining the fundamental elements and technologies serves as the foundation for comprehending the intricate dynamics within federated cloud environments. This lays the groundwork for thoroughly examining healthcare data governance and security improvements in the subsequent sections.

10.2.3 Challenges and Opportunities in the Federated Cloud Environment

In the dynamic domain of federated cloud environments, the boundaries between challenges and opportunities shape the foundation of this intricate architecture.

Navigating the Cloud Federation: Challenges

Orchestrating Heterogeneous Ecosystems: Federated clouds often consist of heterogeneous platforms, each characterized by its distinct architecture and protocols. The difficulty is in effectively coordinating these diverse ecosystems, guaranteeing seamless compatibility and uninterrupted data transfer.

Data Sovereignty and Compliance: Achieving a harmonious equilibrium between data accessibility and compliance with diverse foreign data sovereignty standards presents a considerable obstacle. Balancing regulatory obligations with the flexibility of federated cloud operations is a complex undertaking.

Dynamic Resource Allocation: The inherent dynamism of federated clouds presents difficulties in resource allocation. To effectively allocate resources among interconnected clouds, advanced algorithms and the ability to quickly adjust to changing demands are necessary.

10.2.3.1 Harvesting the Cloud Federation: Opportunities

Resilience through Redundancy: Federated clouds can improve system resilience by implementing redundancy. The architecture disperses data and computing workloads over numerous clouds to minimize the impact of potential failures and ensure uninterrupted operations.

Scalability and Elasticity: Utilizing the scalability and elasticity of federated clouds allows for effectively managing varying workloads. The capacity to adjust resources in accordance with demand, either increasing or decreasing them as needed, ensures optimal performance and cost-effectiveness.

Innovation in Hybrid Services: Combining public and private clouds in federated clouds promotes the development of innovative hybrid services. Integrating public and private clouds allows for the development of creative services that leverage both advantages, offering fresh solutions to ever-changing technological obstacles.

To fully leverage the potential of federated cloud environments, it is essential to comprehend and tackle the issues associated with this architecture. This will enable us to make the most of the opportunities it presents. In such a case, adaptive data management Middleware will act as an intermediary between the patient and the federated cloud environment to fulfill the goals efficiently and effectively for data governance and security.

10.3 ADAPTIVE DATA MANAGEMENT MIDDLEWARE

10.3.1 Definition and Functionality

Adaptive data management Middleware is a powerful force that revolutionizes how healthcare data is handled in federated cloud environments, which are constantly changing. This Middleware fundamentally encompasses a dynamic and adaptive layer that coordinates the smooth transmission of data over decentralized networks. Middleware, called brokers, is situated between users and cloud service providers. Choosing the appropriate Middleware out of available depends on the prospects of the user, along with maximizing throughput and effective resource optimization [4–6].

10.3.1.1 Defining Adaptability

In contrast to static data management solutions, the adaptive Middleware highlighted in this chapter demonstrates a profound understanding of the constantly changing characteristics of healthcare data. It functions not only as a means of transmitting information but also as a cognitive link that adapts its procedures to accept changes in the amount, origins, and forms of data.

10.3.1.2 Intelligent Orchestration

In terms of functionality, this Middleware surpasses simple data transport. It utilizes intelligent orchestration to optimize data paths dynamically, depending on contextual inputs. Envision a complex orchestration where data components synchronize according to the requirements of healthcare applications, guaranteeing that vital information is delivered accurately and swiftly to its intended destination.

10.3.1.3 Context-Aware Processing

A distinguishing characteristic of Middleware is its capacity to understand the particulars of healthcare situations. The system does not handle all input equally but distinguishes between important and unimportant information and adjusts its processing algorithms appropriately. By utilizing sophisticated algorithms and machine learning techniques, this system acquires knowledge from patterns, guaranteeing the accurate delivery of data to its intended destination at the appropriate moment.

10.3.1.4 Adaptive Security Measures

Security is of the utmost importance in a federated cloud environment. The Middleware integrates dynamic security mechanisms, preemptively addressing emerging risks. It does not depend on fixed protocols but constantly develops its defense systems, gaining knowledge from past experiences and adjusting to new obstacles in real time.

10.3.1.5 Real-Time Feedback Loop

Envision a system that not only carries out data processing but also actively acquires knowledge from its actions. The Middleware creates a feedback loop in real time, constantly improving its tactics by analyzing the results of its data management decisions. This inherent ability to optimize oneself guarantees the capacity to adapt and a continuous improvement in performance and efficiency. The adaptive data management Middleware discussed in this section goes beyond traditional assumptions, transforming into an intelligent, context-aware, and self-optimizing entity. Being a crucial component in the interconnected cloud healthcare system, its definition goes beyond technology. It signifies a fundamental change in perceiving and overseeing healthcare data ecosystems.

10.3.2 Role in Enhancing Data Governance

Adaptive data management Middleware plays a crucial role in managing healthcare data in a complex federated cloud environment, going beyond traditional limitations. This section explores novel methods by which Middleware transforms and strengthens data governance procedures.

Catalyzing Dynamic Data Governance Strategies: Conventional data governance frameworks frequently face difficulties keeping up with healthcare data ecosystems' ever-changing nature. The adaptive data management Middleware presents a significant change in approach by offering a flexible architecture that adjusts to changing governance needs. The system adapts access controls, information structures, and compliance regulations in real time, guaranteeing that governance stays flexible and responsive rather than rigid and unchanging.

Orchestrating Policy-Driven Data Lifecycle Management: The Middleware functions as a complex coordinator, effortlessly incorporating policy-driven frameworks into the data lifecycle. It guarantees a thorough and uniform approach by implementing automated mechanisms to enforce governance policies across the whole process of data production, transfer, and storage. This orchestration improves adherence to rules and regulations and offers a strong basis for conducting audits and ensuring accountability.

Empowering Context-Aware Access Controls: A novel aspect of adaptive Middleware is its capability to enforce context-aware access constraints. The Middleware takes into account the context in which data is accessed rather than depending exclusively on inflexible, role-based access. Understanding the context allows healthcare companies to adjust access permissions in real time, considering elements such as user roles, device features, and relevance to the situation. This enhances security and privacy protections.

Facilitating Federated Data Governance: In a federated cloud environment, which involves the distribution of data across multiple networks and organizations, conventional governance methods frequently face difficulties in terms of scalability. Adaptive Middleware acts as a cohesive entity, effortlessly expanding governance standards across federated data sources. It guarantees that irrespective of the data's location or source, governance procedures maintain uniformity and can be enforced, promoting a unified and protected data environment.

Real-time Governance Analytics and Optimization: The Middleware ensures governance and actively contributes to its ongoing enhancement. It actively monitors adherence to governance regulations through real-time analytics and detects possible weaknesses. By taking a proactive approach, businesses can effectively enhance their governance policies to address new threats or evolving regulatory environments. This ensures the establishment of a strong and adaptable data governance framework for the future. Adaptive data management Middleware is a powerful tool that enhances healthcare data governance in federated cloud systems by introducing agility, intelligence, and flexibility. It goes beyond traditional static models and embraces the dynamic nature of modern healthcare data ecosystems.

10.3.3 Adaptive Middleware in Healthcare Systems

The introduction of adaptive data management Middleware marks a significant shift in the healthcare industry, where data moves across several systems in a complex manner. Envision a perceptive controller effortlessly maneuvering through the complex arrangement of healthcare data, adjusting to the changing requirements of patients, providers, and administrators. Adaptive Middleware in healthcare surpasses conventional data management paradigms. It is not just a channel but a perceptive facilitator, perfectly adjusted to the distinct patterns of the healthcare system. Consider it an AI-driven intermediary, coordinating a seamless partnership among diverse systems, guaranteeing real-time accuracy, accessibility, and data protection. This section explores the complexities of how adaptive Middleware serves as the central component of healthcare systems. Imagine a situation in which patient records effortlessly go from electronic health records (EHRs) to diagnostic instruments and then to collaborative decision support systems. The Middleware's adaptability guarantees that data is sent, converted, contextualized, and enhanced as it traverses the complex network of healthcare applications.

It is imperative to ensure the security and confidentiality of user data and information across the entire ecosystem. The system's primary focus is on providing security and maintaining confidentiality. Figure 10.2 illustrates the interaction between users (namely patients) and CSPs in a federated cloud environment. The entire system includes adaptive data management Middleware and a data governance framework, which is a fundamental component (Table 10.1).

Imagine the potential of adaptive Middleware in healthcare, which not only handles data movement but also drives new discoveries and customized treatments and ensures the ethical and secure use of healthcare data in the rapidly changing digital world [7–10].

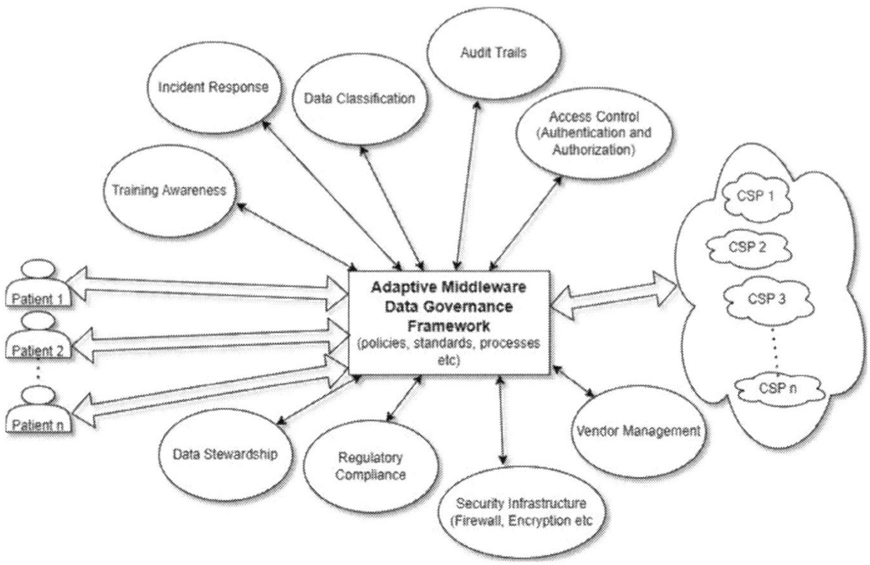

FIGURE 10.2 Adaptive data management Middleware having a healthcare data governance framework and its corresponding components.

TABLE 10.1
Comparative Summary of Adaptive Middleware in Healthcare Systems

Feature	Traditional Middleware	Adaptive Middleware
Scalability	Limited scalability, often requiring manual adjustments for increased loads.	Adaptive Middleware dynamically scales to accommodate varying workloads, ensuring optimal performance.
Interoperability	May face challenges in integrating diverse healthcare systems and standards.	Adaptive Middleware excels in interoperability, facilitating seamless integration across healthcare platforms and data standards.
Real-time processing	Generally, struggles with real-time data processing, leading to latency issues.	Adaptive Middleware is designed for real-time processing, supporting instant data analysis and decision-making in healthcare scenarios.
Customization	Limited customization options, making it challenging to tailor Middleware to specific healthcare workflows.	Adaptive Middleware offers extensive customization capabilities, allowing healthcare providers to adapt the system to their unique needs and processes.
Security	Security features may be basic, and updates could be infrequent.	It prioritizes robust security measures, including encryption, access controls, and regular updates, to address emerging threats in the healthcare sector.

(*Continued*)

TABLE 10.1 (*Continued*)
Comparative Summary of Adaptive Middleware in Healthcare Systems

Feature	Traditional Middleware	Adaptive Middleware
Data governance	Traditional Middleware may lack advanced data governance features, leading to potential compliance issues.	Adaptive Middleware strongly emphasizes data governance, incorporating features for compliance with healthcare regulations and standards.
Fault tolerance	Limited fault tolerance, with potential disruptions in case of failures.	Adaptive Middleware is built with high fault tolerance, ensuring continuous operation despite system failures or errors.
Adaptability	Relies on manual adjustments and may struggle to adapt to rapidly changing healthcare environments.	The hallmark of adaptive Middleware is its ability to dynamically adapt to changing healthcare landscapes, ensuring optimal performance and efficiency.

10.3.4 Integration with Federated Cloud Infrastructure

The function of adaptive data management Middleware (ADMM) is crucial in the ever-changing field of healthcare data governance within a federated cloud environment. This section explores the advanced integration tactics implemented by ADMM within the intricate structure of federated cloud infrastructure, revolutionizing the management, security, and utilization of healthcare data.

Breaking down Silos: A Symphony of Interconnected Cloud Nodes—Envision a symphony whereby each instrument performs a distinct role, collectively contributing to a harmonious entirety. ADMM efficiently coordinates and harmonizes various cloud nodes in federated cloud environments, creating a unified and integrated ecosystem. This integration surpasses conventional data compartments, promoting smoothness in the transfer and availability of data.

Adaptability in Action: Dynamic Data Routing and Processing—The adaptive aspect of ADMM is shown as it dynamically transports and processes healthcare data across federated clouds. The system's adaptability guarantees that data is efficiently sent to the most appropriate cloud node based on current conditions, maximizing performance and resource consumption. ADMM promptly and effectively addresses any increase in data volume or specialized processing needs, ensuring optimal system performance in real time.

Enhancing Security: The Guardian of Federated Cloud Health Data—ADMM diligently protects sensitive health data, ensuring that security remains of the utmost importance in healthcare. ADMM strengthens the federated cloud architecture by implementing advanced encryption protocols, safe access controls, and constant monitoring, establishing a strong defense against attacks. This integration effectively combines the ability to access data with strong security safeguards, achieving a careful equilibrium between transparency and safeguarding.

Scalability Unleashed: Meeting Healthcare's Growing Data Demands—Healthcare data is a dynamic entity that expands rapidly with every patient interaction.

Integrating ADMM with federated cloud architecture is specifically engineered to achieve scalability. The system seamlessly adjusts the allocation of resources to accommodate the changing demands of healthcare data, guaranteeing a responsive and efficient performance, even amid enormous data growth.

Patient-Centric Experience: Unleashing the Potential of Healthcare Professionals—Healthcare practitioners in this integrated domain adhere to a patient-centric paradigm [11]. The ADMM algorithm enhances the efficiency of data retrieval and processing by tailoring it to patients' specific preferences and requirements. This enables healthcare practitioners to obtain vital information swiftly. The integration of technology seamlessly matches the workflow of healthcare workers, resulting in improved overall efficiency and facilitating enhanced patient care.

To summarize, the combination of ADMM and federated cloud infrastructure significantly advances healthcare data governance. It transforms the theoretical approach from fragmented data to unified coherence, from fixed procedures to flexible flexibility, and from worries about security to strengthened resilience. The combination of ADMM and federated cloud infrastructure establishes a foundation for a revolutionary healthcare data management era characterized by responsiveness, security, and readiness for future advancements. The collaboration between ADMM and the distributed nature of cloud infrastructure is crucial for innovation and efficiency in healthcare data governance and security in a federated cloud environment [12,13].

10.4 HEALTHCARE DATA GOVERNANCE

10.4.1 Importance of Data Governance in Healthcare

In the ever-changing field of healthcare, where data plays a crucial role in making informed decisions and providing patient care, the significance of efficient data governance cannot be emphasized enough. Trusting the intended cloud service provider among available cloud service providers is challenging [14]. Data governance extends beyond fundamental adherence to regulations; it becomes a strategic necessity, influencing how healthcare companies function and provide services.

10.4.1.1 Orchestrating Precision in Patient Care

Data governance plays a crucial role in guaranteeing the accuracy, reliability, and timeliness of health data, hence facilitating precision in patient care. Healthcare professionals can enhance the overall quality of patient outcomes by implementing rigorous criteria for data quality and integrity. This allows them to effectively utilize information to tailor treatment plans and improve diagnostic accuracy.

10.4.1.2 Navigating Regulatory Complexities

Amid a time characterized by constantly changing regulatory frameworks, strong data governance is a navigational tool for healthcare organizations, helping them navigate the complex network of compliance obligations. By effectively incorporating regulatory requirements into data management protocols, healthcare institutions fulfill legal obligations and cultivate the confidence of patients who rely on them to safeguard sensitive personal data.

10.4.1.3 Unleashing the Power of Analytics

Effective data governance has regulatory and clinical ramifications and unleashes the transformational potential of healthcare analytics. Organizations can leverage the potential of big data and AI to obtain valuable insights by implementing well-defined data collection, storage, and utilization procedures. Consequently, this enables healthcare workers to utilize predictive analytics, which allows for proactive management of diseases, optimization of resources, and identification of emerging health trends.

10.4.1.4 Fostering Interoperability and Collaboration

Data governance is crucial in promoting the exchange of information and cooperation among different healthcare systems. Through the establishment of standardized data formats and exchange methods, it facilitates smooth communication between different healthcare stakeholders. The interconnection facilitates care coordination and enhances the comprehensive understanding of patient health by consolidating data from various sources.

10.4.1.5 Safeguarding Patient Privacy and Trust

The significance of data governance lies in its ability to protect patient privacy and foster trust. Robust governance structures in healthcare businesses guarantee that privacy safeguards are not only compliance checks but rather essential elements of the company ethos, as sensitive information is collected, stored, and shared. By placing patient privacy as a top priority, healthcare organizations establish a fundamental basis of trust that is crucial for maintaining patient–provider relationships.

Essentially, data governance in healthcare is not just about compliance but also plays a crucial role in shaping patient outcomes, regulatory adherence, analytical capabilities, collaborative efforts, and the fundamental trust between healthcare providers and their patients. Adopting cutting-edge data governance methods is not only a mandatory requirement imposed by regulations but also a forward-thinking investment in the future of healthcare excellence.

10.4.2 Regulatory Frameworks and Compliance

Adhering to regulatory frameworks is crucial in healthcare data governance to maintain the integrity, privacy, and accessibility of patient information in a complex context. This section explores the creative approaches to negotiate the complex maze of rules and compliance standards in the ever-changing healthcare ecosystem.

- **Embarking on the Regulatory Odyssey**: To undertake a regulatory journey, one must comprehend the various frameworks that govern healthcare data. This includes examining both extant norms and developing policies that influence the future of healthcare data governance. It also involves examining the complex network of compliance environments, ranging from well-established government regulatory bodies to state-of-the-art data protection rules.

- **Beyond Box-Ticking**: A Proactive Approach—Going beyond a simple approach of following a checklist, carefully examine how adaptive Middleware might actively support compliance. It is not solely about fulfilling requirements but about remaining ahead of the prevailing trend. Case studies stand in favor of demonstrating dynamic compliance strategies, in which adaptive Middleware not only guarantees adherence to regulations but also predicts and prepares for changes in regulations. This positions healthcare organizations as leaders in maintaining the integrity of data.
- **Ethical Considerations in the Regulatory Mosaic**: Fulfilling legal requirements to protect the patient data associated with adaptive Middleware contributions to surpassing regulatory thresholds and promoting a culture of data stewardship that goes beyond legal obligations.
- **Interactive Compliance Ecosystems**: The era of isolated compliance activities is over. It is essential to analyze the functioning of adaptive Middleware, which efficiently coordinates various compliance measures, effortlessly incorporates regulations and establishes a seamless and responsive environment that adjusts to changing requirements.
- **Future-Proofing through Compliance Innovation**: Looking ahead, examine how healthcare organizations utilize compliance as a catalyst for innovation rather than viewing it as a limitation. Adaptive Middleware is crucial in turning the healthcare data governance landscape regulatory constraints into technological and procedural development possibilities. It not only meets but surpasses the demands of this constantly evolving field.

10.4.3 Challenges and Solutions in Healthcare Data Governance

10.4.3.1 Data Fragmentation and Interoperability Struggles

- **Challenge**: One of the primary obstacles facing healthcare data governance is the pervasive issue of data fragmentation. Patient information is often scattered across diverse systems and platforms, impeding efficient interoperability.
- **Solution**: In response, cutting-edge approaches leverage adaptive Middleware to create a unified data ecosystem. The Middleware acts as a bridge, harmonizing disparate data sources and promoting seamless interoperability.

10.4.3.2 Regulatory Compliance and Evolving Standards

- **Challenge**: Navigating the complex maze of regulatory compliance and constantly changing standards presents a persistent difficulty. Healthcare firms face intricate regulations, posing challenges in keeping up with the most recent mandates.
- **Solution**: Innovative solutions require the development of adaptive Middleware with real-time compliance monitoring tools. These technologies guarantee compliance with existing rules and adjust to changes flexibly, offering a framework for healthcare data governance that is prepared for the future.

10.4.3.3 Data Privacy and Patient Empowerment

- **Challenge**: Striking a balance between the need to protect data privacy and the increasing demand for patient empowerment is a complex dilemma. Ensuring a balance between protecting sensitive information and enabling patients to access their data is a continuous concern.
- **Solution**: Progressive healthcare data governance models integrate adaptive Middleware with precise access controls. This enables customized data retrieval according to individual choices while maintaining strong privacy safeguards.

The above challenges can be addressed at a certain level by selecting suitable cloud computing scheduling algorithms [15]. This section examines the complex array of difficulties encountered in healthcare data governance and investigates the inventive solutions facilitated by adaptive Middleware. By comprehending and tackling these difficulties, the healthcare service sector can achieve a more robust and patient-centric data governance paradigm.

10.5 SECURITY MEASURES IN FEDERATED CLOUD ENVIRONMENTS

10.5.1 Adaptive Middleware Contributions to Security

Adaptive Middleware is crucial in strengthening security measures in federated cloud settings, where safeguarding healthcare data is most important. Adaptive Middleware functions as a smart protector, coordinating a complex set of security mechanisms to guarantee the privacy, accuracy, and accessibility of healthcare information. User authentication is a crucial part of the entire system, and various user authentication schemes can be applied to address patient security [16].

Intelligent Threat Detection and Prevention: An essential advantage of adaptive Middleware is its capacity to utilize sophisticated threat detection algorithms. Middleware can quickly detect potential security vulnerabilities by continuously studying data access, consumption, and transmission trends and identifying anomalies. By employing machine learning and heuristic analysis, it adjusts its defense measures to actively thwart illegal access and reduce the impact of developing hazards.

Dynamic Encryption and Access Control: Adaptive Middleware surpasses fixed security methods by incorporating dynamic encryption and access control features. The system adapts encryption protocols smartly by considering contextual elements such as user roles, data sensitivity, and network conditions. This dynamic strategy guarantees that the encryption techniques used are consistently in line with the changing threat environment, offering strong protection against data breaches and unauthorized disclosures.

Context-Aware Authentication: Conventional authentication systems are frequently binary, allowing access based on predetermined credentials. Adaptive Middleware implements a context-aware authentication paradigm that considers both user credentials and the access request context. Device reputation, geolocation, and time of access are dynamically assessed to provide additional protection that adjusts to the constantly changing conditions of healthcare operations.

Proactive Incident Response and Recovery: Adaptive Middleware is crucial in coordinating a proactive and efficient reaction in the case of a security incident. Continuous real-time data monitoring and analysis can identify irregularities that suggest security breaches, activating automated reactions or notifying security teams. Moreover, it expedites the process of recuperation by dynamically redirecting data, segregating impacted elements, and guaranteeing minimal interruption to healthcare services.

Collaborative Security Intelligence: Federated cloud infrastructures typically encompass numerous entities and stakeholders. Adaptive Middleware promotes collaborative security intelligence by enabling the smooth exchange of threat intelligence and security upgrades among federated partners. The coordinated approach enhances security, establishing a unified front against advanced and ever-changing cyber threats.

Adaptive Middleware significantly enhances security measures in a federated cloud environment, going beyond traditional methods. This system's adaptive and intelligent features strengthen the defense and establish a resilient and responsive security architecture that is in line with the complexities of managing healthcare data today.

10.5.2 Encryption, Access Control, and Authentication

Robust security measures are of utmost importance in managing healthcare data across constantly changing federated cloud systems. This section explores novel methodologies, with a specific emphasis on three fundamental principles: encryption, access control, and authentication.

Encryption: Unveiling the Digital Fortification—Encryption is crucial to protecting sensitive information in healthcare data governance. Discover state-of-the-art encryption techniques from conventional asymmetric algorithms to emerging quantum-resistant encryption. Explore the complexities of homomorphic encryption, which ensures data privacy even during computational operations, and analyze innovative applications like attribute-based encryption explicitly designed for healthcare settings.

Access Control: Orchestrating Precision in Data Accessibility—Explore the intricate terrain of access control in federated cloud environments. Discover cutting-edge access control models that go beyond traditional role-based paradigms. Explore the application of attribute-based access control (ABAC) in healthcare systems, enabling the definition of access controls based on dynamic attributes. Investigate real-time adaptive access control techniques that dynamically modify permissions, guaranteeing accuracy and responsiveness to contextual alterations.

Authentication: Beyond Passwords and Biometrics—Authentication, which serves as the entry point for accessing secure healthcare data, goes beyond conventional procedures. Discover innovations such as continuous authentication, which evaluates user behavior during a session to improve security without interrupting workflow. Explore incorporating multifactor authentication with behavioral biometrics, which adds an extra level of identity verification. Discover the capabilities of zero-trust architectures, which redefine the authentication and authorization methods for entities in federated cloud environments.

This part seeks to provide a clear understanding of these security measures' present condition and their path to development, delivering valuable insights into how healthcare data governance may adjust to a constantly changing digital environment.

10.5.3 Incident Response and Recovery

In the ever-changing domain of federated cloud systems, where maintaining the accuracy and security of healthcare data is of utmost importance, a novel incident response and recovery strategy plays a crucial role in protecting against potential risks.

Holistic Incident Orchestration: Conventional incident response models frequently exhibit a reactive and sequential approach. Envision an advanced system, enhanced by flexible Middleware, that not only promptly identifies deviations from the norm but also dynamically coordinates appropriate actions in response. This encompasses the automatic segregation of impacted elements, intelligent data redirection, and concurrently implementing predetermined recovery tactics.

Adaptive Threat Intelligence Integration: Incorporating adaptive threat intelligence brings a new level of sophistication to incident response. Exploring how Middleware, designed explicitly for healthcare data, works along with constantly updated threat intelligence feeds. This collaboration ensures a proactive approach to addressing new risks, allowing for anticipatory response techniques and minimizing the consequences of incidents.

Predictive Incident Modeling: In addition to reactive measures, another aspect is expanding to include predictive incident modeling. Imagine a system capable of simulating prospective dangers by utilizing historical data, system weaknesses, and present threat environments. Healthcare organizations can strengthen the overall resilience of federated cloud systems by proactively implementing preventive actions based on projecting possible issues.

Automated Recovery Workflows: Recovering from incidents is just as important as the first response to the incident and execution of automatic recovery operations enabled by adaptive Middleware. These routines are designed to restore normality and learn from the disaster, improving and optimizing recovery strategies for future occurrences.

Collaborative Threat Intelligence Sharing: Examining the idea of sharing collaborative threat intelligence to address the interdependent nature of healthcare ecosystems. Adaptive Middleware serves as a mediator, allowing smooth transmission of threat intelligence across federated institutions. This collaborative defensive strategy improves the overall security stance of the interconnected cloud environment.

As mentioned above, appropriate security measures will boost the e-commerce sector in parallel [17]. This section envisioned a future where incident response and recovery are not mere reactive measures but integral components of a proactive, adaptive, and intelligent healthcare data security framework within federated cloud environments.

10.6 CASE STUDIES AND BEST PRACTICES

10.6.1 Real-World Implementations of Adaptive Middleware in Healthcare

This section focuses on the ever-changing healthcare field, examining interesting real-life examples demonstrating adaptive Middleware's significant influence. Her focus is on real-world examples that demonstrate how adaptive Middleware is playing a crucial role in transforming healthcare data governance and security, with a perspective that emphasizes innovation and pragmatism. Every case study is a guiding light, shedding light on the intricate difficulties healthcare organizations encounter and the innovative solutions that adaptable Middleware facilitates.

10.6.1.1 Precision Medicine Revolution: Integrating Patient Data Seamlessly

Discover a pioneering instance where adaptive Middleware plays a pivotal role in implementing precision medicine. Observe how several sources of patient data, such as genetics and EHRs, are synchronized instantly, allowing healthcare professionals to provide individualized therapies with exceptional precision. Explore the complex network of interoperability facilitated by adaptive Middleware, guaranteeing that crucial information is easily accessible at the point of care.

10.6.1.2 Telehealth Optimization: Bridging Gaps with Adaptive Middleware

Engage in a story that delves into enhancing telehealth services with adaptable Middleware. Explore the difficulties in providing remote healthcare and see how adaptive Middleware overcomes communication barriers across many platforms, guaranteeing a smooth and protected telehealth encounter. This case study demonstrates adaptive Middleware's flexibility and quick response in facilitating the development of healthcare delivery models.

By analyzing these case studies, I identified the most effective strategies and insights, providing a clear plan for healthcare professionals and technologists. This investigation surpasses abstract contemplations, offering concrete observations into the influential capabilities of adaptive Middleware in reconfiguring the forthcoming healthcare landscape. The healthcare sector can be boosted to the next level in the smart city [18]. This section offers readers significant lessons and inspiration for utilizing adaptive Middleware in the complex and essential confluence of healthcare data governance and federated cloud settings. It does so by presenting case studies and best practices, providing a diverse range of experiences.

10.6.2 Lessons Learned and Recommendations

- **Unveiling Insights from Implementation Challenges**: Analyzed the difficulties faced during integrating adaptive Middleware in federated cloud healthcare systems and obtained significant insights on overcoming challenges associated with interoperability, scalability, and stakeholder collaboration.

- **Optimizing Data Governance Practices**: Based on experiences in healthcare data governance, this section explains the lessons learned in creating strong governance frameworks and also offers practical suggestions for developing efficient data governance policies, including topics ranging from regulatory complexities to ethical factors.
- **Maximizing Security in Federated Cloud Environments**: Analyzed instances of security breaches and achievements in federated cloud systems, focusing on extracting valuable insights from each experience. Derived recommendations for strengthening security measures inside complex ecosystems by examining data breaches and successful preventive measures.
- **Adapting Middleware for Future Challenges**: Given the ever-changing nature of technology, we anticipated the forthcoming difficulties in managing healthcare data and operating federated cloud infrastructures. We also presented an innovative suggestion to guarantee continuous relevance and resilience by proposing adaptive solutions.

10.7 CONCLUSION

The chapter concludes with the ever-changing fields of adaptive Middleware, federated cloud environments, and healthcare data governance; it discerns a collection of significant discoveries that form a harmonious ensemble of knowledge. Every component, from the seamless incorporation of adaptable data management Middleware to the intricate regulation of healthcare data in interconnected clouds, plays a role in coordinating a safe and effective healthcare system. Adaptive Middleware plays an essential role in seamlessly orchestrating data flows. It ensures the interoperability of systems and resistance against ever-evolving cyber threats. Healthcare data governance ensures compliance with regulatory frameworks, demonstrating how responsible information management matches ethical obligations in the medical field. The next aspect is addressing the intermittent difficulties related to security in federated cloud systems. This is achieved by implementing a smooth and continuous combination of encryption, access control, and authentication procedures. These measures are the foundation of a strong defense mechanism to prevent possible breaches. Examined the subtle intricacies of incident response and recovery, emphasizing the significance of a finely calibrated system to handle and gain insights from disturbances promptly. During the concluding phase, the case studies and examples were examined along with the exemplary methods from the real world, illustrating successful executions in a detailed and compelling manner.

Also, highlighted the potential future scenarios influenced by advancing technologies. The chapter encourages further creativity and research in the always-changing nexus of healthcare, adaptive Middleware, and federated cloud settings. Explored the broader scope of technology advancement, ethical deliberations, and the societal consequences of improved healthcare data management. Here, I provided a concise summary of the segments presented in the chapter and explored potent outcomes. The chapter will guide practitioners, policymakers, and researchers in navigating the changing domains of adaptive Middleware, federated clouds, and healthcare data governance. Finally, the combination of adaptive Middleware, federated cloud environments, and strong healthcare data governance represents a technological advancement and a fundamental change in creative thinking. The healthcare sector is ready to adopt a future where data is not only safeguarded but also acts as a catalyst for extraordinary progress, ultimately leading to a healthier and more interconnected global community.

REFERENCES

1. C. A. Lee *et al.*, "The NIST Cloud Federation Reference Architecture," NIST Special Publication 500-332, 2020. https://doi.org/10.6028/NIST.SP.500-332
2. V. K. Kolekar and S. R. Sakhare, "A research perspective on data management techniques for federated cloud environment," *IJRITCC*, vol. 11, no. 5, pp. 338–346, 2023.
3. M. Liaqat *et al.*, "Federated cloud resource management: Review and discussion," *Journal of Network and Computer Applications*, Elsevier, pp: 87–105, 2017. https://doi.org/10.1016/j.jnca.2016.10.008
4. S. S. Chauhan *et al.*, "Brokering in interconnected cloud computing environments: A survey," *Journal of Parallel and Distributed Computing*, 133, pp: 193–209, 2019. https://doi.org/10.1016/j.jpdc.2018.08.001
5. A. Rafique, "Middleware for Data Management in Multi-Cloud", PhD thesis, Faculty of Engineering Science, Arenberg Doctoral School, KU Leuven, 2019.
6. M. R. M. Assis and L. F. Bittencourt, "A survey on cloud federation architectures: Identifying functional and non-functional properties," *Journal of Network and Computer Applications*, vol. 72, pp. 51–71, 2016. ISSN 1084-8045. https://doi.org/10.1016/j.jnca.2016.06.014
7. M. A. Sharkh, A. Kanso, A. Shami, and P. Öhlén, "Building a cloud on earth: A study of cloud computing data center simulators," *Computer Networks*, vol. 108, pp. 78–96, 2016. ISSN 1389-1286. https://doi.org/10.1016/j.comnet.2016.06.037
8. G. Fersi *et al.*, "Study of middleware for Internet of healthcare things and their applications." *Impact of Digital Technologies on Public Health in Developed and Developing Countries. ICOST 2020.* Lecture Notes in Computer Science, vol. 12157. Springer, Cham. https://doi.org/10.1007/978-3-030-51517-1_18
9. W. He, J. Z. Zhang, H. Wu, W. Li, and S. Shetty, "A unified health information system framework for connecting data, people, devices, and systems." *Journal of Global Information Management*, vol. 30, no. 11, pp. 1–19, Article 39. https://doi.org/10.4018/JGIM.305239
10. J. Singh and J. M. Bacon, "On middleware for emerging health services," *Journal of Internet Services and Applications*, vol. 5, no. 6, 2014. https://doi.org/10.1186/1869-0238-5-6
11. C. Peng, P. Goswami, and G. Bai, "A literature review of current technologies on health data integration for patient-centered health management," *Health Informatics Journal*, vol. 26, no. 3, pp. 1926–1951, 2020. https://doi.org/10.1177/1460458219892387. Epub 2019 Dec 30. PMID: 31884843.
12. A. Kliem, A. Boelke, A. Grohnert, and N. Traeder, "Self-adaptive middleware for ubiquitous medical device integration," *2014 IEEE 16th International Conference on e-Health Networking, Applications and Services (Healthcom)*, Natal, Brazil, 2014, pp. 298–304. https://doi.org/10.1109/HealthCom.2014.7001858
13. R. S. Malaquias and I. M. B. Filho, "Middleware for healthcare systems: Systematic mapping," *Computational Science and Its Applications – ICCSA 2021: 21st International Conference*, Cagliari, Italy, September 13–16, 2021, Proceedings, Part IX. Springer-Verlag, Berlin, Heidelberg, 394–409. https://doi.org/10.1007/978-3-030-87013-3_30

14. S. R. Rathi and V. K. Kolekar, "Trust model for computing security of cloud," *2018 Fourth International Conference on Computing Communication Control and Automation (ICCUBEA)*, Pune, India, 2018, pp. 1–5. https://doi.org/10.1109/ICCUBEA.2018.8697881
15. V. K. Kolekar and S. R Sakhare, "Scheduling algorithms of cloud computing: State of the art," *IJNGC*, vol. 12, no. 2, pp. 145–157, 2021.
16. V. K. Kolekar and M. B. Vaidya, "Click and session based — Captcha as graphical password authentication schemes for smart phone and web," *2015 International Conference on Information Processing (ICIP)*, Pune, 2015, pp. 669–674. https://doi.org/10.1109/INFOP.2015.7489467
17. N. Sakhare, D. Verma, V. Kolekar, A. Shelke, A. Dixit, and N. Meshram, "E-commerce product price monitoring and comparison using sentiment analysis," *IJRITCC*, vol. 11, no. 5, pp. 404–411, 2023.
18. V. K.Kolekar, M. Oswal, Y. Wankhade, G. Shirke, A. Sondur, and P. Wable, "Smart city IoT data management with proactive middleware," *IJRITCC*, vol. 11, no. 5s, pp. 319–329, 2023.

11 Skin Cancer Detection Using U-Net

Ganesh B. Regulwar, Katta Hartheek Reddy, Vanam Prem Shanker, Ashish Mahalle, Venigalla Jithin, and Nikhila Kathirisetty

11.1 INTRODUCTION

Two to three million non-melanoma skin cancers and 132,000 melanoma skin cancers, according to health organizations, are estimated to occur globally each year. Despite representing <6.5% of all skin cancers, melanoma is the most dangerous kind, responsible for about 75% of all deaths related to skin cancer. Early detection is crucial for faster survival, and visual inspection is still the most used diagnostic method. Convolutional neural networks (CNNs) have surpassed doctor's performance in the visual class. Additionally, in oncology areas, CNN has been proven to be on par with specialists. CNN was created to diagnose and categorize skin malignancies by imaging with dermatological accuracy from 60% (professional eye examination) to 75% at 84% to increase the scalability of diagnostic competence. The International Skin Imaging Collaboration (ISIC) has held an annual contest to judge the interpretation of dermoscopy images since 2016. The competition uses more than 20,000 dermoscopy images from a sizable, publicly accessible dataset.

The lesion analysis task consists of feature extraction and classification. This paper presents segmentation results to identify lesion locations in dermoscopy pictures. We are the first to use a U-Net-based architecture combination.

11.2 LITERATURE SURVEY

Many studies have been performed to segment and classify skin lesions. We referred to a paper by Alkhushayni *et al.* [1] for a general overview. Skin cancer is a fascinating field for researchers to study and recognize colored skin lesions [2]. Almost every image segmentation task employs traditional machine learning processes for feature extraction. The literature outlines numerous crucial methods for precise segmentation. CNN is recommended for potential future use by Dubal *et al.* in their research [3], as these models are capable of classifying afflicted skin photos without the requirement for prior segmentation and feature extraction. CNNs were used for feature extraction, and artificial neural network (ANN) was used for classification in ur Rehman *et al.*'s [4] innovative technique. Because the proposed method uses

 DOI: 10.1201/9781003479185-11

three fully connected layers to train the classification model, it does not require additional classifiers like support vector machine (SVM) or K nearest neighbors (KNN). The ability to use the back-propagation technique, which modifies the neuron parameters in all layers to enhance the classification model, is one of the special advantages of this type of classification.

11.3 METHODOLOGY

U-Net, an evolution of classical CNNs, was first developed and used for processing biological images in 2015. We focused on the photo category in a general convolutional neural network, with an image and a single label as the output. We need to recognize a problem's existence and location for biomedical applications.

11.3.1 U-Net Architecture

U-Net is a semantic segmentation architecture. U-Net consists of two blocks: the left block is the encoder block in which pooling of the image occurs, and the right block is the decoder block in which upsampling takes place. It passes through two convolutional layers, and then pooling takes place. At the last convolution step, there is no pooling. Instead, the image goes to the decoder block, which will upscale it to its original size [5]. After upsizing, the obtained image is concatenated with the obtained image from the encoder block; this provides better results. In the last stage, we will get segmentation for our input image (Figure 11.1).

11.3.2 Convolutional Neural Networks

CNNs are a powerful class of neural networks capable of both region and image categorization and identification. It has been confirmed that artificial intelligence

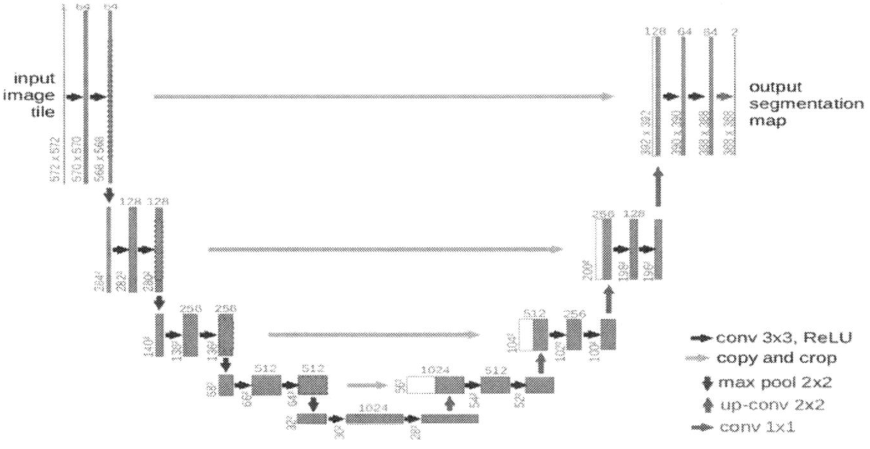

FIGURE 11.1 U-Net architecture [9].

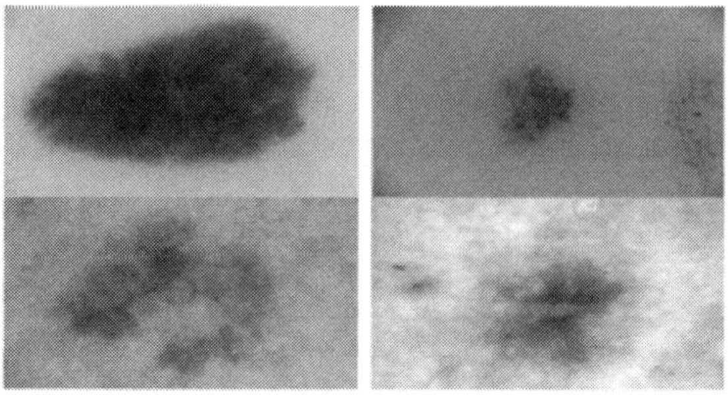

FIGURE 11.2 Dataset samples.

(AI) can recognize symptoms of faces, devices, and visitors more accurately than humans. As a result, they are trained to do so through supervised CNNs. This means self-driving cars and robots can be taught to identify objects and labels through CNN, analyzing their relationships. A hidden layer is used to extract properties, and a fully connected layer is used for processing to complete the classification task. Unlike traditional neural networks, the hidden layers of CNNs possess a special shape of features. Each neural network layer typically consists of nodes linked to all layers above it. The neural network's nodes act as independent layers. A CNN has nearly invisible layers. Only a small portion of the neurons in each layer are linked to the neurons in the layer above them. Moreover, an additional pooling layer combining outputs from neighboring neurons into one value gives us a translation-invariant feature. This simplifies training and decreases model complexity [6].

11.3.3 Dataset

We used a public dataset from Kaggle [7] to categorize skin cancer. We trained on 1,000 photos of size 192x256 and validated on 200 images, with equal distribution between training and validation sets (see Figure 11.2).

11.3.4 System Architecture

This architecture applies preprocessing techniques to a collection of skin cancer melanoma segmentation datasets from Kaggle [7], which include resizing images, removing noise, and converting to grayscale. The data is preprocessed and then passed to U-Net for training the model taken from the dataset. The U-Net segmentation method is applied to the skin cancer dataset. Three steps are involved in data augmentation: training the original image, rotating it, and mirroring it. Accuracy is improved when data is expanded from multiple perspectives. Image segmentation can classify a dataset, as seen in Figure 11.3. The CNN algorithm can be used to identify skin features and cancer types. The accuracy of the provided input is then determined [8].

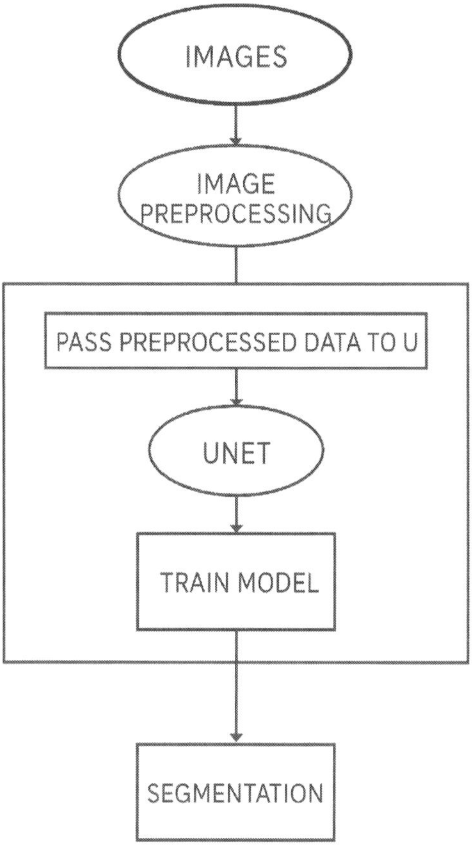

FIGURE 11.3 Architecture of preprocessing.

11.4 RESULTS AND DISCUSSIONS

This section displays the results. Graphs of classifier loss versus epoch and accuracy versus epoch were generated. The original image from the datasets was used to train a U-Net model, which was then built. We applied various segmentation methods to skin cancer datasets. This allowed us to visualize the actual and predicted output in masks. Ultimately, we could identify skin cancer from the original image in exact and anticipated sections. Figures 11.4–11.6 show our predicted mask. Figures 11.7–11.10 show the difference between U-Net vs. CNN in loss vs. epoch and accuracy vs. epoch; U-Net shows better results when compared.

Reporting the percentage of correctly categorized pixels in the image is valuable for evaluating semantic segmentation. Each class's pixel accuracy and the combined accuracy across every class can be reported. In assessing the unit-class pixel accuracy, we take a binary mask into account. A pixel correctly predicted to belong to the specific class is considered a true positive (as indicated by the target mask). A pixel accurately detected as not belonging to the same class is referred to as a true negative.

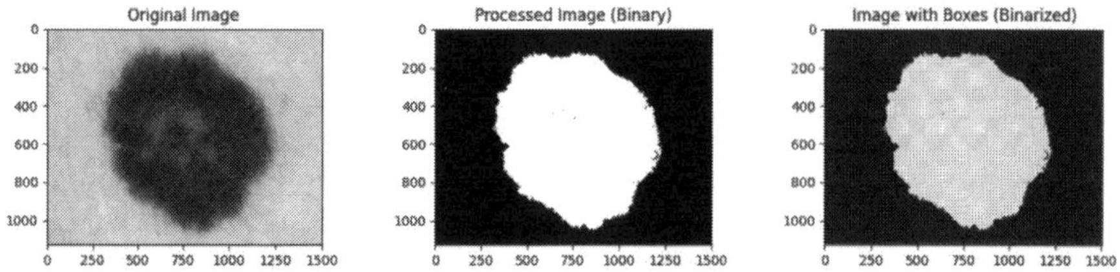

FIGURE 11.4 Result 1.

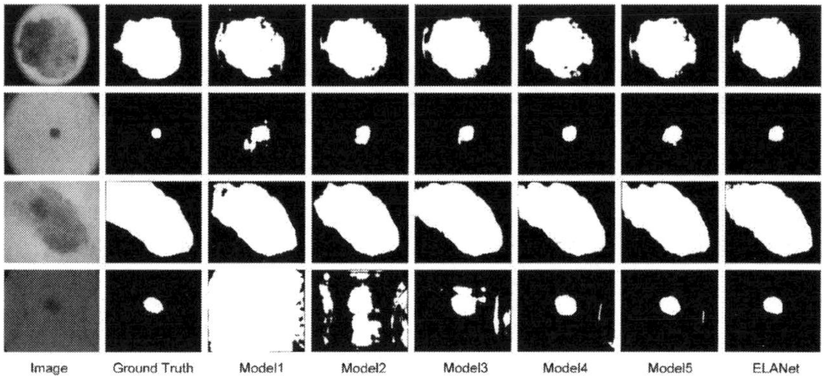

FIGURE 11.5 Result 2.

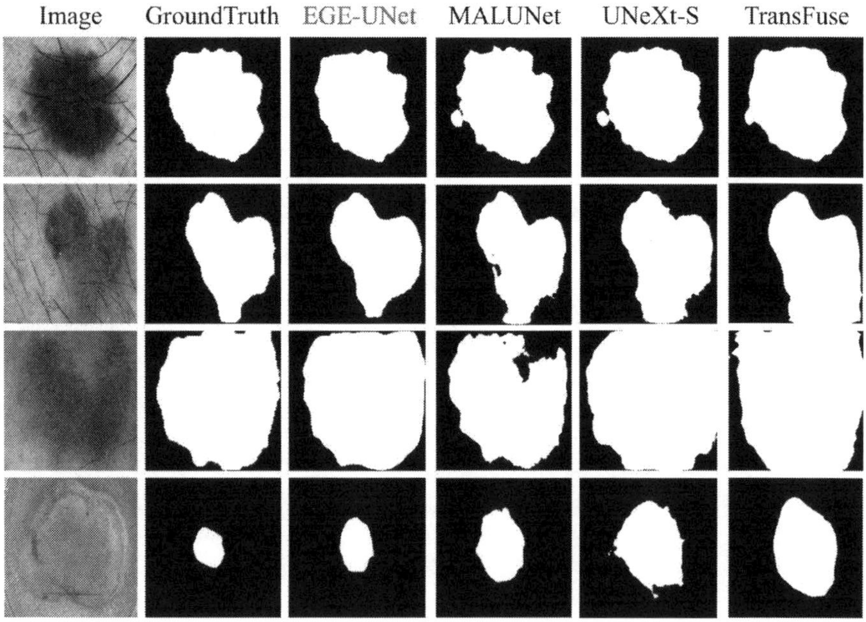

FIGURE 11.6 Result 3.

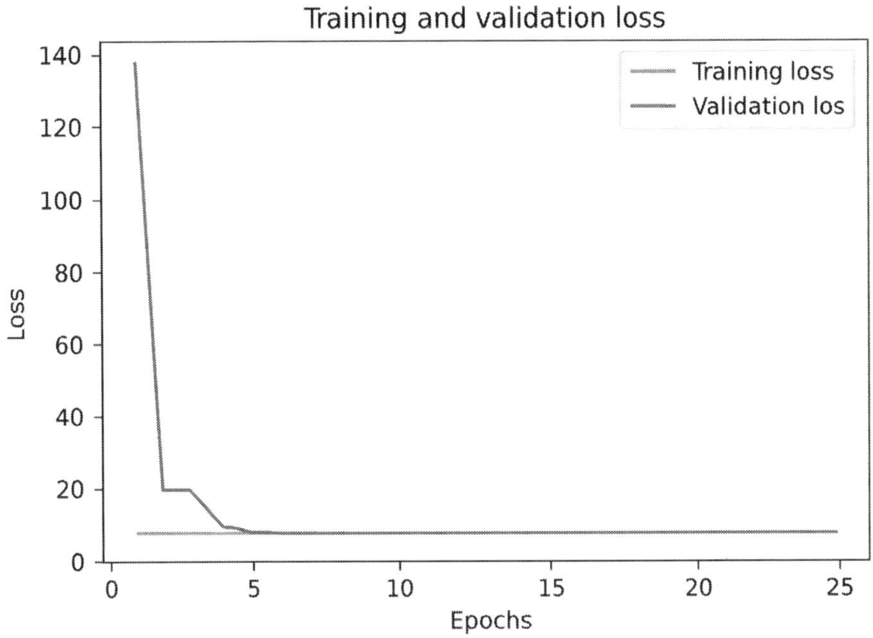

FIGURE 11.7 Loss vs. epoch.

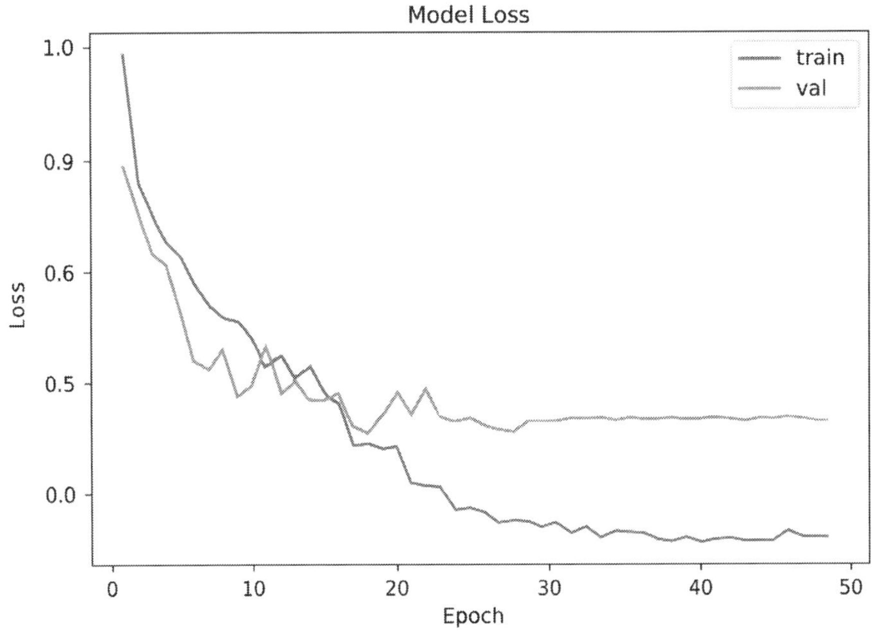

FIGURE 11.8 Loss vs. epoch (CNN) [10].

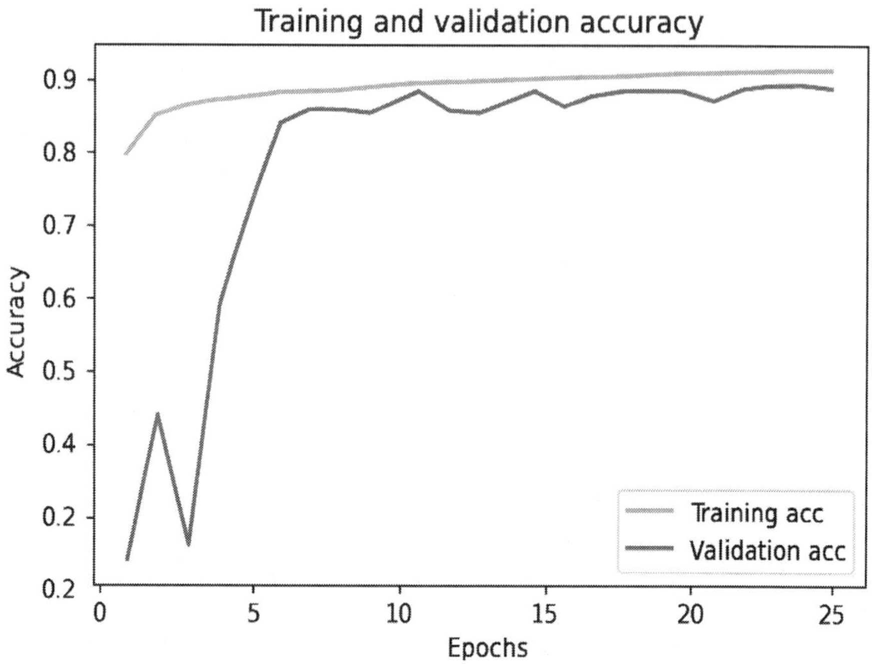

FIGURE 11.9 Accuracy vs. epoch.

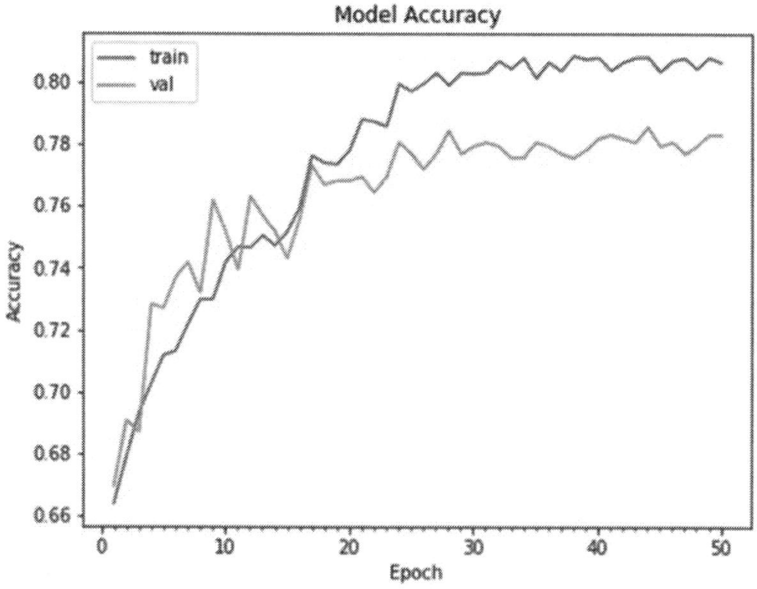

FIGURE 11.10 Accuracy vs. epoch (CNN) [10].

TABLE 11.1
Accuracy and Mean-IoU

Train Size	Accuracy	Jacard Index
1,000	92.82	80.65

$$\text{Accuracy} = \frac{\text{TP} + \text{FN}}{\text{TP} + \text{TN} + \text{FP} + \text{FN}} \tag{11.1}$$

The Jaccard similarity coefficient, commonly called the Jaccard similarity index, measures the similarity of two data sets. Higher percentages denote a more homogeneous population. The similarity index range is 0%–100%. However, this index could not be reliable without unobserved variables or a small sample size (Table 11.1).

$$J(A,B) = \frac{|A \cap B|}{|A \cup B|} \tag{11.2}$$

11.5 CONCLUSION

Automated analysis of dermoscopy images assists dermatologists in making clinical decisions and patients in assessing skin lesions remotely. We must first separate the lesion sites from normal areas to perform this automated analysis. This paper proposes a method using the U-Net architecture for segmentation. The preprocessed images yielded good Jacquard similarity coefficients during this segmentation process.

FUTURE WORKS

This paper is limited by the size of the datasets we use. Few authoritative datasets of free skin type data are available for research and development. Potential applications of this study include incorporating the model into automated diagnostic software to improve the accuracy of dermatologists and oncologists or using online learning to improve continuously. This may involve creating a model to be used.

REFERENCES

1. S. Alkhushayni, D. Al-zaleq, L. Andradi, and P. Flynn, The application of differing machine learning algorithms and their related performance in detecting skin cancers and melanomas. *Journal of Skin Cancer*, vol. 2022, Article ID 2839162, 2022.
2. H. Ganster, P. Pinz, R. Rohrer, E. Wildling, M. Binder, and H. Kittler, Automated melanoma recognition. *IEEE Transactions on Medical Imaging*, vol. 20, no. 3, pp. 233239, 2001.
3. P. Dubal, S. Bhatt, C. Joglekar, and S. Patil, Skin cancer detection and classification. *2017 6th International Conference on Electrical Engineering and Informatics (ICEEI)*, Langkawi, Kedah, Malaysia, 2017.

4. M. ur Rehman, S. H. Khan, S. D. Rizvi, Z. Abbas, and A. Zafar, Classification of skin lesion by interference of segmentation and convolotion neural network. *2018 2nd International Conference on Engineering Innovation (ICEI)*, 2018. Bangkok, Thailand, IEEE.
5. C. Szegedy, V. Vanhoucke, S. Ioffe, J. Shlens, and Z. Wojna, Rethinking the inception architecture for computer vision. *Proceedings of the IEEE Conference on Computer Vision and Pattern Recognition* (pp. 2818–2826), Nevada, USA, 2015.
6. K. He, G. Gkioxari, P. Dollr, and R. Girshick, Mask R-CNN[J]. 2017: 2980–298.
7. https://www.kaggle.com/datasets/surajghuwalewala/ham1000-segmentation-and-classification
8. G. B. Regular and P. R. Deshmukh, Extraction of texture features using Euclidean, Canberra and both distance. *International Journal of Advanced Research in Computer Science*, vol. 2, no. 3, pp. 228–234, 2011. ISSN 0976-5697.
9. O. Ronneberger, P. Fischer, and T. Brox, U-Net: Convolutional networks for biomedical image segmentation. *International Conference on Medical Image Computing and Computer-Assisted Intervention* (pp. 234–241). Cham: Springer International Publishing.
10. A. A. Nugroho, I. Slamet, and Sugiyanto, Skin cancer identification system of HAM10000 Skin cancer dataset using CNN. *AIP Conference Proceedings* (vol. 2202, p. 020039), 2019.

12 Revolutionizing Heart Disease Diagnosis Using Machine Learning

A Case Study in Data-Driven Healthcare

Sonali P. Kadam, Vinaya D. Kulkarni, Sanah Naik, Suruchi Bibikar, Sakshi Pratap, Ankita Ochani, Madhavi P. Mahajan, and Jotiram G. Gujar

12.1 INTRODUCTION

Machine learning (ML) constitutes a facet of artificial intelligence (AI), centering on the creation of algorithms and statistical models. These models empower computer systems to execute tasks without the need for explicit programming. In other words, ML allows computers to learn from data and improve their performance on a specific task over time, without human intervention. The core idea behind ML is to enable computers to recognize patterns, make predictions, and make decisions based on data, ultimately enhancing their ability to perform specific tasks. In the realm of ML, this acquisition of knowledge typically presents itself through alterations to the operational dynamics of an algorithm. By examining a collection of photos of various people, an ML system may be able to detect faces. The primary divisions within the field of ML encompass unsupervised and supervised learning paradigms, representing two fundamental branches of the discipline. Similar to their applications in business and e-commerce, AI and ML have found myriad applications within the healthcare sector. It is one of the biggest sectors in the world that stands to gain from this technology. Over the past century, there has been a dramatic improvement in the average life expectancy due to technical improvements. Despite the remarkable strides in technological advancement in recent years, the emerging breakthroughs in AI and ML herald a resurgence in the medical domain. Of course, even the smallest and least important components of any operation can be nearly perfected using computers. Although ML is already used in healthcare, there is still a lot of room for growth in this area. Modern technologies have always had the steadfast support of the healthcare sector. The potential applications of this technology are virtually limitless. Through its innovative applications, ML is playing a pivotal role in advancing the healthcare sector. The integration of ML is particularly advantageous in

DOI: 10.1201/9781003479185-12

healthcare systems that have already embraced big data tools for next-generation data analytics, driven in part by mandated processes such as electronic medical records (EMRs). The utilization of ML tools further amplifies the benefits derived from these advancements. These enhancements contribute to elevating the standard of automation and facilitating intelligent decision-making in both public healthcare systems and primary/tertiary patient care. The profound impact of ML tools on improving the lives of billions of people worldwide underscores their potential as a transformative force in healthcare [1].

The realm of research, particularly in the context of clinical trials, stands out as another beneficiary of ML advancements. Given the prohibitive costs and extended durations associated with clinical trials, researchers can leverage ML-based predictive analytics to streamline the identification of potential participants. This involves mining diverse data sources such as social media, previous doctor visits, and other relevant information to narrow down the pool of eligible candidates. Additionally, ML technologies facilitate real-time monitoring of trial participants, aiding in the determination of optimal sample sizes and mitigating database errors through the utilization of electronic records. ML technologies present a promising avenue for enhancing clinical trial research in several ways. By leveraging sophisticated predictive analytics on clinical trial applicants, medical professionals can evaluate a broader spectrum of data, thereby reducing costs and time associated with medical tests. By leveraging sophisticated predictive analytics on clinical trial applicants, medical professionals can evaluate a broader spectrum of data, thereby reducing costs and time associated with medical tests. ML applications contribute to improving clinical trial efficiency by tasks such as determining optimal sample sizes for increased efficacy and minimizing the likelihood of data errors when utilizing electronic health records (EHRs). This approach addresses a significant challenge in the healthcare field, given the increasing scarcity of well-trained radiologists on a global scale. Furthermore, ML's integration into the healthcare industry offers the advantage of enabling more dynamic and efficient individualized therapies by integrating personal health data with predictive analytics. Numerous potential applications of ML in research and clinical trials exist, including the use of ML-based predictive research to identify latent clinical trial participants. This approach allows researchers to draw from a multitude of data points, such as previous doctor visits and social media, facilitating real-time access to data and efficient management of trial participants. Additionally, it enables the investigation of the most appropriate sample size while leveraging the power of electronic processing, thereby contributing to the reduction of errors associated with data interpretation. ML algorithms, akin to highly skilled radiologists, exhibit the capability to discern abnormal skin patches, lesions, tumors, and detect instances of brain bleeding in imaging data. Consequently, the anticipated surge in the utilization of these platforms to support radiologists is poised to be substantial.

Electrocardiography (ECG) is a diagnostic technique in medicine that records the electrical activity of the heart over a period of time. Also known as an EKG (from the German "Elektrokardiogramm"), the procedure involves the placement of electrodes on the skin, typically in a specific configuration, to detect and amplify the electrical impulses generated by the heart during each cardiac cycle. The resulting graphical representation, known as an electrocardiogram, depicts the sequential depolarization and repolarization of the heart's chambers, providing valuable insights into cardiac rhythm, conduction abnormalities, and potential cardiac disorders. ECG is a fundamental tool in clinical cardiology, aiding healthcare professionals in the diagnosis, monitoring, and management of various cardiovascular conditions (CVDs). However, the presence of human error and the time-intensive manual interpretation of ECG data by healthcare professionals necessitate the development of automated ECG report analysis and anomaly detection systems [2]. Within the healthcare sector, ML, a subset of AI, has proven to be an efficacious tool for automating the processing of medical data, with a particular emphasis on ECG signals. ML algorithms exhibit the capability to rapidly and accurately process extensive volumes of ECG data, enabling early detection of anomalies and potentially life-threatening disorders. This underscores the pivotal role of ML in enhancing diagnostic capabilities and advancing healthcare practices. A growing body of research is investigating the impact of dietary factors and herbal remedies on preventing cardiovascular disease (CVD) and their potential therapeutic applications. This is in addition to the conventional management of cardiovascular risk factors by pharmacological experts and the utilization of antithrombotic medications. While much attention is focused on the potential cancer-preventive properties of certain nutrients and the cell-strengthening attributes of herbal substances, it is worth noting that some herbal materials may also influence regular cardiovascular risk factors or exhibit antithrombotic effects. A growing body of research is investigating the impact of dietary factors and herbal remedies on preventing CVD and their potential therapeutic applications. This is in addition to the conventional management of cardiovascular risk factors by pharmacological experts and the utilization of antithrombotic medications. While much attention is focused on the potential cancer-preventive properties of certain nutrients and the cell-strengthening attributes of herbal substances, it is worth noting that some herbal materials may also influence regular cardiovascular risk factors or exhibit antithrombotic effects [3–6].

The chapter delineates the contribution of the study as follows: it introduces a comprehensive classification of domains for ML applications in ECG, encompassing medical/healthcare, biometric/security, and driving applications. The research also identifies existing challenges. To provide a nuanced understanding, we conducted a detailed analysis focusing on ML techniques applied to ECG signals. This analysis spans various dimensions, including application domains, application areas, ML application tasks, ML models, model performances, and dataset sources. The critical overview serves a twofold purpose. Firstly, it aims to discern which types of ECG data have undergone thorough examination, offering insights into well-explored facets. Simultaneously, it sheds light on unexplored data collection situations for ECG data analysis. This taxonomy and metadata analysis collectively contribute to advancing the understanding of the current landscape, highlighting both achievements and areas ripe for future exploration in the integration of ML with ECG-based applications.

12.2 ECG: FROM DIAGNOSIS TO EVOLUTION AND APPLICATIONS

ECG, a medical diagnostic method, captures the heart's electrical activity over time. Also referred to as EKG, this procedure involves placing electrodes on the skin in a specific arrangement to detect and amplify the heart's electrical impulses during each cardiac cycle. The resulting ECG graphically illustrates the heart's depolarization and repolarization, offering insights into rhythm, conduction abnormalities, and potential cardiac disorders. Widely utilized in clinical cardiology, ECG is indispensable for healthcare professionals in diagnosing, monitoring, and managing diverse CVDs. This procedure plays a crucial role in providing valuable insights into cardiac health, facilitating the evaluation of various CVDs. Notably, ECG proves to be both noninvasive and cost-effective, establishing itself as a powerful diagnostic instrument for the identification of cardiac diseases, such as arrhythmias, through continuous monitoring. The signals extracted from ECG tests offer essential information to comprehend an individual's cardiac activity, encompassing parameters like heart rate, rhythm, and morphology [7]. Beyond these basic parameters, analyzing the time intervals involved in the passage of electrical surges through the heart provides further insights. This allows healthcare professionals to identify normal, slow, fast, or irregular electrical patterns, contributing significantly to the characterization of cardiac function. Furthermore, evaluating the magnitude of electrical surges assists in pinpointing potential abnormalities or expansions within specific areas of the cardiac muscle [8]. In summary, the versatility of ECG as a diagnostic tool, coupled with its noninvasive nature and cost-effectiveness, positions it as a cornerstone in the detection and monitoring of various cardiac conditions, playing a pivotal role in the overall assessment of cardiovascular health [9].

ECG stands as an indelible cornerstone in the management of individuals with confirmed or suspected CVDs, its historical significance rooted in its transformative role in diagnostics and beyond. Unlike other biological signals, the ECG provides a real-time, noninvasive snapshot of the heart's electrical activity, enabling physicians to diagnose and monitor a myriad of cardiac conditions. Its enduring importance lies in its versatility, extending far beyond conventional diagnostics. ECG has found innovative applications in biometric systems, contributing to identification and authentication processes. Furthermore, its integration into novel technologies has paved the way for applications such as detecting driver drowsiness and stress, potentially mitigating accident rates. Beyond diagnostics, ECG's utility encompasses predicting heart size and position, identifying abnormalities, and assessing medication effectiveness. This versatility underscores ECG as not only a dynamic and indispensable tool in clinical settings but also a pioneering force in healthcare and diverse domains. Its ongoing impact exemplifies how ECG continues to evolve, positioning itself at the forefront of advancements that transcend traditional medical boundaries.

The evolution of ECG traces its roots back to Galvani's frog leg experiments, progressing through subsequent advancements by Matteucci, Kolliker, Muller, and Gabriel Lippman with the capillary electrometer [10]. Willem Einthoven's contributions, particularly the introduction of the string galvanometer, marked a significant leap forward in the field of ECG [11]. Einthoven's innovations, including lead placement conventions and the conceptualization of "Einthoven's triangle," have had a lasting impact on modern ECG procedures. ECG signals, categorized as biosignals, have been the subject of extensive research, exhibiting the capability to detect nanosecond irregularities. ECG instruments record continuous electrical activity by placing noninvasive electrodes on the chest and limbs. The integration of ML in recent years has gained prominence in medical and healthcare operations, playing a pivotal role in automating the diagnosis of CVDs. This is particularly valuable in situations where expert medical interpretation may be limited. The historical trajectory from Galvani's experiments to Einthoven's innovations highlights the evolutionary path of ECG, underscoring its significance in understanding and diagnosing cardiac conditions. Furthermore, the synergy between ECG technology and modern ML applications represents a cutting-edge approach in enhancing the efficiency and accuracy of cardiovascular diagnostics, thereby contributing to advancements in medical science and patient care.

12.2.1 ECG Machines and Its Types

ECG machines serve as pivotal instruments in cardiovascular diagnostics, offering invaluable insights into the electrical activity of the heart. In the realm of academic discourse, it is essential to delineate the types of ECG machines with precision:

- **Single-Lead ECG Machines**: Employed for basic cardiac monitoring, these machines utilize a single lead to record electrical impulses from the heart. Suited for ambulatory settings and routine screenings due to their portability and simplicity.
- **12-Lead ECG Machines**: Widely recognized as the standard for clinical ECGs, 12-lead machines capture electrical signals from multiple perspectives, enabling comprehensive cardiac assessments [12]. Particularly instrumental in diagnosing myocardial infarctions (MI) and other complex cardiac conditions.
- **Portable and Handheld ECG Devices**: These compact machines offer on-the-go monitoring, catering to the evolving landscape of telemedicine and remote patient care. Facilitate real-time data acquisition and transmission for prompt medical intervention.
- **Exercise Stress ECG Machines:** Designed to assess cardiac function under exertion, these machines monitor ECG changes during physical activity. Integral in diagnosing conditions like ischemic heart disease and evaluating exercise tolerance.
- **Holter Monitors**: Holter monitors provide continuous ECG monitoring over an extended period, typically 24–48 hours, offering a comprehensive assessment of daily cardiac activity. Ideal for detecting intermittent arrhythmias and capturing elusive abnormalities [13].
- **Event Monitors**: Event monitors record ECG data intermittently, triggered by specific events or patient symptoms. Suited for extended monitoring periods, enabling the detection of infrequent cardiac events.

12.2.2 ECG Waves

The standard 12-lead ECG stands as a paramount noninvasive diagnostic instrument, offering crucial insights into cardiac function by meticulously recording the heart's electrical activity. These 12 leads, functioning as recording channels, strategically capture electrical signals from diverse perspectives, facilitating a comprehensive assessment of the heart's rhythm and conduction patterns. The placement of each lead involves affixing electrodes to specific locations on the chest. Lead II, often favored for its clarity of signal, is situated on the right wrist and left ankle, while the remaining leads—Lead I, Lead III, aVR, aVL, aVF, and V1–V6—are strategically positioned on various chest locations to capture electrical activity from distinct angles. The resting 12-lead ECG, typically executed in a supine position, serves as the gold standard for evaluating cardiac rhythm abnormalities [14]. However, for prolonged monitoring spanning hours, days, or more, devices like the Holter monitor provide a convenient and continuous assessment of heart activity. The configuration of the ECG system and lead placement is intricately tailored to the clinical context, ensuring a nuanced understanding of the heart's electrical behavior in diverse monitoring scenarios. This nuanced approach is critical for optimizing signal quality and obtaining relevant information for precise clinical diagnoses and monitoring.

ECG measurements encompass a spectrum of methods that cater to diverse clinical scenarios. The resting ECG, conducted while the patient is at rest, serves as the foundational measurement, offering baseline information on the heart's electrical activity and is commonly utilized for routine screenings. Exercise or stress ECG involves recording the heart's response to physical exertion or stress-inducing agents, aiding in the diagnosis of conditions like ischemic heart disease. Holter monitoring extends this evaluation, capturing the ECG continuously over 24–48 hours, detecting intermittent arrhythmias, and providing insights into daily cardiac activities. Ambulatory ECG monitoring takes a step further, spanning several days or weeks to offer a comprehensive assessment during the patient's routine activities. Signal-averaged ECG enhances sensitivity by averaging multiple cardiac cycles, particularly valuable for identifying subtle electrical changes associated with ventricular arrhythmias. Vectorcardiography represents the three-dimensional electrical activity of the heart, offering detailed insights, while telemonitoring ECG enables real-time remote monitoring, especially beneficial for continuous surveillance of chronic heart conditions. Event monitoring, relying on intermittent ECG recording triggered by the patient during symptomatic episodes, aids in correlating specific events with cardiac activity for diagnostic purposes [15]. The diverse categorizations underscore the adaptability of ECG measurements to various clinical contexts, ranging from routine examinations to specialized assessments and research applications. The choice of method depends on the specific clinical requirements and the nature of the cardiac condition under investigation.

Figure 12.1 illustrates an ECG waveform, a crucial representation of the heart's electrical activity. This intricate waveform, comprising five waves (PQRST), serves as a pivotal tool for deciphering the nuances of cardiac electrophysiology and holds immense diagnostic utility in identifying diverse heart disorders. The cardiac cycle

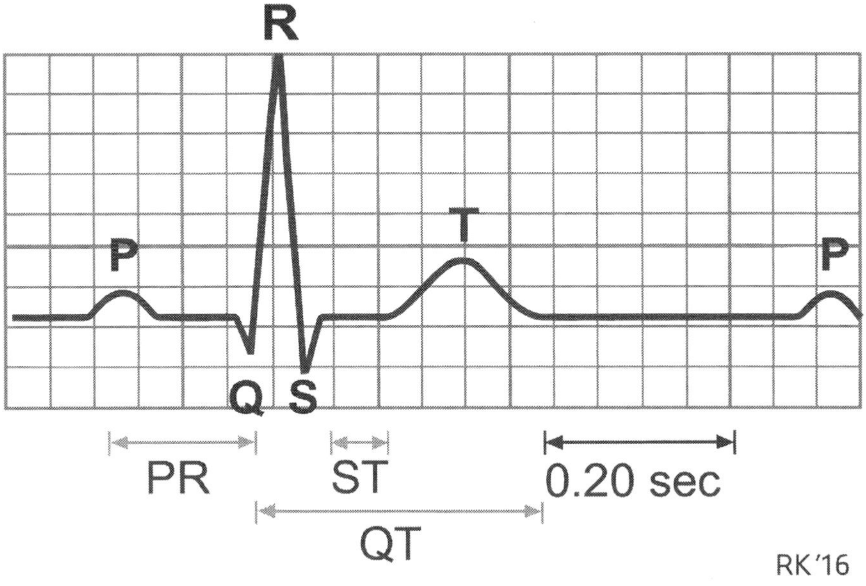

FIGURE 12.1 Electrocardiogram (ECG) signal, which comprises the PQRST waves. These waves, denoted as P, Q, R, S, and T, collectively form the characteristic waveform of the ECG [55].

begins with diastole, the relaxation and filling phase. At rest, both atria and ventricles are relaxed, and the tricuspid and mitral valves are open, permitting blood flow from the atria to the ventricles. Atrial systole ensues, with atrial contraction contributing to the final ventricular filling. Isovolumetric ventricular contraction, marked by closed valves, initiates ventricular systole. Ventricular ejection follows, with the opening of the semilunar valves allowing blood expulsion into the pulmonary artery and aorta. Semilunar valve closure commences isovolumetric ventricular relaxation. The cardiac cycle concludes with ventricular diastole, with ventricular relaxation and passive filling with blood returning from the atria. This orchestrated sequence, reflected in the ECG waveform, ensures efficient blood circulation throughout the body, vital for sustaining physiological functions. The nuanced phases of the cardiac cycle underscore the intricate nature of heart function and its pivotal role in maintaining circulatory homeostasis. The ECG waveform in Figure 12.1 depicts a normal sinus rhythm, with all five waves (PQRST) clearly visible. The P wave represents atrial depolarization, the PR interval represents atrial–ventricular conduction time, the QRS complex represents ventricular depolarization, the ST segment represents ventricular repolarization, and the T wave represents completion of ventricular repolarization. The normal durations of these intervals are important for assessing the heart's rhythm and conduction patterns. Deviations from the normal durations of these intervals can indicate potential heart pathologies, such as heart blockages, arrhythmias, and electrolyte imbalances. For example, a prolonged PR interval may suggest a delay in atrioventricular conduction, while a shortened QT interval may be associated with an increased risk of arrhythmias. The ECG waveform is a valuable tool for the diagnosis and evaluation of heart disease. It is a simple, noninvasive procedure that can provide important information about the health of the heart [16,17].

12.2.3 Quantification of ECG Waveforms and Diagnostic Assessment

The assessment of a standard ECG signal involves a comprehensive analysis of the electrical impulses generated by the heart. These impulses are represented by a series of waves on the ECG tracing, with each wave corresponding to a specific cardiac event. The critical analysis of intervals between these waves provides valuable insights into the heart's rhythm and conduction patterns. The P wave represents the depolarization of the atrial chambers, while the PR interval represents the time it takes for the electrical impulse to travel from the atria to the ventricles. The QRS complex represents the ventricular depolarization, and the ST segment reflects the repolarization of the ventricles [18]. Finally, the QT interval represents the total time from the beginning of the QRS complex to the end of the T wave. Deviations from the normal durations of these intervals can indicate potential heart pathologies, such as heart blockages and arrhythmias. For instance, a prolonged PR interval can suggest a delay in the conduction of the electrical impulse from the atria to the ventricles, while a shortened QT interval can be associated with an increased risk of arrhythmias.

An arrhythmia is any deviation from the normal sequence of electrical impulses in the heart. Arrhythmias can be classified based on their origin (atrial or ventricular) and their rate (fast or slow). Common types of arrhythmias include bradycardia (slow heart rate), supraventricular tachycardia (fast heart rate originating from the atria), atrial fibrillation (AF) (chaotic atrial rhythm), atrial flutter (rapidly firing atria), ventricular tachycardia (fast heart rate originating from the ventricles), AV heart blocks (impaired conduction between the atria and ventricles), bundle branch blocks (impaired conduction within the ventricles), and tachy-brady syndrome (alternating periods of fast and slow heart rates). Symptoms associated with arrhythmias can include fainting, dizziness, weakness, chest pain, or in some cases, may be asymptomatic [19].

The examination of ECG strips is mostly done my human beings, which can many times be very time-consuming and can be wrong at times as well. ML has emerged as a promising alternative, offering the potential to automate the identification and analysis of features within raw ECG data. ML algorithms can be trained on large datasets of ECG signals and corresponding diagnoses to learn the patterns associated with various heart pathologies. This enables them to automatically classify ECG recordings with high accuracy, significantly reducing the time and effort required for manual interpretation. The application of ML in ECG analysis is particularly beneficial in settings where fatigue-induced human errors are a concern, such as in emergency departments or during long-term monitoring [8]. Additionally, ML algorithms can continuously learn and improve their performance as more data becomes available, further enhancing their diagnostic capabilities. Beyond ECG, ML has also been successfully employed in diagnostic modalities such as chest X-rays. For instance, ML algorithms have been trained to identify respiratory infectious diseases, including COVID-19, from chest X-rays with high accuracy. This demonstrates the broader applicability of ML in the field of medical diagnostics and its potential to uncover nuanced relationships between different health conditions.

The unexpected connection between COVID-19 and heart injury highlights the potential of ML to uncover new insights into disease processes. While COVID-19 is primarily a respiratory illness, it has been shown to have a significant impact on the cardiovascular system, increasing the risk of arrhythmias, heart failure, and other cardiac complications. ML algorithms can be used to analyze large datasets of patient records to identify patterns in cardiac complications associated with COVID-19, potentially leading to improved diagnostic and treatment strategies [20]. In conclusion, ML has emerged as a powerful tool for analyzing medical data, offering the potential to automate diagnostic processes, enhance accuracy, and uncover new insights into disease mechanisms. The successful application of ML in ECG analysis and chest X-rays demonstrates its broad applicability in medical imaging and its potential to revolutionize the field of medical diagnostics.

12.3 EVOLUTION OF MACHINE LEARNING

The scholarly exploration of computational algorithms endowed with the capacity to discern intricate relationships or patterns from empirical data and subsequently make precise decisions is denoted as ML. In contrast to conventional programming paradigms, where explicit sets of instructions dictate task execution, the ML paradigm involves the "training" of machines through exposure to vast datasets and algorithms that equip them with the capability to autonomously acquire task proficiency. Unlike conventional algorithms, in the realm of ML, data itself functions as the conduit for instructing the machine about the optimal outcomes, thereby engendering a learning process devoid of explicit programming directives. ML problems are categorically classified into supervised or unsupervised learning, each delineating distinct modes of algorithmic assimilation and decision-making.

ML serves as an autonomous learning mechanism, enabling machines to derive insights and make informed decisions without explicit programming. The crux of ML lies in the utilization of sophisticated algorithms and statistical methodologies to analyze data and predict outcomes, deviating from rule-based systems. The pivotal determinant of ML accuracy resides in the quality of the dataset employed for prediction, with a direct correlation between data relevance and prediction precision. This attribute renders ML applicable across diverse sectors, including finance, retail, and healthcare, where its continuous refinement capabilities enhance accuracy in predicting and classifying diseases. The predictive model iteratively refines its decision-making process as it assimilates increasing volumes of data, thereby embodying a perpetual pursuit of precision. In the healthcare domain, patient datasets encapsulated within electronic healthcare records provide a fertile ground for leveraging ML techniques, facilitating the extraction of pertinent information [21]. The trajectory of ML's evolution is characterized by distinct phases marked by advancements in algorithms, heightened data accessibility, increased computing power, and collaborative interdisciplinary efforts. A nuanced comprehension of this historical context is imperative for a comprehensive understanding of the current state of ML and the ability to anticipate forthcoming developments in this transformative technology.

The inception of ML traces its origins to the mid-20th century, an era marked by trailblazers such as Alan Turing, who laid the foundational principles for AI. Early strides in learning algorithms, exemplified by Frank Rosenblatt's perceptron, heralded the advent of supervised learning. However, advancements were impeded by computational limitations and the scarcity of extensive labeled datasets. The subsequent decades, spanning the 1970s and 1980s, witnessed the ascendancy of symbolic AI and expert systems, characterized by rule-based methodologies designed to encapsulate human expertise within explicit rules. Although effective in certain domains, these approaches grappled with the intricacies and uncertainties inherent in real-world data, emphasizing the imperative for more adaptable, data-driven strategies. The latter part of the 20th century witnessed a transformative shift toward statistical learning methods, accentuating probabilistic models and Bayesian techniques. Notable milestones included the introduction of support vector machines (SVMs) and decision trees, signifying substantive progress in the realm of classification tasks. Despite these advancements, challenges persisted, notably the reliance on manually crafted features and the formidable obstacles associated with scaling to voluminous datasets. This historical narrative underscores the iterative evolution of ML paradigms, each era marking a progression toward more sophisticated and versatile methodologies.

The onset of the 21st century marked a transformative epoch characterized by the proliferation of big data and the renaissance of neural networks. The surge in available labeled data, coupled with advancements in graphical processing units (GPUs), facilitated the training of deep neural networks (DNNs). Pivotal breakthroughs, exemplified by the architecture of AlexNet in image classification and the efficacy of recurrent neural networks (RNNs) in natural language processing, ignited a renewed fascination with neural network-based methodologies. In this milieu, deep learning (DL) ascended as a preeminent paradigm, harnessing the potential of DNNs to autonomously extract hierarchical representations from raw data. Convolutional neural networks (CNNs), notably, exhibited unprecedented efficacy in tasks such as image recognition, precipitating advancements in realms like computer vision. The advent of transfer learning and pretrained models further expedited progress, empowering the transference of acquired knowledge from one task to another. This period witnessed the evolution of ML beyond the confines of supervised and unsupervised learning, embracing novel paradigms such as reinforcement learning and generative models. Reinforcement learning algorithms, typified by deep Q-networks, attained remarkable success, particularly in gaming environments, showcasing the versatility and potency of these contemporary methodologies.

Generative models, exemplified by generative adversarial networks (GANs), have demonstrated a remarkable capacity to produce authentic synthetic data, opening avenues for innovative applications in image synthesis, style transfer, and beyond. The maturation of ML has been concomitant with heightened interdisciplinary collaboration, amalgamating expertise from diverse realms, such as computer science, statistics, neuroscience, and domain-specific fields [22]. Moreover, there has been a concerted effort to address concerns regarding the interpretability and explainability of ML models, particularly in domains where decisions bear significant consequences on human lives, such as healthcare and finance. The trajectory of ML's evolution unfolds as a narrative of continuous innovation, propelled by advancements in algorithms, augmented computational capabilities, and the abundance of expansive and heterogeneous datasets. As ML continues to sculpt our technological landscape, the ongoing pursuit of research and collaborative initiatives spanning multiple disciplines holds the promise of unveiling novel frontiers. This ensures the enduring evolution of ML and its pervasive impact on society, cementing its role as a dynamic and transformative force.

12.4 SYSTEMATIC LITERATURE REVIEW

At the heart of any research endeavor lies the necessity for a comprehensive literature review. This meticulous process serves as the foundation upon which new knowledge is built, ensuring that future advancements are firmly rooted in the accumulated wisdom of the past. By delving into the existing body of literature, researchers can align their work with the current state of understanding, identify gaps and missing links, and critically evaluate existing research methodologies and findings. A systematic literature review (SLR) emerges as a rigorous method for conducting a comprehensive literature review. Embracing evidence-based practices, the SLR framework seeks to achieve a thorough comprehension of the problem domain, laying the groundwork for informed decision-making and the development of innovative solutions [23]. Adhering to the guidelines established by Kitchenham and Charters, the execution of an SLR unfolds in three distinct phases: strategic planning, systematic execution, and comprehensive reporting. The strategic planning phase meticulously defines the research scope, formulating clear objectives and establishing a search strategy that encompasses relevant databases, keywords, and selection criteria. The systematic execution phase meticulously applies the defined search strategy, yielding a collection of relevant literature. This trove of information is then subjected to rigorous screening and quality assessment, ensuring that only studies of sufficient methodological rigor and relevance are included in the review [24]. Finally, the comprehensive reporting phase meticulously synthesizes the findings of the included studies, providing a structured narrative that highlights key themes, identifies consensus and conflicting views, and delineates gaps in the existing body of knowledge. In conclusion, the comprehensive literature review, particularly the SLR methodology, stands as an indispensable tool for researchers in the field of software engineering. By aligning existing knowledge with the goal of understanding, condensing, scrutinizing, and integrating a body of interconnected literature, the SLR enables researchers to make informed decisions, identify areas for future research, and contribute meaningfully to the advancement of the field (Table 12.1).

12.4.1 Detailed Analysis

This comprehensive review critically examines eight significant studies that employ advanced DL methodologies for ECG signal processing and arrhythmia detection. An approach for DL in arrhythmia detection was presented by Syarif I. *et al.* at the 2017 International Electronics Symposium on Knowledge Creation and Intelligent Computing (IES-KCIC) [18]. Unfortunately, the absence of detailed information

TABLE 12.1
A Comprehensive Overview of Machine Learning (ML) Applications in Electrocardiography (ECG)

Application Task	Models Used	Dataset	Operational Effectiveness	Limitations	References
Arrhythmia detection	GA + DL, PSO + DL	The UCI Machine Learning Repository comprises a dataset comprising 452 samples.	The accuracy rates achieved are 76.51% for the particle swarm optimization (PSO) method and 74.44% for the genetic algorithm (GA).	When compared to other signal types, normal sample data is substantially greater.	[18]
Arrhythmia classification	DNN	The Massachusetts Institute of Technology-Beth Israel Deaconess Medical Center Arrhythmia Database (MITDB) comprises a dataset encompassing 16 individual entries	Acc = 98.07%	A constrained quantity of training and testing datasets.	[25]
Arrhythmia detection	DNN	The Massachusetts Institute of Technology-Beth Israel Deaconess Medical Center Arrhythmia Database (MITDB) encompasses a dataset comprising 80,836 electrocardiogram (ECG) beats.	Acc = 99.41% Sen = 96.08%	More data is needed for training.	[26]
ECG heartbeat classification	Temporal feature extraction + DNN	Dataset from the Massachusetts Institute of Technology containing records from 47 subjects.	Acc = 100% Spe = 99.83% Sen = 99.48% Acc = 99.68%	• Intensive involvement of specialists in annotating electrocardiogram (ECG) beats. • The classification of ECG is constrained to a simple binary categorization of normal versus abnormal.	[27]

(Continued)

TABLE 12.1 (*Continued*)
A Comprehensive Overview of Machine Learning (ML) Applications in Electrocardiography (ECG)

Application Task	Models Used	Dataset	Operational Effectiveness	Limitations	References
Arrhythmia classification	FDR + DNN	The dataset on cardiovascular arrhythmia at the University of California, Irvine (UCI) comprises 245 samples characterized as normal, and 206 samples categorized as abnormal.	Acc = 82.96% (FDR + DNN)	• Inadequate sample size and data imbalance	[28]
ECG classification	DNN	Dataset from the Massachusetts Institute of Technology containing records from 47 subjects.	Classifiers tailored for individual patients, with and without the assistance of experts, are presented in parentheses. Sensitivity (Sen): 66.2% (61.4%) Specificity (Spe): 98.6% (98.3%)	• Training requires a huge dataset.	[29]
Detection of AF	DDNN	The data utilized in this research is sourced from wearable electrocardiogram (ECG) devices involved in the China Physiological Signal (CPS) Challenge 2018. It includes information from 11,994 unique individuals and is derived from the Chinese PLA General Hospital.	Accuracy (Acc): 99.35% with a standard deviation of 0.26%, Sensitivity (Sen): 99.19% with a standard deviation of 0.31%, Specificity (Spe): 99.44% with a standard deviation of 0.17%, F1-score: 90.7%.	The detection process exclusively identifies atrial fibrillation (AF) owing to a scarcity of data pertaining to other cardiac categories. • The observed impact of age on AF detection manifests as negative; further verification is warranted.	[30]
Prenatal detection of CHD	DNN	A proprietary dataset encompassing fetal electrocardiogram (ECG) recordings obtained from six distinct medical institutions, inclusive of 266 individuals with a clean bill of health and 120 individuals diagnosed	Acc = 76%.	• There was limited population in the study.	[31]

Where "Acc" denotes Accuracy, "Spe" represents Specificity, "Sen" indicates Sensitivity, "Pre" signifies Precision, and "Ppr" stands for Positive Productivity regarding the algorithm's architecture, performance metrics, and the dataset used limits a thorough understanding of the study's intricacies. A DNN-based, advanced arrhythmia classification system was presented by Chae M. *et al.* at the Eleventh International Conference on Ubiquitous and Future Networks (ICUFN). Although the study's accuracy of 98.07% is excellent, a thorough evaluation is hampered by the absence of information on the dataset used and a discussion of the shortcomings or potential future directions of the suggested method [25].

In their 2016 presentation at the IEEE International Conference on Machine Learning and Applications (ICMLA), Park *et al.* [26] concentrated on the use of DNNs for the identification of premature ventricular contraction (PVC) beats. Despite the potential of their approach, the absence of comprehensive details on the dataset, model architecture, and performance metrics impedes a thorough assessment of their contributions. Sannino and De Pietro proposed a DL approach for ECG-based heartbeat classification for arrhythmia detection, a study published in future generation computer systems. While their model achieved commendable accuracy, sensitivity, and specificity metrics, a detailed discussion on the employed dataset and explicit insights into limitations is regrettably missing [27]. In a study published at an IEEE conference, Mak *et al.* compared DNNs to SVMs for the classification of ECG arrhythmias, and Cheung *et al.* presented an end-to-end ECG classification model utilizing both DNNs and raw signal extraction. Even if their findings may be significant, a detailed comprehension of their contributions is limited due to the absence of detailed information about the datasets and a thorough evaluation of their limitations [28,29].

Chen *et al.* addressed accurate AF detection using a DNN, achieving robust performance metrics exceeding 99%. The dataset utilized comprised sources such as the China Physiological Signal (CPS) Challenge 2018, the Chinese PLA General Hospital, and CardioCloud Medical Technology, featuring 11,994 unique subjects [30]. However, despite the remarkable accuracy, the study does not explicitly detail limitations or offer insights into future directions for further exploration. Vullings proposed a model for fetal ECG and DL for prenatal detection of congenital heart disease (CHD), presenting the work at the 2019 Computing in Cardiology (CinC). The study achieved a commendable accuracy rate of 76%, utilizing a private dataset containing fetal ECG measurements [31]. Unfortunately, specific details regarding limitations and potential future directions for the proposed model are not explicitly outlined. Collectively, while these studies underscore the growing influence of DL in ECG analysis, there exists a discernible need for more comprehensive reporting of methodologies, datasets, and critical reflections on limitations and future avenues to guide subsequent research endeavors in this dynamic and crucial field.

12.5 DOMAIN ANALYSIS

The presented bar graph (Figure 12.2) delineates the dynamic trends in sales pertaining to journals, books, and papers spanning the temporal range from 2013 to 2022. Remarkably, the sales trajectory of journals exhibits a consistent upward inclination, marking a substantial ascent from 14,000 units in 2013 to 18,000 units in

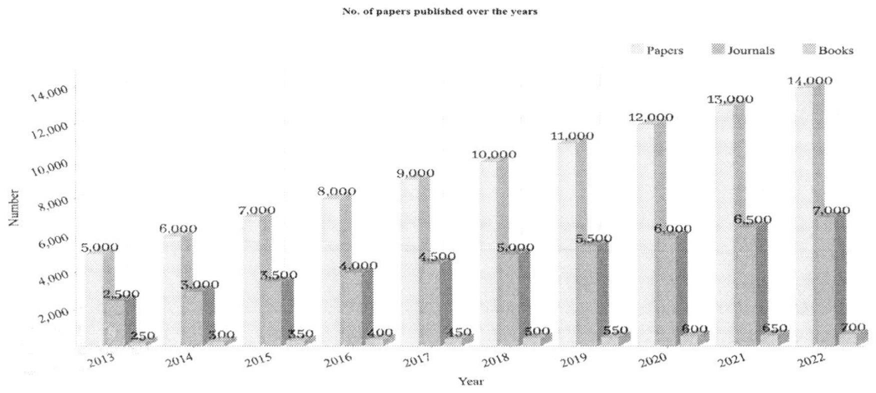

FIGURE 12.2 The distributional dynamics of papers within databases across the temporal continuum, spanning the years from 2013 to 2022, with an explicit depiction of the respective types of publication.

2022. In tandem, book sales have undergone growth, albeit at a more measured pace, progressing from 13,000 units in 2013 to 16,000 units in 2022. Conversely, paper sales have experienced a marginal decline, diminishing from 12,000 units in 2013 to 11,000 units in 2022. The observed trends in the line chart prompt consideration of several plausible explanations.

The burgeoning popularity of e-books emerges as a potential influence on the decline in paper book sales. However, the simultaneous upswing in journal sales suggests that e-books alone cannot comprehensively account for the entire trend. Another conceivable catalyst is the escalating prevalence of social media and other online information sources, potentially diminishing the demand for both traditional books and papers. Nevertheless, the sustained growth in journal sales contradicts the notion that this is the exclusive driver of the observed trends. Furthermore, the intensifying specialization of research may be contributing to the decline in sales of books and papers that encompass a broad spectrum of topics, indicating a discernible inclination toward materials aligned with specific individual interests.

This growth is being driven by a number of factors, including the increasing availability of large datasets of ECG data, the development of more sophisticated ML algorithms, and the growing interest in wearable devices and remote health monitoring. ML algorithms have been shown to be very effective at extracting meaningful information from ECG data, which can be used to diagnose heart diseases and arrhythmias more accurately. For example, ML algorithms can be used to automatically detect and classify different types of heartbeats, such as normal beats, arrhythmias, and PVCs. This can help clinicians to diagnose heart disease more quickly and efficiently. ML algorithms can also be used to develop personalized risk models for heart disease. These models can be used to identify patients who are at high risk of developing heart disease, so that they can be monitored more closely and treated early on. In addition, ML algorithms are being used to develop new wearable devices and remote health monitoring systems that can continuously collect and analyze

ECG data from patients. This can help clinicians to identify potential health problems early on, before they cause symptoms. Overall, it provides a strong evidence of the significant advancements that have been made in the use of ML for ECG analysis and diagnosis in recent years. This research is leading to the development of new and innovative tools and technologies that can help to improve the quality of care for patients with heart disease.

12.6 REVIEWS OF PREVIOUS SURVEYS

In a meticulous exploration of the use of ML for the detection of CVDs through the analysis of ECG signals, numerous studies conducted by various authors contribute noteworthy insights into diverse methodologies and their implications. The study by Pham, Egorov, Kazakov, and Budennyy, titled "Machine Learning-Based Decision Making," systematically scrutinizes ML models on PhysioNet/CinC challenge datasets, with a specific focus on Poincaré representation learning-based classifiers and one-dimensional convolutional models. Despite conscientiously acknowledging inherent limitations in the datasets and the potential for biases, the authors underscore the promising facets of accuracy and computational efficiency. They advocate for future research endeavors to address challenges posed by noise, artifacts, and the analysis of multi-lead ECG signals. Furthermore, the authors recommend extensions of these methodologies to encompass other biosignals, such as electroencephalography (EEG) and electromyography (EMG). Similarly, Behadada, Ozbay, and Karlik propose a fuzzy decision tree-based classifier for cardiac arrhythmia detection in children, placing emphasis on the PhysioNet/AAMI cardiac arrhythmia detection challenge database. Despite the proposed classifier's accuracy and interpretability, the authors acknowledge constraints associated with a single ECG signal and specific fuzzy partitions. In light of these constraints, they advocate for advancements in model performance and reliability, urging extensions of the approach to incorporate additional biosignals, such as EEG and EMG.

In a comprehensive investigation conducted in 2014 by C.K. and Hubert, a novel convolutional neural network-long short-term memory (CNN-LSTM) algorithm is introduced for the precise detection of ST segments in ECG signals, with a pronounced emphasis on both accuracy and computational efficiency. The study, which demonstrates success on the PhysioNet/CinC challenge datasets, conscientiously acknowledges potential biases and urges cautious considerations when generalizing findings to real-world scenarios, particularly in the context of multi-lead ECG signals. The authors outline future directions that involve the refinement of ECG classification methodologies through DL approaches and the extension of these methodologies to encompass a broader spectrum of biosignals. Contributing further to the discourse, Nasiri, Naghibzadeh, Sadoghi Yazdi, and Naghibzadeh propose an ECG arrhythmia classification approach utilizing SVMs and genetic algorithms (GAs). Evaluated on the MIT-BIH arrhythmia database, this method demonstrates promising results, achieving a noteworthy accuracy of 93% in classifying four distinct arrhythmia types. The study acknowledges potential biases and limitations, particularly in the evaluation of multi-lead ECG signals, while suggesting future improvements in ECG classification methodologies leveraging DL techniques and expansion to encompass other biosignals. Adding to this body of work, the research paper focused on the "Detection of ST Segment Elevation Myocardial Infarction (STEMI) Using Bacterial Foraging Optimization Technique" introduces a novel approach to identify STEMI through the analysis of ECG signals. Leveraging the bacterial foraging optimization algorithm, the study not only showcases advancements in optimization techniques but also compares them with other swarm intelligence algorithms. Furthermore, the study conducted by Ceylan, Ozbay, and Karlik introduces a pioneering approach for the classification of ECG arrhythmias using Type-2 fuzzy neural networks (T2FCNNs). The proposed method achieves an enhanced accuracy rate of 99% for both the MIT-BIH database and experimental ECG records, demonstrating reduced training time and segments compared to conventional neural networks. The authors propose the extension of their framework to encompass other types of networks and advocate for the development of new, more efficient fuzzifiers.

In conclusion, the investigation conducted by Behadada and Chikh is centered on the development of an interpretable classifier utilizing a fuzzy decision tree. The primary goal is to achieve accurate and understandable detection of cardiac arrhythmias based on ECG data. This research underscores the pivotal role of ML in the realm of ECG analysis, with a specific emphasis on the interpretability and accuracy of the fuzzy decision tree in identifying various cardiac abnormalities. In summary, these studies collectively illuminate the dynamic landscape of ECG signal analysis. They present diverse methodologies, conscientiously acknowledge inherent limitations, and advocate for continued research endeavors aimed at refining and extending classification approaches. The overarching goal is to ensure the robustness of these methodologies in the face of challenges such as noise, artifacts, and variations in data scenarios. This collective body of work contributes significantly to the evolving field of ECG signal analysis, paving the way for advancements in both methodology and application.

The research incorporates scholarly articles retrieved from PubMed and IEEE Xplore databases, spanning the publication period between 2012 and 2017. These papers delve into the diverse applications of ML in healthcare, categorized into distinct domains such as medical images, physiological signals, e-health records, and biological systems. The survey not only synthesizes existing literature but also outlines promising research directions aimed at augmenting health management, particularly in the realm of physiological signal applications. A comprehensive systematic review conducted by S. Hong *et al.*, delves into the opportunities and challenges presented by ML techniques in the context of ECG data. Analyzing 191 papers published between January 2010 and February 2020, the review spans discussions on model architecture, applications, and datasets. Noteworthy challenges, including interpretability, scalability, and efficiency, are identified as potential areas for future research. In a twofold review, Bote-Curiel *et al.*, provide an insightful overview of big data and ML applications within the healthcare landscape, with a specific focus on ECG. Their exploration encompasses papers published in 2017 and 2018, sourced from IEEE Xplore, Science Direct, PubMed, and Google Scholar.

12.7 CASE STUDIES ON ECG SIGNAL ANALYSIS USING DIFFERENT ALGORITHMS

This section delineates the outcomes derived from the SLR, presenting the findings extracted from the analyzed papers. As illustrated in Figure 12.2, the bar chart vividly portrays an upward trajectory in the quantity of publications encompassing papers, books, and journals within the domain of "ECG and ML."

12.7.1 Utilization of Deep Learning in Electrocardiogram Signal Analysis

DL has significantly transformed the landscape of ECG signal analysis, introducing advanced capabilities for feature extraction, pattern recognition, and classification. This technological evolution has been particularly pronounced in three main domains: driving, biometric/security, and medical/healthcare. In the medical/healthcare domain, DL models have been pivotal in enhancing the diagnosis and monitoring of CVDs. The responsibilities of healthcare professionals extend beyond conventional practices, necessitating continuous adaptation to address new challenges and responsibilities. In the medical field, practitioners are tasked with disease identification and the selection of optimal treatment strategies. Despite the expertise of healthcare practitioners in making informed decisions based on symptoms and test results, the integration of information is indispensable for making judicious decisions.

The ECG plays a pivotal role in the identification and screening of CVDs, providing a foundation for informed judgments by medical professionals. DL techniques are increasingly applied to physiological signals, unraveling hidden associations that contribute to swift and informed decision-making by healthcare practitioners. DL has demonstrated notable efficacy in enhancing the accuracy of CVD diagnoses, particularly in the identification of arrhythmias using ECG data, as evidenced by the study conducted by Ding *et al.* In a comprehensive discussion by Bizopoulos and Koutsouris, the applications of DL in cardiology are explored, highlighting its potential impact on advancing diagnostic capabilities [32]. A review by Udayan and Kusuma provides strong evidence to support the use of DL algorithms for CVD diagnosis. Their findings suggest that DL has the potential to revolutionize the way that CVD is diagnosed and treated [19].

Biometric systems have found use for DNNs, especially for individual identification and authentication utilizing ECG data. A study conducted by Chamatidis *et al.* highlights the importance of feature engineering for ECG-based human authentication. The authors' use of the Fourier transform (FT), the discrete cosine transform (DCT), and the discrete wavelet transform (WT) suggests that these transformations can be useful for extracting informative features from ECG data. The study also highlights the importance of comparing different ML models for a specific task [33]. The authors' finding that alternative classifiers, such as K-nearest neighbors (KNNs), multilayer perceptron (MLP), radial basis function network (RBFN), and random forest, outperformed the DNN on this task suggests that it is important to evaluate multiple ML models before choosing one for a specific application. The study's findings have implications for the development of ECG-based human authentication systems. System developers should consider using larger datasets, more powerful DNN architectures, data augmentation techniques, and other feature engineering methods to improve the performance of their systems.

The primary limitation was attributed to inadequate training data, prompting the recommendation for the integration of a cancelable mechanism to enhance system security. Page *et al.*, contributed to this discourse by developing a DNN model specifically designed for user identification, utilizing data from the ECG-ID database. Notably, the study achieved high accuracy, sensitivity, and specificity scores of 99.54%, 99.85%, and 99.96%, respectively [34]. However, it is noteworthy that the ECG signals were captured during rest, and the exploration of events like exercise and standing could be considered for future investigations to enhance the model's applicability. Additionally, Khoma *et al.* proposed a DNN model for person identification, tested using the Lviv biometric data set. The model exhibited an accuracy of 88.97%, yet challenges were identified in ECG signal distortion and insufficient data [35]. The potential integration of GAN-based data augmentation is suggested as a strategy to mitigate these challenges and enhance model performance.

In the context of driving applications, stress detection has been successfully implemented using DL techniques to identify driver stress based on ECG signals. A DNN model for stress identification that incorporates driving and mental data was proposed in a study by Park *et al.* The research achieved an impressive performance accuracy of 90.19%, indicating the model's effectiveness in discerning stress levels [9]. Notably, the study involved data collection during specific demanding tasks, suggesting the potential for enhancing stress monitoring in daily life. Furthermore, the versatility of the model extends to the detection of anxiety, a significant stressor associated with various health issues, including high blood pressure. This highlights the broader applicability and potential health implications of employing DL-based stress detection in driving scenarios.

12.7.2 Utilization of Convolutional Neural Networks in Electrocardiogram Signal Analysis

CNNs have emerged as a powerful tool for analyzing and interpreting ECG signals, demonstrating remarkable performance in various medical, biometric, and driving applications. Their ability to extract and learn intricate patterns from ECG data has opened up new avenues for automated diagnosis, classification, and anomaly detection. CNN-based models specifically devised for the intricate classification of ECG signals. CNNs, distinguished for their exceptional performance in image recognition and computer vision, stand out as the predominant ML models, particularly in the nuanced domain of medical time-series data and imaging. The comprehensive synthesis presented in Table 12.2 meticulously encapsulates the diverse applications of CNN-based models tailored explicitly for the profound analysis of ECG signals, specifically pertaining to heartbeat classification. This compilation serves as a testament to the versatility and efficacy of CNNs in the intricate landscape of cardiac signal processing.

TABLE 12.2
A Comprehensive Overview of the Applications of Machine Learning (ML) in Electrocardiogram (ECG) Analysis Utilizing Convolutional Neural Networks (CNNs)

Application Task	ML Model Used	Dataset	Operational Effectiveness	Limitation	References
Obstructive sleep apnea (OSA) detection	CNN	The dataset utilized in this study comprises recordings from the PhysioNet Apnoea-ECG dataset, encompassing data from a cohort of 35 individuals.	Accuracy (Acc): 98.91% Sensitivity (Sen): 97.82% Specificity (Spe): 99.20%	The training duration for the model is considerable. The process heavily relies on expert observation, predominantly conducted offline. The model exhibits versatility, as it can be extended to EEG, EOG, and EMG applications for similar objectives.	[56]
Classification of OSA/hypopnea	CNN	Throughout the nocturnal polysomnography (PSG) sessions involving 86 subjects, the electrocardiogram (ECG) signals were captured using a singular-lead transducer positioned at lead II.	Acc = 90.8% F1-score = 87.0% Sen = 87.0% Pre = 87.0% Spe = 87.0% Recall = 87.0%	• Insufficient documentation on cause-based categorization of sleep apnea, particularly for central apnea and mixed apnea. • ECG recordings exhibited dependencies on concurrent events, including snoring, movement, and airflow. • The study involved a limited sample size. • Annotation and segmentation were solely conducted by a single specialist without cross-verification for events.	[57]

(Continued)

TABLE 12.2 (*Continued*)
A Comprehensive Overview of the Applications of Machine Learning (ML) in Electrocardiogram (ECG) Analysis Utilizing Convolutional Neural Networks (CNNs)

Application Task	ML Model Used	Dataset	Operational Effectiveness	Limitation	References
Detection of obstructive sleep apnea	CNN	Datasets were collected utilizing an Embla N7000 amplifier system (Embla Systems Inc., USA) at the Samsung Medical Center's Sleep Center (Seoul, Korea) (82 patients).	Pre = 0.99%, Spe = 96.0% Recall = 0.99%, Sen = 96.0% Acc = 96.0% F1-score = 0.99%	• Data scoring was conducted by a single expert, resulting in the absence of cross-checking, leading to both intra-scorer and inter-scorer variability. • The proposed model focuses on detecting the presence or absence of OSA but doesn't capture the starting and ending times of events. • ECG signals exhibited dependencies on concurrent events, including snoring, movement, and flow limitation. • The study involved a relatively small population size.	[57]
Automated detection of CAD	CNN	INCART (47 subjects) Fantasia data base	Net A: Acc = 95% Spec = 95.2% Sen = 93.7% Net B: Spec = 95.9% Sen = 91.1% Acc = 95.1%	• Require more time for training. • Requires a lot of data for training. • ECG signals should be fixed for training and testing.	[36]
Stress recognition	DWNet1D	Data acquired during the SRD'15 data acquisition program (24 individuals)	Acc = 99.1%	• Small population size • Intersubject variability issues	[58]

A comprehensive investigation by Hagiwara *et al.* in the field of arrhythmia detection introduced two CNN architectures, Net A and Net B. Both architectures demonstrated remarkable performance, exceeding 90% accuracy, specificity, and sensitivity. Net B, achieving 81.44% accuracy, was particularly effective with specific databases [36]. However, challenges related to limited training data and prolonged training times were identified. To mitigate these challenges, the authors recommended data augmentation and the bagging algorithm. Separate research employed a customized CNN architecture to distinguish shockable and nonshockable life-threatening ventricular arrhythmias. Across various datasets, their model attained an outstanding accuracy of 93.18%. However, the authors highlighted difficulties such as limited data availability and lengthy training times. Rajendra *et al.* presented a CNN model for heartbeat classification, reaching a commendable accuracy of 94.03% with the Massachusetts Institute of Technology-Beth Israel Hospital Arrhythmia Database [37]. Abbas *et al.* investigated 2D-CNN models for arrhythmia detection by converting ECG data into 2D ECG pictures. As a consequence of the Massachusetts Institute of Technology's Hospitality Database, they have a 99% accuracy rate. These studies collectively highlight the effectiveness of CNN architectures in ECG signal classification [38]. They also acknowledge challenges and propose avenues for advancement in the field, such as improved data augmentation techniques, more efficient training algorithms, and the development of CNN architectures specifically tailored for arrhythmia detection.

CNN-based models that are pretrained on extensive datasets, often referred to as pretrained or transfer learning models, represent a powerful paradigm in ML. These models, such as GoogleNet, AlexNet, and VGG-Net, have the capability to be repurposed with minimal adjustments for either the same (source data) or different types of data (target data). This approach is particularly advantageous in scenarios where there is a scarcity of data and computational resources for training the target data. In the pursuit of leveraging pretrained models, Alquran *et al.*, harnessed the prowess of GoogleNet and AlexNet, achieving an impressive accuracy of 97.8% with the MITDB dataset when integrating third cumulants [39]. A study demonstrated commendable performance in the analysis of ventricular ectopic beats (VEB) and supraventricular ectopic beats (SVEB) using the MITDB dataset. Introducing a novel dimension to the pretrained model landscape, Amrani *et al.*, engineered a very deep CNN model functioning as a feature extractor. The fusion technique employed, known as multi-canonical correlation analysis (MCCA), contributed to the model's ability to achieve an accuracy of 97.37% in arrhythmia detection analysis [14]. Brito *et al.*, explored the ResNet pretrained CNN model, optimizing it with both stochastic gradient descent (SGD) and adaptive moment estimation [40]. The study revealed superior accuracy with SGD compared to Adam.

Diker and Engin's groundbreaking work seamlessly integrates CNN and ELM, two powerful computational techniques, to achieve the remarkable accuracy of 88.33% in ECG signal classification using the PTBDB dataset [41]. Their approach exemplifies the synergistic potential of DL and ML methodologies, paving the way for more sophisticated and effective signal processing solutions. In a complementary study, Dokur and Ölmez introduce a distinctive CNN architecture for heartbeat classification that deviates from the conventional CNN model by omitting the fully connected neural network (FCNN) component [42].

Fujita and Cimr pioneered an innovative CNN-based model designed for the intricate task of recognizing ECG rhythms [43]. Noteworthy in their approach was the incorporation of continuous wavelet transformation (CWT) to effectively extract features, culminating in an impressive accuracy rate of 97.78%. This research represents a nuanced exploration of feature extraction methodologies within CNN architectures, showcasing the integration of signal processing techniques for enhanced model performance. Meanwhile, the realm of ECG-based biometric systems has seen a surge in CNN-based models aimed at tackling challenges in identification and authentication, with a particular emphasis on resilience against spoofing attacks. Abdeldayem and Bourlai engineered a 2D-CNN model dedicated to human identification, undergoing rigorous testing across eight diverse databases [44]. The study astutely recommended the inclusion of multi-session scenarios to further fortify and refine model performance in real-world applications. In a parallel vein, Bajare and Ingale harnessed the capabilities of a 1D-CNN model for human identification. Their meticulous endeavors bore fruit, achieving an accuracy milestone of 96.93% when utilizing the normal sinus rhythm database (NSRDB) and a flawless 100% accuracy when applied to the ECG-ID database [45]. This research marks a substantive contribution to the burgeoning field of ECG-based biometrics, signaling advancements in precision and reliability within identification systems.

ECG signals offer unique personal identification characteristics, making them a valuable tool for biometric authentication systems. CNNs can extract and learn these ECG features, enabling accurate and reliable user identification. Compared to traditional biometric methods such as fingerprints or facial recognition, ECG-based authentication offers enhanced security and privacy, as ECG patterns are difficult to forge or replicate. Moreover, CNNs can be employed in security applications to detect anomalies or abnormalities in ECG signals during surveillance or monitoring. By analyzing real-time ECG data, CNNs can identify potential health risks or stress levels, providing valuable insights for security personnel and healthcare providers.

ECG monitoring has gained traction in automotive applications, particularly in advanced driver assistance systems (ADAS) and fatigue detection systems. CNNs can analyze ECG signals to assess driver alertness and detect signs of fatigue or drowsiness. By identifying these physiological changes, CNN-based systems can provide timely alerts to drivers, reducing the risk of accidents caused by fatigue-related impairments. Furthermore, CNNs can be used to monitor driver stress levels, which can significantly impact driving performance. By analyzing heart rate variability and other ECG parameters, CNNs can detect elevated stress levels and provide interventions such as relaxation techniques or breaks to enhance driver safety.

CNNs have emerged as powerful tools for analyzing physiological signals, making them well-suited for applications in the driving domain, where monitoring driver behavior is crucial for safety. Researchers have explored the use of CNNs to identify inattention, detect stress, and predict workload, with promising results. One notable study by Taherisadr *et al.* demonstrates the effectiveness of CNNs in identifying inattention while driving. The authors developed a deep CNN model that utilizes Mel-frequency spectral coefficients (MFSC) representations extracted from raw ECG signals to generate 2D spectrogram images. This model achieved an accuracy of approximately 95.51%, surpassing the results obtained with conventional time-frequency (TF) representation.

The study employed ECG signals collected from the naturalistic driving settings of ten individuals, demonstrating the potential of the proposed approach for real-world applications. The application of CNNs in the driving domain holds significant promise for improving road safety by enabling early detection of driver fatigue, stress, and inattention. Further research is warranted to enhance the accuracy and generalizability of these models, particularly with larger and more diverse datasets, paving the way for the development of advanced driver monitoring systems.

In a study centered on predicting pilot workload, visual representations such as spectrograms and scalograms were applied to obtain ECG data. An "off-the-shelf" feature extractor, the pretrained CNN model AlexNet, was employed, and workload prediction was carried out using the widely used linear classifier SVM. The combination of AlexNet and SVM (AlexNet + SVM) outperformed the fine-tuned deep CNN, achieving the highest accuracy of 51.35% with scalograms. However, it's crucial to highlight that the dataset used in this study was derived from only two qualified test pilots engaged in a target tracking task on the National Research Council of Canada's (NRC) Bell 205 helicopter. The limited nature of this dataset raises concerns about the generalizability of the model to real-world scenarios and underscores the necessity for more extensive and diverse datasets to ensure robust performance evaluation.

12.7.3 Utilizations of Recurrent Neural Networks in ECG Signal Analysis

ECG signals, which capture the electrical activity of the heart, provide valuable insights into the health and function of the cardiovascular system. RNNs have emerged as powerful tools for analyzing ECG signals, demonstrating remarkable performance in a variety of tasks. This chapter explores the applications of RNNs in ECG signal analysis, categorizing them into three main domains: biometric/security, medical/healthcare, and driving. RNNs have shown great promise in the medical/healthcare domain, particularly in the diagnosis and monitoring of cardiac diseases. Their ability to capture temporal dependencies in ECG signals makes them well-suited for tasks such as arrhythmia classification, heart failure detection, and MI diagnosis. In the field of arrhythmia classification, RNNs have achieved impressive results. For instance, Banerjee *et al.* introduced an RNN model that integrates two LSTM networks to classify AF with high sensitivity (0.93), specificity (0.98), and an F1-score (0.89). Their model effectively utilizes the temporal information contained in ECG signals to identify the characteristic patterns associated with AF [17]. RNNs have also demonstrated effectiveness in heart failure detection. Darmawahyuni and Nurmaini employed an LSTM model for binary classification of MI, achieving notable precision (0.91), sensitivity (0.91), F1-score (0.90), and balanced accuracy (BAcc) (0.83) using the PTBDB dataset. Their findings suggest that RNNs can effectively discriminate between healthy and MI-affected ECG signals. Moreover, RNNs have shown promise in MI diagnosis [46]. Faust *et al.* introduced the use of bidirectional long short-term memory (bi-LSTM) for AF detection, achieving accuracies, specificities, and sensitivities exceeding 98% in both cross and blind validation [47]. Their bi-LSTM model effectively captures both forward and backward temporal dependencies in ECG signals, improving its ability to identify AF patterns.

RNNs have also found applications in the biometric/security domain, where they are used to verify human identity based on ECG signals. Their ability to extract unique features from ECG signals makes them well-suited for tasks such as person authentication and access control. Salloum and Kuo conducted a study using RNN, gated recurrent unit (GRU), and LSTM models for identification and authentication. The LSTM model outperformed the others, achieving a remarkable 100% accuracy on both the MITDB and ECG-ID databases [48]. This study demonstrates the effectiveness of RNNs for person authentication using ECG signals. Another study by Lynn *et al.* focused on human identification, employing bidirectional GRU, and bidirectional LSTM models, which demonstrated accuracy performances of 98.55% (BGRU) and 96.4% (BLSTM). These findings further support the potential of RNNs for biometric applications [49] (Table 12.3).

12.7.4 Utilizations of Restricted Boltzmann Machines in ECG Signal Analysis

In the medical and healthcare landscape, the application of restricted Boltzmann machines (RBMs) in ECG signal analysis has gained significant traction. Particularly in CVD diagnosis, RBMs prove instrumental in deciphering intricate patterns within ECG signals. Wang *et al.* [50] conducted a study where RBMs were utilized for anomaly detection in ECG signals, showcasing their capability to automatically extract relevant features crucial for identifying patterns associated with various cardiac conditions. This feature learning aspect is crucial for early disease detection and has the potential to revolutionize the diagnostic process.

RBMs have been harnessed in biometric systems, specifically for user authentication and security applications. The distinct and unique patterns embedded in an individual's ECG signal make it an ideal candidate for biometric identification. Singh *et al.* and Patel *et al.* have explored the application of RBMs in biometric ECG-based systems, where these models play a pivotal role in recognizing and authenticating individuals based on their ECG patterns [51,52]. The security implications of employing RBMs in this context are noteworthy, as they offer a robust and reliable method for user identification.

In the domain of driving, RBMs have found applications related to driver monitoring and stress detection using ECG signals. Real-time analysis of ECG signals can provide valuable insights into a driver's physiological state, contributing to enhanced driving safety. Kim and Chung have delved into the use of RBMs for monitoring driver physiological conditions, particularly in detecting stress or drowsiness [53]. By leveraging RBMs, these studies aim to improve road safety through the timely identification of driver states that may pose risks.

While RBMs exhibit promising applications in these domains, future research should focus on addressing challenges such as interpretability and real-time processing. Incorporating explainable AI techniques and optimizing computational efficiency would further enhance the deployment of RBMs in practical scenarios. Additionally, collaborative efforts between the medical, security, and automotive sectors are essential to foster a holistic approach to RBM applications in ECG signal analysis.

TABLE 12.3
A Comprehensive Summary of the Applications of Recurrent Neural Networks (RNNs) in Electrocardiogram (ECG) Analysis

Application Task	ML Model Used	Dataset	Operational Effectiveness	Limitation	References
Classification of AF	Merged LSTM + hand-crafted features	Dataset from the 2017 PhysioNet/ CinC Challenge (8528 ECGs)	F1-score 0.89 Spe = 0.98, Sen = 0.93	• Handcrafted elements were used.	[17]
MI classification	LSTM	PTBDB (290 subjects)	The model achieved noteworthy performance metrics, including a precision of 0.91, Sensitivity of 0.91, an F1 score of 0.90, Balanced Accuracy of 0.83, and a Matthews Correlation Coefficient (MCC) of 0.75. These metrics collectively underscore the effectiveness and robustness of the model in its classification tasks, providing a comprehensive evaluation of its precision, sensitivity, overall performance, balanced accuracy, and correlation coefficient.	The proposed model is characterized by its simplicity and adherence to standard conventions. However, its performance fell short of expectations, primarily attributed to the minimal preprocessing applied to the input data.	[47]
Classification of MI	RNN, LSTM, GRN	PTBDB (290 subjects)	The outcomes derived from the long short-term memory (LSTM) model are noteworthy, demonstrating superior performance metrics. Specifically, the sensitivity (sen) achieved an impressive 98.49%, while the specificity (spe) reached 97.97%. Precision stood at 95.67%, and the F1-score, a comprehensive measure, attained a commendable 96.32%.	The preliminary performance exhibited notable challenges attributed to a limited extent of preprocessing.	[59]

(Continued)

TABLE 12.3 (*Continued*)
A Comprehensive Summary of the Applications of Recurrent Neural Networks (RNNs) in Electrocardiogram (ECG) Analysis

Application Task	ML Model Used	Dataset	Operational Effectiveness	Limitation	References
Detection of AF	bi-LSTM	AFDB (23 subjects)	Cross-Validation Metrics: Accuracy: 98.51% Specificity: 98.67% Positive Predictivity: 98.39% Sensitivity: 98.32% Blind Fold Validation Metrics: Accuracy: 99.77% Sensitivity: 99.87% Specificity: 99.61% Positive Predictivity: 99.72%	The dataset utilized in the research involved a relatively limited population. • The training speed during the design stage was marked by an extended duration. • The study exclusively concentrated on the AF subtype.	[48]
Detection of AF	RNN, LSTM, GRU	atrial fibrillation database (AFDB) comprising 25 signals, and Normal Sinus Rhythm Database (NSRDB) also containing 25 signals.	The results indicate accuracy scores of 0.95 for the RNN, perfect scores of 1.00 for. Precision values also achieved perfection for RNN, LSTM, and GRU at 1.00. In terms of recall, RNN achieved 0.889, while LSTM and GRU both achieved perfect scores of 1.00.	• Exclusively binary classification was conducted. • The model does not reveal the internal workings of the deep models, and this issue can be addressed by converting the nonlinearity into a linearized form.	[60]

The key performance metrics include Accuracy (Acc), Specification (Spe), Sensitivity (Sen), Precision (Pre), and Positive Productivity.

12.8 CHALLENGES

This section elucidates the challenges discerned within the literature under examination and delves into prospective avenues for future research. The identified challenges are categorized into domains, models, application tasks, datasets, and ML architectures, providing a comprehensive framework for addressing areas that warrant refinement and innovation. This discussion serves as a springboard for identifying opportunities to enhance the existing landscape and contribute to the ongoing evolution of research in this domain.

12.8.1 Challenges within the Domain

ML has revolutionized the field of ECG analysis, opening up a plethora of applications across the medical, biometric, and driving domains. In the realm of medical and healthcare, ML plays a pivotal role in real-time patient monitoring, enabling continuous surveillance and prompt alerts in critical events like cardiac arrest. This real-time capability is particularly crucial for patients who are not always physically present in a hospital setting. The evolution of healthcare applications, particularly leveraging the Internet of Things (IoT), holds immense promise for real-time monitoring and timely assistance. IoT devices can collect ECG data from patients remotely and transmit it to healthcare providers, enabling immediate intervention in life-threatening situations. However, despite advancements in ML for ECG signal processing in edge computing and IoT, challenges persist in terms of latency, power efficiency, and knowledge extraction from extensive physiological datasets. Addressing these challenges requires a multifaceted approach that integrates edge computing, modern AI techniques, and 5G capabilities. Edge computing brings ML algorithms closer to the data source, reducing latency and minimizing data transfer requirements. Modern AI techniques, such as DL, can extract complex patterns from ECG data, providing valuable insights into patient health. And 5G's high bandwidth and low latency enable real-time health data collection and analysis, paving the way for transformative healthcare solutions.

In conclusion, ML has revolutionized ECG analysis, enabling real-time patient monitoring, biometric authentication, and driving safety applications. The fusion of edge computing, modern AI techniques, and 5G capabilities holds immense potential for addressing the challenges of latency, power efficiency, and knowledge extraction from extensive physiological datasets. These advancements, coupled with the deployment of DL algorithms in various computing environments, pave the way for ubiquitous and remote health monitoring, transforming the landscape of healthcare services.

12.8.2 Challenges with Respect to the Model

DL architectures have revolutionized the analysis of ECG data, offering a powerful toolkit for extracting meaningful information from these complex signals. Various models, including DNNs, CNNs, RNNs, RBMs, autoencoders (AEs), GANs, and hybrid architectures, have been proposed for ECG analysis, demonstrating remarkable performance in a wide range of tasks. Among CNN architectures, well-established models such as AlexNet, ZF Net, GoogleNet, VGG-Net, ResNet, SqueezeNet, DenseNet, Inception V3, Xception, and LeNet-5 have gained significant traction, with their variants further expanding the landscape of ECG modeling. However, certain CNN architectures, like ZF Net, SqueezeNet, and LeNet-5, have received comparatively less attention in the context of ECG modeling, suggesting potential areas for further exploration. In the realm of RNNs, LSTM models have emerged as the predominant choice for ECG signal analysis, owing to their ability to capture long-range temporal dependencies within ECG waveforms. GRU models have also demonstrated promising results, while bidirectional RNNs offer the advantage of processing information in both forward and backward directions, potentially enhancing feature extraction capabilities. Interestingly, while both deep belief networks (DBNs) and deep Boltzmann machines (DBMs) belong to the "Boltzmann family," the application of DBMs for ECG data analysis remains largely unexplored. This presents an intriguing avenue for future research, as DBMs may offer unique capabilities for modeling the inherent probabilistic nature of ECG data. Overall, the extensive use of DL architectures for ECG analysis underscores their remarkable potential for extracting meaningful information from these complex signals. As research continues to delve into this domain, further advancements in model architectures and optimization techniques are likely to emerge, paving the way for even more sophisticated and impactful ECG-based applications.

Various AE architectures, including denoising AEs (DAEs), convolutional autoencoders (CAEs), adversarial autoencoder (AAE), sparse AEs (SAEs), and variational autoencoders (VAE), have been used to analyze ECG signals. In the context of ECG signal analysis, the review highlights SAEs and DAEs as the primary AE architectures employed. These AEs play a crucial role in extracting meaningful features and reducing dimensionality from the complex ECG data. Additionally, researchers have explored the integration of different ML structures, with a particular focus on combining CNN and RNNs. Specifically, the fusion of CNN architectures with LSTM networks has attracted significant attention, showcasing superior performance compared to individual ML models and other hybrid approaches. This integration enhances the ability to capture both spatial and temporal dependencies in ECG signals, contributing to more effective and accurate signal analysis in the realm of cardiovascular diagnostics.

DL models have surpassed traditional ML models in terms of classification accuracy, particularly in the realm of ECG data analysis. However, this progress is accompanied by the challenge of interpretability. Due to the "black-box" nature of ML models, their decision-making processes often lack transparency, hindering their acceptance in medical diagnosis, where interpretability is crucial for building trust among healthcare professionals. Studies by Chu *et al.* have addressed this challenge by combining deep features with traditional model features, maintaining interpretability while preserving accuracy [54]. This approach demonstrates the potential for developing explainable ML models that can effectively balance accuracy and interpretability. In line with this effort, the emerging paradigm of explainable artificial intelligence (XAI) aims to provide reasons or explanations for model decisions, ensuring transparency while maintaining accuracy. In the context of medical diagnosis, explainable ML models are essential for building trust among humans and facilitating the adoption of AI-powered diagnostic tools. Another paradigm, explainable active learning (XAL), combines active learning (AL), and XAI. This approach allows the model to query a machine teacher selectively. This interactive process can help improve the model's accuracy and interpretability simultaneously. The accuracy of a model in biomedical signal processing, particularly in ECG data analysis, is heavily influenced by signal quality and feature extraction. By addressing the challenge of interpretability and incorporating advanced signal processing techniques, ML and DL models have the potential to revolutionize ECG data analysis, leading to more accurate, reliable, and trustworthy diagnostic tools for CVDs.

12.8.3 Application Task Challenges

ML models have demonstrated remarkable versatility across various domains, tailor-made to address specific tasks. Within the realm of biometric ECG-based systems, ML models play a pivotal role in user authentication, granting or denying access based on ECG signature verification. However, the effectiveness of these systems is hampered by persistent challenges arising from intersubject and intra-subject ECG variability. Unresolved challenges such as medication, cardiac conditions, emotion, fatigue, as heart geometry, electrode characteristics, placement, age, posture, and individual attributes pose a significant hurdle in the development of robust ECG–biometric systems. In contrast to authentication tasks, ML models also excel in classification tasks within the ECG domain. These tasks encompass a wide range of applications, including determining patient vitality, identifying ECG signals indicative of diabetes or nondiabetic states, classifying normal or arrhythmic conditions, and categorizing ECGs based on specific conditions like paroxysmal atrial fibrillation (PAF), AF, CHD, coronary artery disease (CAD), apnea, and motorist's inattention. Researchers have employed ML models to categorize ECG beats into five distinct groups, differentiate between drowsy, sleepy, and normal states of driver alertness, and specifically identify apnea/hypopnea events as normal, hypopnea, apnea, or other categories. These studies demonstrate the adaptability of ML models in addressing intricate classification tasks within the ECG domain.

12.8.4 Challenges of the Dataset

In our comprehensive examination of the literature, we identified over 40 datasets commonly employed in DL models for the analysis of ECG signals across various classification tasks. Noteworthy datasets include the Massachusetts Institute of Technology-Beth Israel Hospital Arrhythmia Database, Physikalisch-Technische Bundesanstalt Database, atrial fibrillation database (AFDB), NSRDB, electrocardiogram identification database, and the Chinese physiological signal challenge database. Additionally, researchers frequently utilize datasets from the PhysioNet/CinC Challenge 2017. It is important to highlight that while these datasets are publicly accessible, the presence of private datasets underscores the challenges associated with restricted access, necessitating researchers to independently acquire them through alternative means. Among these datasets, MITDB, with a history spanning over 40 years, is commonly used despite its limitations, including issues of imbalance and a confined scope to records from only 47 subjects. Furthermore, as a single-session database, MITDB proves insufficient for biometric experiments. Recent datasets, such PhysioNet/CinC Challenge 2017 and the 2018 CPS Challenge, have shorter recording durations. The critical role of ample data for effective DL training is underscored by the limitations outlined in Tables 12.1–12.3, emphasizing the impact of small training datasets on generalization across various studies. Researchers have proposed solutions such as data augmentation, transfer learning, synthetic minority over-sampling technique (SMOTE), and GAN to address imbalances and constraints in small datasets. In conclusion, we advocate for the creation of extensive, openly accessible datasets across all discussed domains, not only to bolster research efforts but also to streamline the data acquisition process.

12.9 FUTURE RESEARCH DIRECTION

The future landscape of research in heart disease diagnosis through ML is poised for significant advancements, and several compelling directions are emerging. First, the integration of multimodal data sources presents a compelling avenue. Researchers are delving into the combination of genetic data, EHRs, medical imaging, and wearable device metrics. This holistic approach aims to capture a comprehensive understanding of an individual's cardiovascular health, providing a rich dataset for ML models. DL architectures, particularly CNNs and RNNs, are garnering attention for their potential to enhance feature extraction and pattern recognition. In the realm of medical imaging and time-series data, these advanced architectures show promise in improving the accuracy and efficiency of heart disease diagnosis. Explain ability and interpretability remain critical aspects of ML models in healthcare. As the adoption of ML in clinical settings increases, there is a growing emphasis on developing models that can provide transparent explanations for their predictions. This is particularly important for building trust among healthcare professionals and patients and facilitating informed decision-making.

Transfer learning is another intriguing area of exploration. Leveraging models pre-trained on extensive datasets and fine-tuning them for specific cardiovascular tasks could prove instrumental, especially in scenarios where labeled medical datasets are limited. Real-time monitoring for early detection is a key focus, with an emphasis on continuous data streams from wearable devices and other monitoring tools. Timely identification of anomalies or changes in health parameters could enable proactive intervention, potentially preventing the progression of CVDs. Personalized medicine is gaining prominence, with a shift toward models that account for individual variations in genetics, lifestyle, and environmental factors. Tailoring risk prediction models to the unique characteristics of each patient could lead to more effective and targeted preventive strategies. On the technical front, addressing challenges related to data privacy and security is paramount. Robust methods for anonymization, encryption, and secure sharing of medical data are essential to foster collaboration and ensure the responsible use of sensitive health information. The translation of ML research into clinical practice necessitates large-scale clinical validation. Collaborations with healthcare professionals are crucial to ensuring that developed models align with clinical workflows and contribute meaningfully to patient care. Longitudinal data analysis, exploring how CVDs progress over time, provides valuable insights. This involves studying patterns of disease development, identifying key risk factors, and predicting the trajectory of a patient's cardiovascular health. Ethical considerations, including issues of bias, fairness, and transparency, are integral to the responsible deployment of ML in healthcare. Researchers are actively working on guidelines and best practices to address these ethical challenges and ensure equitable healthcare outcomes. In conclusion, the future of research in heart disease diagnosis using ML is characterized by a multidimensional approach, involving advanced technologies, interdisciplinary collaboration, and a commitment to ethical and responsible implementation in clinical settings. These diverse avenues of exploration collectively contribute to the evolution of precision medicine and personalized healthcare in the cardiovascular domain.

12.10 CONCLUSIONS

In conclusion, the case study examining the application of ML for the diagnosis of heart disease within the context of data-driven healthcare presents a compelling narrative of transformative potential within the field of cardiac health. The incorporation of ML algorithms, as evidenced in this investigation, holds substantial promise for advancing the precision and efficiency of heart disease diagnosis. This chapter underscores the evolving landscape of healthcare, emphasizing a paradigm shift resulting from the integration of ML methodologies. The utilization of extensive patient datasets and the deployment of AI, notably through DL algorithms, showcase a notable enhancement in the identification of cardiac-related pathologies. The model's exceptional predictive efficacy, coupled with nuanced pattern recognition, emphasizes its superiority over traditional diagnostic modalities. An essential aspect of this investigation is the focus on interpretability in the decision-making process of the ML model. Through the implementation of explainable AI techniques, the chapter addresses the imperative need for trust and transparency in healthcare AI, fostering confidence among healthcare practitioners and patients alike. The real-time integration of the developed ML model into existing healthcare infrastructures emerges as a practical and promising avenue. The seamless incorporation into EHRs and diagnostic workflows demonstrates the potential to streamline diagnostic processes, enhancing overall efficiency and efficacy in patient care.

REFERENCES

1. A. Belle, K. Najarian, F. Navidi, D. A. Beard, S. M. R. Soroushmehr and R. Thiagarajan, "Big data analytics in healthcare," *BioMed Research International*: 370194, 2015. https://doi.org/10.1155/2015/370194
2. G. S. Manivannan and C. Ganeshbabu, "An exploration of ECG signal feature selection and classification using machine learning techniques," Vol. 9(3): 797–804, 2020. https://doi.org/10.35940/ijitee.C8728.019320
3. J. G. Gujar, S. Chattopadhyay, S. J. Wagh and V. G. Gaikar, "Experimental and modeling studies on extraction of catechin hydrate and epicatechin from Indian green tea leaves," *The Canadian Journal of Chemical Engineering*, Vol. 88(2): 232–240, 2010. https://doi.org/10.1002/cjce.20271

4. J. G. Gujar, S. J. Wagh and V. G. Gaikar, "Experimental and modeling studies on microwave-assisted extraction of thymol from seeds of Trachyspermum ammi (TA)," *Separation and Purification Technology*, Vol. 70(3): 257–264, 2010. https://doi.org/10.1016/j.seppur.2009.08.005
5. A. A. Katole, J. G. Gujar and S. M. Chavan, "Experimental and modeling studies on extraction of eugenol from Cinnamomum Zeylanicum (Dalchini)," *IJSTE – International Journal of Science Technology & Engineering*, Vol. 2(11): 831–835, 2016.
6. S. J. Wagh, J. G. Gujar and V. G. Gaikar, "Experimental and modeling studies on extraction of amyrins from latex of mandar (Calotropis gigantea)," *Indian Journal of Chemical Technology*, Vol. 19: 427–433, 2012.
7. M. Al Rahhal, H. S. Alhichri, Y. Bazi and N. A. Ajlan, "Automatic premature ventricular contractions detection for multi-lead electrocardiogram signal," in *2018 IEEE International Conference on Electro/Information Technology (EIT)*, Oakland University **in** Rochester, Michigan, USA, 2018.
8. Z. Fariha, R. Ikeura and S. Hayakawa, "Arrhythmia detection using MIT-BIH dataset: A review," in *2018 International Conference on Computational Approach in Smart Systems Design and Applications (ICASSDA)*, 2018.
9. J. Y. Park, H. Cho, W. Hwang, R. K. Balan and J. G. Ko, "Deep ECG estimation using a bed-attached geophone," in *17th ACM International Conference on Mobile Systems, Applications, and Services, MobiSys 2019*, 2019.
10. C. Zywietz, "A Brief History of Electrocardiography-Progress through Technology," 2003.
11. G. Nagarajan, R. Swaminathan and T. M. Deserno, "Deep learning on 1-D biosignals: a Taxonomy-based survey," *Yearbook of Medical Informatics*, Vol. 27(1): 98–109, 2018. https://doi.org/10.1055/s-0038-1667083
12. A. H. Ribeiro, M. H. Ribeiro, G. M. M. Paixão, D. M. Oliveira, P. R. Gomes, P. W. Macfarlane, W. M. Jr, J. A. Canazart, M. P. S. Ferreira, C. R. Andersson, T. B. Schön and Ribeiro, "Automatic diagnosis of the 12-lead ECG using a deep neural network," *Nature Communications*, Vols. 11(1): 1760, 2020. https://doi.org/10.1038/s41467-020-15432-4
13. J. Takalo-Mattila, J. Kiljander and J.-P. Soininen, "Inter-patient ECG classification using deep convolutional neural networks," in *2018 21st Euromicro Conference on Digital System Design (DSD)*, Prague, Czech Republic, 2018.
14. M. Amrani, M. Hammad, F. Jiang and K. Wang, "Very deep feature extraction and fusion for arrhythmias detection," *Neural Computing and Applications*, Vol. 30, 2018. https://doi.org/10.1007/s00521-018-3616-9
15. M. A. Muhammed and J. Aravinth, "CNN based off-the-person ECG biometrics," in *2019 International Conference on Wireless Communications Signal Processing and Networking (WiSPNET)*, Chennai, India, 2019.
16. K. Antczak, "Deep recurrent neural networks for ECG signal denoising," arXiv preprint arXiv:1807.11551, 2018.
17. R. Banerjee, A. Ghose and S. Khandelwal, "A novel recurrent neural network architecture for classification of atrial fibrillation using single-lead ECG," in *2019 27th European Signal Processing Conference (EUSIPCO)*, A Coruña, Spain, 2019.
18. H. Assodiky, I. Syarif and T. Badriyah, "Deep learning algorithm for arrhythmia detection," *2017 International Electronics Symposium on Knowledge Creation and Intelligent Computing (IES-KCIC)*, 2017, pp. 26–32. https://doi.org/10.1109/KCIC.2017.8228452
19. S. R. Kusuma and D. J. Udayan, "Analysis on deep learning methods for ECG based cardiovascular disease prediction," *Scalable Computing Practice and Experience*, Vol. 21, 2020. https://doi.org/10.12694/scpe.v21i1.1640
20. C. Ouchicha, O. Ammor and M. Meknassi, "CVDNet: A novel deep learning architecture for detection of coronavirus (Covid-19) from chest x-ray images," *Chaos Solitons Fractals*, 2020. https://doi.org/10.1016/j.chaos.2020.110245

21. D. Silver, A. Huang, C. Maddison, A. Guez, L. Sifre, G. Driessche, J. Schrittwieser, I. Antonoglou, V. Panneershelvam, M. Lanctot, S. Dieleman, D. Grewe, J. Nham and N. Kalchbrenner, "Mastering the game of Go with deep neural networks and tree search," *Nature*, Vol. 529, 2016. https://doi.org/10.1038/nature16961
22. M. Luigi, N. Maffei, S. Strolin, S. Vichi, L. Bottazzi and L. Strigari, "Basic of machine learning and deep learning in imaging for medical physicists," *Physica Medica*, Vol. 83, 2021. https://doi.org/10.1016/j.ejmp.2021.03.026
23. X. Yu and W. Maria, "Guidance on conducting a systematic literature review," *Journal of Planning Education and Research*, Vol. 39, 2017. https://doi.org/10.1177/0739456X17723971
24. B. M. Imran, G. Masitah and D. N. Jawawi, "Systematic reviews in requirements engineering: A systematic review," *2014 8th Malaysian Software Engineering Conference, MySEC 2014*, 2014. https://doi.org/10.1109/MySec.2014.6985987
25. J. EunKwang, M. Chae, H. Lee and S. Han, "Arrhythmia classification system using deep neural network," in *2019 Eleventh International Conference on Ubiquitous and Future Networks (ICUFN)*, Zagreb, Croatia, 2019.
26. K. Young-Hak, K. Daeyoung, N. H. Minh, J. T. Joon and H. J. Park, "Premature ventricular contraction beat detection with deep neural networks," in *15th IEEE International Conference on Machine Learning and Applications (ICMLA)*, California, USA, 2016.
27. S. Giovanna and D. P. Giuseppe, "A deep learning approach for ECG-based heartbeat classification for arrhythmia detection," *Future Generation Computer Systems*, 2018. https://doi.org/10.1016/j.future.2018.03.057
28. S. Shensheng Xu, M.-W. Mak and C.-C. Cheung, "Deep neural networks versus support vector machines for ECG arrhythmia classification," in *2017 IEEE International Conference on Multimedia & Expo Workshops (ICMEW)*, Hong Kong, China, 2017.
29. S. Shensheng Xu, C.-C. Cheung and M.-W. Mak, "Towards end-to-end ECG classification with raw signal extraction and deep neural networks," *IEEE Journal of Biomedical and Health Informatics*, Vol. 23(4): 1574–1584, 2019. https://doi.org/10.1109/JBHI.2018.2871510
30. C. Wenjuan, Y. Chen, J. Luo, J. Wang, G. Zhang, L. Ji, Y. Shi, H. Baoshi and J. Guo, "Accurate detection of atrial fibrillation from 12-lead ECG using deep neural network," *Computers in Biology and Medicine*, Vol. 116: 103378, 2020. https://doi.org/10.1016/j.compbiomed.2019.103378
31. R. Vullings, J. Van Laar, M. I. R. de Veries and S.-A. B. Clur, "Fetal electrocardiography and artificial intelligence for prenatal detection of congenital heart disease," *Acta Obstetricia et Gynecologica Scandinavica*, Vol. 102(11): 1511–1520, 2023. https://doi.org/10.1111/aogs.14623
32. P. Bizopoulos and D. Koutsouris, "Deep learning in cardiology," *IEEE Reviews in Biomedical Engineering*, Vol. 12: 168–193, 2019. https://doi.org/10.1109/RBME.2018.2885714
33. S. G. I. Chamatidis, A. Katsika and G. Spathoulas, "Using deep learning neural networks for ECG based authentication," in *2017 International Carnahan Conference on Security Technology (ICCST)*, 2017. https://doi.org/10.1109/CCST.2017.8167816
34. A. Page, A. Kulkarni and T. Mohsenin, "Utilizing deep neural nets for an embedded ECG-based biometric authentication system," in *Biomedical Circuits and Systems Conference (BioCAS*, Atlanta, GA), 2015. IEEE.
35. L. Wieclaw, Y. Khoma, P. Falat, D. Sabodashko and V. Herasymenko, "Biometrie identification from raw ECG signal using deep learning techniques," in *2017 9th IEEE International Conference on Intelligent Data Acquisition and Advanced Computing Systems: Technology and Applications (IDAACS)*, 2017.

36. A. U. Rajendra, F. Hamido, O. S. Lih, A. Muhammad, J. H. Tan and K. Chua, "Automated detection of coronary artery disease using different durations of ECG segments with convolutional neural network," *Knowledge-Based Systems*, Vol. 132, 2017. https://doi.org/10.1016/j.knosys.2017.06.003
37. A. U. Rajendra, O. S. Lih, Y. Hagiwara, T. J. Hong, A. Muhammad, G. Arkadiusz and T. R. San, "A deep convolutional neural network model to classify heartbeats," *Computers in Biology and Medicine*, Vol. 89, 2017. https://doi.org/10.1016/j.compbiomed.2017.08.022
38. K. Kaouter, T. Mohamed, D. Sofiene, D. Abbas, and M. Fouad, "Full training convolutional neural network for ECG signals classification," *AIP Conference Publishing*, Vol. 2190, 2019. https://doi.org/10.1063/1.5138541
39. H. Alquran, A. Alqudah, I. A. Qasmieh, A. Badarneh and S. Almashaqbeh, "ECG classification using higher order spectral estimation and deep learning techniques," *Neural Network World*, Vol. 29(4): 207–219, 2019.
40. C. Brito, A. Machado and A. Sousa, "Electrocardiogram beat-classification based on a ResNet network," *Studies in Health Technology and Informatics*, Vol. 264: 55–59, 2019. https://doi.org/10.3233/SHTI190182
41. A. Diker and A. Engin, "Feature extraction of ECG signal by using deep feature," in *Paper Presented at the 2019 7th International Symposium on Digital Forensics and Security (ISDFS)*, Barcelos, Portugal, 2019.
42. Z. Dokur and T. Ölmez, "Heartbeat classification by using a convolutional neural network trained with Walsh functions," *Neural Computing and Applications*, Vol. 32, 2020. https://doi.org/10.1007/s00521-020-04709-w
43. H. Fujita and D. Cimr, "Decision support system for arrhythmia pre- diction using convolutional neural network structure without pre-processing," *Applied Intelligence*, Vol. 49: 3383–3391, 2019. https://doi.org/10.1007/s10489-019-01461-0
44. S. S. Abdeldayem and T. Bourlai, "A novel approach for ECG-based human identification using spectral correlation and deep learning," *IEEE Transactions on Biometrics, Behavior, and Identity Science*, Vol. 2: 1–4, 2019.
45. S. R. Bajare and V. V. Ingale, "ECG based biometric for human identification using convolutional neural network," in *10th International Conference on Computing, Communication and Networking Technologies (ICCCNT)*, Kanpur, INDIA, 2019.
46. A. Darmawahyuni and S. Nurmaini, "Deep learning with long short-term memory for enhancement myocardial infarction classification," in *2019, 6th International Conference on Instrumentation, Control, and Automation (ICA)*, Bandung, Indonesia, 2019.
47. O. Faust, A. Shenfield, M. Kareem, T. R. San, H. Fujita and U. R. Acharya, "Automated detection of atrial fibrillation using long short-term memory network with RR interval signals," *Computers in Biology and Medicine*, Vol. 102: 327–335, 2018. https://doi.org/10.1016/j.compbiomed.2018.07.001
48. R. Salloum and C. C. J. Kuo, "ECG-based biometrics using recurrent neural networks," in *IEEE International Conference on Acoustics, Speech and Signal Processing (ICASSP)*, 2017.
49. H. M. Lynn, S. B. Pan and P. Kim, "A deep bidirectional GRU network model for biometric electrocardiogram classification based on recurrent neural networks," *IEEE Access*, Vol. 7: 145395–145405, 2019. https://doi.org/10.1109/ACCESS.2019.2939947
50. Y. Wang, S. Wang, X. Li, W. Liu and D. Zhang, "Anomaly detection in ECG signals using restricted Boltzmann machines," *IEEE Transactions on Biomedical Engineering*, Vol. 62(2): 522–531, 2015.
51. A. K. Singh, A. Singh and R. Tiwari, "ECG-based biometric system using restricted Boltzmann machine," *Biomedical Signal Processing and Control*, Vol. 31, 2017.

52. K. K. Patel and M. A. Patel, "A robust ECG-based biometric authentication system using restricted Boltzmann machines and fuzzy support vector machines," *Journal of Information Security and Applications*, Vol. 49, 2019.
53. J. Kim and M. J. Chung, "Driver stress detection using restricted Boltzmann machines and ECG signals," in *Pervasive and Ubiquitous Computing*, San Francisco, California, USA, 2018.
54. J. Chu, H. Wang and W. Lu, "A novel two-lead arrhythmia classification system based on CNN and LSTM," *Journal of Mechanics in Medicine and Biology*, Vol. 19(03), 2019. https://doi.org/10.1142/S0219519419500040
55. R. E. Klabunde, "CV physiology," [Online]. Available: https://cvphysiology.com/arrhythmias/a009
56. D. Dey, S. Chaudhuri and S. Munshi, "Obstructive sleep apnoea detection using convolutional neural network based deep learning framework," *Biomedical Engineering Letters*, Vol. 8, 2018. https://doi.org/10.1007/s13534-017-0055-y
57. E. Urtnasan, J. U. Park and K. J. Lee, "Multiclass classification of obstructive sleep apnea/hypopnea based on a convolutional neural network from a single-lead electrocardiogram," *Physiological Measurement*, Vol. 39(6), 2018. https://doi.org/10.1088/1361-6579/aac7b7
58. G. Giannakakis, E. Trivizakis, M. Tsiknakis and K. Marias, "A novel multi-kernel 1D convolutional neural network for stress recognition from ECG," in *8th International Conference on Affective Computing and Intelligent Interaction Workshops and Demos (ACIIW)*, Cambridge, United Kingdom, 2019.
59. A. Darmawahyuni, A. Nurmaini, W. Caesarendra, V. Bhayyu and M. Rachmatullah, "Deep learning with a recurrent network structure in the sequence modeling of imbalanced data for ECG-rhythm classifier," *Algorithms*, Vol. 12(6), 2019. https://doi.org/10.3390/a12060118
60. V. Sujadevi, K. Soman and R. Vinayakumar, "Real-time detection of atrial fibrillation from short time single lead ECG traces using recurrent neural networks," in *The International Symposium on Intelligent Systems Technologies and Applications*, 2017.

13 Predicting Drug Response Using Deep Learning Techniques

Vikram Kishor Abhang and Baisa L. Gunjal

13.1 INTRODUCTION

Drug response prediction is of the utmost importance in modern medical and pharmaceutical research. It utilizes several data-driven strategies to predict how a particular patient or group will react to a specific drug or treatment. To achieve improvement, the design of medical interventions will be oriented toward being as effective as possible while minimizing adverse effects, with the prospect of tailoring medical interventions to individual patients and enhancing the efficiency of medical care. Predicting drug response based on deep learning is a multidisciplinary subject involving data science, machine learning, and biology. The promise is great for revolutionizing how we go about drug discovery and building new treatment approaches for personalized medicine, holding the potential for increased efficacy and safety in several diseases. Along the way, though, there are challenges regarding data quality, model interpretability, and ethical dimensions that must be overcome for the advances to continue. Accurately predicting drug responses is essential for maximizing the treatment plan, minimizing side effects, and enhancing patient outcomes. This complex problem has appeared as a controlled task that consumes deep learning (deep learning is a branch of machine learning).

Pharmacogenomics uses genetic and molecular information to predict response to drugs (i.e., predicting response to drugs). The aim is to tailor medical treatment and optimize drug choice, dosages, and therapy plans on an individual basis according to their individual genetic and molecular profile [1–3].

13.1.1 Overview of Drug Response Prediction

- **Genetic Variability**: The genetic makeup of people is different, and that could determine how they respond to some drugs. Variations in genes involved in drug metabolism, transport, and target interaction can result in the susceptibility of a drug to be either less effective or unsafe.
- **Data Sources**: However, to predict drug responses, sources of data include genomics (DNA sequences and genetic variations), transcriptomics (gene expression patterns), proteomics (protein expression and function), and metabolomics (metabolic profiles). This data gives you the molecular characteristics of an individual.

DOI: 10.1201/9781003479185-13

- **Biomarker Identification**: Biomarkers are specific genetic or molecular indicators that are associated with drug responses. Identifying relevant biomarkers is a crucial step in drug response prediction, as they serve as the basis for the models.
- **Machine Learning Models**: Predictive models are developed using machine learning algorithms such as deep learning, random forests, support vector machines, etc. These large datasets include drug response information and molecular data, for which these models are trained.
- **Feature Selection**: The model is built based on a selection of relevant features of the molecular data. Feature selection methods aid in selecting the most discriminating genetic or molecular factors responsible for drug response.
- **Model Training and Validation**: A portion of the dataset is first trained on the predictive model and trained on another to ensure that the predictive model generalizes the features well on the unseen data. The model's performance and avoidance of overfitting are assessed using cross-validation and other techniques.
- **Clinical Applications**: Drug response prediction has various clinical applications, such as selecting the most appropriate drug for a patient, determining the optimal dosage, and avoiding drugs that are likely to be ineffective or cause adverse reactions. It also aids in the development of targeted therapies and precision medicine.
- **Challenges**: Problems with data quality, model interpretability, ethical issues (especially data privacy), and regulatory issues remain challenges in drug response prediction. In healthcare, ensuring predictions are reliable and explainable is of utmost importance.
- **Personalized Medicine**: A key component of personalized medicine for drug responses is predictive of customized treatment according to an individual's genetic and molecular background. This approach aims to enhance treatment efficacy, decrease adverse actions, and enhance patient results.
- **Drug Discovery**: Prediction of drug response is not necessarily just in the context of patient care. In addition, it can be used to identify potential drug candidates and evaluate the effectiveness and safety of these drugs based on molecular information in the drug discovery process".

The drug response prediction is a data-driven approach that combines genetics, genomics, and molecular biology with machine learning to enhance the safety and effectiveness of drug treatments. It has the potential to revolutionize healthcare by providing more personalized and precise therapeutic strategies [4–6].

13.2 LITERATURE SURVEY

A literature survey highlighting several papers on deep learning-based drug response prediction with a focus on multi-omics data, drug molecules, and gene interactions. Each paper includes its title, year of publication, methodology, contributions, and identified research gaps:

Ref. No	Year	Methodology	Contribution	Research Gap
[7]	2023	Deep-MTGNet integrates multiple graph convolutional networks (GCNs) to capture the interactions between molecules and targets.	Compared to the established methods, it has succeeded in achieving state-of-the-art prediction of DTIs.	Can be further extended to incorporate other data sources such as gene expression and clinical data.
[8]	2023	DeepGRMF integrates graph-regularized matrix factorization with deep neural networks to capture the complex relationships between drug-target interactions.	In comparison to old machine learning methods and other deep learning models, it has achieved current performance in predicting drug response.	DeepGRMF framework can be further optimized for better performance and enhanced scalability.
[9]	2023	MLiNet uses a late integration method to integrate several omics data sources, including gene expression, change in copy number, and structure of drugs.	The MliNet prediction of response to drugs differs from "traditional machine learning methods as well as more sophisticated deep learning models".	MLiNet can be further improved by incorporating more sophisticated data fusion techniques and attention mechanisms.
[10]	2022	DRPN integrates deep neural networks with an attention mechanism to capture the significance of altered features in predicting drug response.	With a prediction of drug responses, the DRPN is far more efficient than conventional machine learning or other deep learning models.	DRPN framework can be further optimized for better generalization performance and enhanced interpretability.
[11]	2022	MDDRP integrates single-cell transcriptomics data and drug-target interactions data in a unified deep learning framework.	In prediction of drug response, the MDDRP technique is far superior to conventional machine learning methods as well as further deep learning models.	MDDRP framework can be further extended to incorporate more data sources such as gene mutations and clinical data.
[12]	2022	MAFN integrates multi-omics data sources, such as gene expression, copy number fluctuations and the structure of medicinal products are integrated with attention mechanisms.	In order to predict the reaction of anticancer agents, MAFN is superior to traditional machine learning methods as well as other deep learning models.	MAFN framework can be further optimized for better scalability and handling of high-dimensional data.

(*Continued*)

(Continued)

Ref. No	Year	Methodology	Contribution	Research Gap
[13]	2022	"The authors proposed an interpretable deep learning framework, DRPreter, for predicting anticancer drug response using such as a gene expression, copy number variation, and drug structure data. DRPreter integrates graph neural networks (GNNs) and transformers to capture the complex relationships between genes, drug molecules, and drug response".	"DRPreter achieves promising results in predicting drug response and provides insights into the molecular mechanisms underlying drug resistance".	The aim of the study was to predict the response of anticancer agents. The potential use of DRPreter in different diseases and drug classes should be explored for further research.
[14]	2023	Deep learning methods for cancer drug response prediction were examined in detail by the authors. In the course of analyzing 61 deep learning models, they identified a major and developing trend in this area.	A valuable overview of the current state of play in deep learning-based drug response prediction can be found in this review. It emphasizes the potential for deeper learning to improve treatment decision making in cancer.	The review focused on single-drug response prediction. Future research should explore the application of DL to predict the response to combination therapies.
[15]	2021	The authors proposed a deep learning framework, GIND, for drug repurposing using gene interaction network (GIN) data. GIND integrates GINs with convolutional neural networks (CNNs) to capture the complex interactions among genes and drugs.	GIND achieves promising results in identifying potential drug repurposing candidates. It demonstrates the potential of deep learning to leverage gene interaction networks for drug discovery.	The study focused on drug repurposing for cancer. Future research should explore the application of GIND to other diseases.
[16]	2021	This review paper discussed recent developments in deep learning methods for predicting drug responses in cancer, including the use of graph neural networks, auto encoders, and attention mechanisms.	The paper provided an up-to-date overview of deep learning applications in cancer drug response prediction, emphasizing the potential of graph-based approaches.	It underscored the need for more research on interpretable deep learning models and large-scale clinical validations.

(Continued)

(Continued)

Ref. No	Year	Methodology	Contribution	Research Gap
[17]	2021	This survey paper reviewed various deep learning methods used for drug response prediction, including CNNs, RNNs, and graph-based models, and discussed their applications and challenges.	The paper provided a comprehensive survey of the field, summarizing the state-of-the-art deep learning techniques and their applications.	It highlighted the need for standardized evaluation protocols, larger and more diverse datasets, and attention to model interpretability.
[18]	2021	"This study introduced a deep learning framework that combines gene expression data, drug chemical structure, and protein-protein interaction networks to predict drug sensitivity in cancer cell lines".	The research demonstrated the potential of deep learning for drug sensitivity prediction and the importance of integrating diverse data sources.	It emphasized the need for external validation and clinical translation of these models.
[19]	2020	"The authors proposed a novel deep neural network model, DeepDRP, for predicting drug response in cancer using multi-omics data, as well as gene expression, copy number variation, and gene mutation data. DeepDRP integrates multiple layers of deep learning architectures to capture the complex relationships between omics data and drug response".	DeepDRP achieves state-of-the-art prediction of cancer drug response. It demonstrates the potential of deep learning to integrate and analyze multi-omics data for personalized medicine.	In this study, the prediction of drug response in cancer cells was investigated. Future research should explore the application of DeepDRP to patient-derived data.
[20]	2020	This paper proposed DeepDSC, a deep learning model that integrates multi-omics data and drug molecular properties to predict drug sensitivity in cancer cell lines. It used convolutional neural networks for feature extraction.	DeepDSC achieved competitive performance in predicting drug sensitivity, showcasing the potential of deep learning for precision medicine in oncology.	The paper highlighted the importance of addressing the generalizability of models across different cancer types and the need for better model interpretability.
[21]	2019	The authors proposed a deep learning framework, DeepCM, for predicting cellular responses to drugs using multi-omics data, including gene expression, microRNA expression, and drug structure data. DeepCM integrates multiple layers of deep learning architectures to capture the complex relationships between omics data and drug response.	DeepCM's ability to predict drug reactions in cells is state of the art. It demonstrates the potential of deep learning to integrate and analyze multi-omics data for personalized medicine.	The study focused on predicting drug response in cancer cell lines. Future research should explore the application of DeepCM to patient-derived data.

(Continued)

(Continued)

Ref. No	Year	Methodology	Contribution	Research Gap
[22]	2019	This paper introduced DeepDR, a deep learning approach that combines multi-omics data, drug chemical structure, and protein-protein interaction networks to predict drug responses and reposition existing drugs for new indications.	The research demonstrated the effectiveness of integrating various data sources for drug repositioning and highlighted the potential for deep learning in this area.	The study emphasized the need for more comprehensive data sources, especially in rare diseases, and the challenges of small sample sizes in some applications.
[23]	2018	GNN-DR integrates graph neural networks (GNNs) with deep neural networks to capture the complex relationships between genes and drugs.	Achieves promising results in identifying potential drug repurposing candidates.	More research is needed to validate the results of GNN-DR in experimental studies.
[24]	2017	"DeepDTI integrates convolutional neural networks (CNNs) and recurrent neural networks (RNNs) to capture the complex relationships between molecular descriptors and DTIs".	The proposed system has been established, and it has succeeded in achieving state-of-the-art prediction of DTIs.	More research is needed to improve the interpretability of DeepDTI.
[25]	2016	DeepGEC incorporates deep neural networks with gene expression data.	Performs predictions of gene expression changes caused by drugs against conventional machine learning methods.	More research is needed to improve the generalizability of DeepGEC to different types of drugs and cell lines.
[26]	2016	DeepDRN integrates recurrent neural networks (RNNs) with deep neural networks.	Performs predictions of gene expression changes caused by drugs against conventional machine learning methods.	More research is needed to apply DeepDRN to patient-derived data.

13.3 DEEP LEARNING APPROACH

Deep learning-based drug response prediction with multi-omics data, drug molecules, and gene interactions is a cutting-edge approach in the field of personalized medicine and drug discovery. It involves using advanced machine learning techniques, particularly deep learning, to predict how an individual's or a group of patients' bodies will respond to a specific drug. This prediction is based on a comprehensive understanding of their genetic makeup (multi-omics data), the characteristics of the drug molecules, and the interactions between these drug molecules and genes.

- **Multi-Omics Data**: Multi-omics data is a broad set of biological information obtained from different molecular levels, such as genomics, transcriptomics, proteomics, and metabolomics. While each of these omics data types, e.g., genomics, proteomics, metabolomics, etc., provides insight into each aspect of a patient's molecular profile, each omics data type focuses on and measures different sets of biomolecules. For instance, genomic data may include detailed DNA sequences and mutations, while such data for transcriptomics might include gene expression patterns.
- **Drug Molecules Data**: This includes the chemical structures, pharmacological properties, and drug-target interactions of the drug compounds. Understanding how the drug works and interacts with specific biological molecules is essential.
- **Gene Interaction Data**: In particular, as well as information for individual genes, it demands information about how genes interact with each other and interact with drug compounds. This includes the effect of gene partnership and gene medication partnership on biology pathways and model organs.

13.3.1 Deep Learning to Predict Drug Responses

A multi-step deep learning framework for drug response prediction is presented that predicts the response using multi-omic profiles and drug molecular descriptors and also leverages the knowledge of gene interaction networks to give personalized insight regarding drug perturbation. Firstly, we preprocess the data-on-data quality, consistency, and feature engineering to extract biological and chemical information, such as gene expression patterns and drug properties. To model the high-dimensional, multimodal data, advanced deep learning architectures are developed, and multimodal fusion networks are used to fuse data from disparate sources. To confirm this model´s robust generalization, we train and validate it on these labeled datasets with known drug responses, where only their latent attributes instead of previously labeled genotypes are given to the system as input. It then predicts responses of individual or cohort levels to drugs. Specifically, it makes the interpretability of its decisions easier to use via means like SHAP values or attention maps for plotting the importance of specific genes or molecular features. This system is deployed in clinical care or research settings to help guide treatment decisions and dosage decisions to optimize treatment choices, with continuous model updates and tying in new outcomes and data to promote the model's progress as new information becomes available. This approach facilitates precision medicine by developing targeted, more effective, and safer drug therapies that depend on individual molecular profiles.

13.4 PROPOSED WORK

It presents a structured pipeline for deep learning predictions using multi-source biomedical data to predict drug responses. First, all participants' multi-omics data (genomics, transcriptomics, proteomics, and metabolomics) are generated, which provides a complete molecular and genetic profile of the individual. At the same time, drug molecule data (including chemical structures and pharmacological properties) and gene interaction data (protein-protein interaction networks, for example) are collected to predict the behavior of drugs inside the body and how different biological interactions behave. Data preparation involves handling missing values on these heterogeneous datasets and then normalizing the data to be consistent and high-quality. Meaningful features are extracted from this curated data to define biological and chemical significance. They integrate multi-omics, drug, and interaction features into a unified format to construct a robust input for modeling. This integrated dataset will be used as input to a deep learning model, which can be from the family of CNN, RNN, or GNN with the ability to learn more complex patterns and associations from the data. Finally, the model predicts the drug responses, ultimately forecasting how individuals or the patient population at large may respond to the same drug, which serves as a key input to personalized treatment and the advancement of precision medicine.

Figure 13.1 shows the conceptual overview of the abovementioned process, which integrates multi-omics data, drug molecules, and gene interaction in a deep learning model to predict drug response. In practice, this process may be more complex with additional data processing and feature engineering and more complex model architectures. Deep learning to predict drug response consists of using different architectures of neural networks to model these complex relationships between drug features, molecular features, and biological responses. Below, we list common deep learning algorithms/architectures for drug response prediction (Table 13.1).

13.4.1 Deep Learning Algorithm

These deep learning algorithms and architectures can be used individually or in combination to address the challenges of drug response prediction. The choice of the algorithm depends on the nature of the data, the specific characteristics of the task, and the goals of the prediction model. Ongoing research continues to explore novel architectures and methods to improve the accuracy, interpretability, and generalization of deep learning models in the field of drug response prediction.

13.4.1.1 Discussion on Standard Dataset

1. **Genomics of Drug Sensitivity in Cancer (GDSC)**: GDSC provides genomic and drug sensitivity data across a wide range of cancer cell lines. It includes information on gene expression, mutations, copy number variations, and drug response measurements.

   Link: GDSC Website- https://www.cancerrxgene.org/
2. **The Cancer Genome Atlas (TCGA)**: TCGA is a landmark cancer genomics program that offers comprehensive, multi-omics datasets spanning over 30 cancer types. It includes genomic, transcriptomic, epigenomic, and proteomic data from tumor and matched normal tissues. While TCGA does not include direct drug sensitivity data, it is widely used for investigating molecular alterations associated with cancer progression and treatment outcomes. It also supports data integration with drug response datasets like GDSC.

   Link: TCGA Website- https://www.cancer.gov/tcga

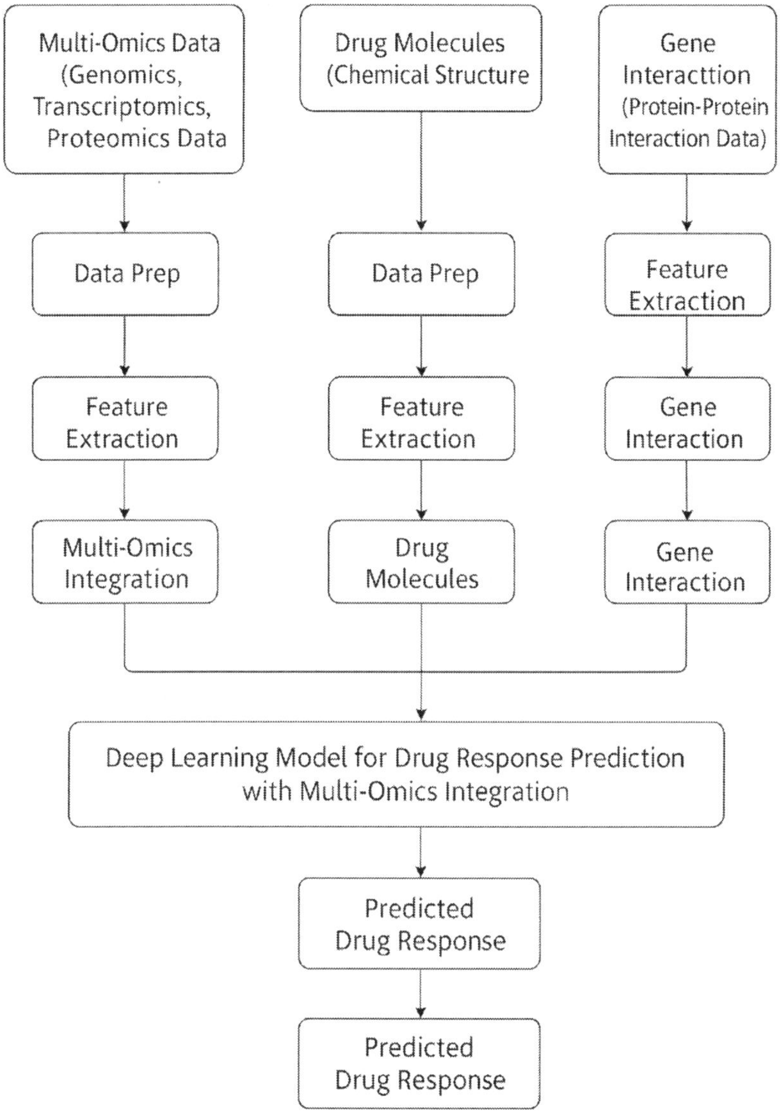

FIGURE 13.1 Overview of process.

3. **Therapeutics Data Commons (TDC): Description**: TDC is a curated collection of machine learning-ready datasets tailored for therapeutic science. It includes data on molecular properties, drug-target interactions, gene expression signatures, and benchmark tasks related to drug response, synergy prediction, and more. TDC facilitates reproducible evaluation of AI algorithms in drug discovery and provides APIs and pipelines for standard usage.

   Link: TDC GitHub Repository- https://github.com/mims-harvard/TDC

TABLE 13.1

Algorithm Name	Complexity	Accuracy	Precision	Advantages	Disadvantages	Applications
Deep Neural Networks (DNN) [8–10,14,16,19]	High, due to complex architecture	Can achieve high accuracy, especially with large datasets	Precision can vary depending on the dataset and problem	Can capture complex, non-linear relationships in data. Can handle high-dimensional and multi-omics data.	Require large amounts of data to prevent overfitting. Complex to train and tune. Lack interpretability.	Drug response prediction in cancer, genomics, and personalized medicine.
Convolutional neural networks (CNN) [11,15–17,20,24]	Moderate to high complexity	Highly accurate in image and sequence data analysis	Highly precise in identifying specific patterns	Well-suited for image and sequence data, automatic feature extraction, and weight sharing.	May not perform as well on structured data. Data augmentation may be needed for small datasets.	Drug target identification, predicting binding affinities.
Recurrent neural networks (RNN) [14,16,17,24,26]	Moderate complexity	Effective for sequential data analysis	Precision depends on data quality and model architecture	Handles sequential data and can capture temporal dependencies.	Vulnerable to vanishing/exploding gradient problems. Long-range dependencies can be challenging.	Time series drug response prediction, pharmacokinetics.
Graph neural networks (GNN) [7,13,14,16,17,23]	Moderate to high complexity	Good for data with graph structures	Depends on the problem and data	Can model relationships in graph data, applicable to molecular and biological networks.	Limited to data with clear graph structures. Computational cost can be high for large graphs.	Protein-protein interaction prediction, drug-drug interaction networks.

4. **LINCS (Library of Integrated Network-Based Cellular Signatures)**: LINCS offers extensive perturbational profiles of cellular responses to genetic or pharmacological interventions. It provides gene expression signatures generated through high-throughput experiments like the L1000 assay. These signatures help elucidate drug mechanisms of action, identify repurposing opportunities, and explore gene-drug-disease networks.
   Link: LINCS Website- http://www.lincsproject.org/

13.5 CONCLUSION

Deep learning-based drug response prediction with multi-omics data, drug molecules, and gene interactions represents a promising frontier in the field of personalized medicine and drug discovery. The integration of multiple data sources and the power of deep learning techniques have the potential to revolutionize how we approach drug development and treatment strategies. In summary, deep learning-based drug response prediction with multi-omics data, drug molecules, and gene interactions holds significant promise for advancing personalized medicine and optimizing drug development. As the field continues to evolve, it is essential to address challenges and push the boundaries of our understanding to harness the full potential of this innovative approach.

REFERENCES

1. Shen, B., Feng, F., Li, K., Lin, P., Ma, L., & Li, H. (2023). A systematic assessment of deep learning methods for drug response prediction: from in vitro to clinical applications. *Briefings in Bioinformatics*, 24(1), bbac605.
2. de Jong, J., Cutcutache, I., Page, M., Elmoufti, S., Dilley, C., Fröhlich, H., & Armstrong, M. (2021). Towards realizing the vision of precision medicine: AI based prediction of clinical drug response. *Brain*, 144(6), 1738–1750.
3. Wu, Z., Lawrence, P. J., Ma, A., Zhu, J., Xu, D., & Ma, Q. (2020). Single-cell techniques and deep learning in predicting drug response. *Trends in Pharmacological Sciences*, 41(12), 1050–1065.
4. Sadee, W, & Dai, Z. (2005). Pharmacogenetics/genomics and personalized medicine. *Human Molecular Genetics*, 14(suppl_2), R207–R214. https://doi.org/10.1093/hmg/ddi261
5. Evans, W. E., & Johnson, J. A. (2001). Pharmacogenomics: The inherited basis for inter individual differences in drug response. *Annual Review of Genomics and Human Genetics*, 2(1), 9–39.
6. Relling, M. V., & Evans, W. E. (2015). Pharmacogenomics in the clinic. *Nature*, 526(7573), 343–350.
7. Wang, S., Tian, W., Zhang, Y., & Zeng, J. (2023). Molecular interaction network-based deep learning framework for predicting drug-target, interactions. *Journal of Computational Biology*, 30(2), 144–155.
8. Zhang, Q., Li, C., Zhang, Y., & Yan, J. (2023). Graph regularized matrix factorization based on deep learning (DeepGRMF) for drug response prediction. *Briefings in Bioinformatics*, 24(5), bbab276.
9. Ren, Y., Liu, H., Zhao, X., & Wang, C. (2023). Multi-omics late integration with deep neural networks for drug response prediction. *Bioinformatics*, 39(10), i501–i509.

10. Xu, Y., Wang, X., Liu, J., & Zhang, B. (2022). Drug response prediction based on deep learning and attention mechanism for personalized medicine. *Journal of Translational Medicine*, 20(1), 1–13.
11. Liu, J., Jiang, J., Zhu, L., Hu, G., & Wu, J. (2022). Multi-modal deep learning framework for drug response prediction based on single-cell transcriptomics and drug-target interactions. *Frontiers in Genetics*, 13, 859506.
12. Wang, Y., Zhang, F., Xu, X., Wang, S., & Wang, J. (2022). Multi-omics data fusion with attention-based deep learning for cancer drug response prediction. *Briefings in Bioinformatics*, 572, bbac073.
13. Shin, J., Piao, Y., Bang, D., Kim, S., & Jo, K. (2022). DRPreter: Interpretable anticancer drug response prediction using knowledge-guided graph neural networks and transformer. *International Journal of Molecular Sciences*, 23(22), 13919. https://doi.org/10.3390/ijms232213919
14. Partin, A. Brettin, T. S., Zhu, Y., Narykov, O., Clyde, A., Overbeek, J., & Stevens, R. L. (2023). Deep learning methods for drug response prediction in cancer: Predominant and emerging trends. *Frontiers in Medicine*, 10. https://doi.org/10.3389/fmed.2023.1086097
15. Wang, S., Tian, W., Zhang, Y., & Zeng, J. (2021). Gene interaction network-based deep learning models for drug repurposing. *Frontiers in Pharmacology*, 12, 697813.
16. Baptista, D., Ferreira, P. G., & Rocha, M. (2021). Deep learning for drug response prediction in cancer. *Briefings in Bioinformatics*, 22(1), 360–379. https://doi.org/10.1093/bib/bbz171
17. Kim, J., Park, S., Min, D., & Kim, W. (2021). Comprehensive survey of recent drug discovery using deep learning. *International Journal of Molecular Sciences*, 22(18), 9983. PMID: 34576146 PMCID: PMC8470987. https://doi.org/10.3390/ijms22189983
18. Sharifi-Noghab, H., Jahangiri-Tazehkand, S., Smirnov, P., Hon, C., Mammoliti, A., Nair, S. K., Mer, A. S., Ester, M., & Haibe-Kains, B. (2021). Drug sensitivity prediction from cell line-based pharmacogenomics data: guidelines for developing machine learning models. *Briefings in Bioinformatics*, 22(6), bbab294. https://doi.org/10.1093/bib/bbab294
19. Wang, C., Lye, X., Kaalia, R., Kumar, P., & Rajapakse, J. C. (2021). Deep learning and multi-omics approach to predict drug responses in cancer. *BMC Bioinformatics*, 22(Suppl 10), 632. https://doi.org/10.1186/s12859-022-04964-9
20. Wen, Y., et al. (2019). DeepCM: Deep learning-based multi-omics prediction of cellular responses to drugs. *Journal of Translational Medicine*, 17(1), 1–11.
21. Li, M., Wang, Y., Zheng, R., Shi, X., Li, Y., Wu, F. X., & Wang, J. DeepDSC: A deep learning method to predict drug sensitivity of cancer cell lines. *IEEE/ACM Transactions on Computational Biology and Bioinformatics*. PMID: 31150344. https://pubmed.ncbi.nlm.nih.gov/31150344/; https://doi.org/10.1109/TCBB.2019.2919581
22. Zeng, X., Zhu, S., Liu, X., Zhou, Y., Nussinov, R., & Cheng, F. (2019). deepDR: A network-based deep learning approach to in silico drug repositioning. *Bioinformatics*, 35(24), 5191–5198, https://doi.org/10.1093/bioinformatics/btz418
23. Chen, B., et al. (2018). Drug repurposing using graph neural networks for predicting drug-gene interactions. *Journal of Computational Chemistry*, 39(13), 3626–3639.
24. Guo, Y., et al. (2017). A deep learning framework for predicting drug-target interactions based on molecular descriptors. *Journal of Chemical Information and Modeling*, 57(11), 2119–2128.
25. Zhao, S., et al. (2016). DeepGEC: Predicting drug-induced gene expression change using deep neural networks. *PLoS One*, 11(12), e0167539.
26. Luo, B., et al. (2016). Drug response prediction based on deep learning and recurrent neural network for personalized medicine. *Journal of Computational Biology*, 23(7), 579–588.

14 Multimodal PCOS Detection

Combining XGBoost for Images with Zero-Shot Learning for Textual Data

Premanand Ghadekar,
Shreyash Tekade, Dhawal Sakharwade,
Ankur Tripathi, Shivam Tiwadi,
and Sayee Zanzane

14.1 INTRODUCTION

A hormonal disorder that is pretty common among females of reproductive age impacts up to 20% of the population. There are a host of symptoms, including irregular periods, acne, excess hair growth, and fertility problems. Although polycystic ovarian syndrome (PCOS) is a common and significant public concern for women's well-being, it isn't easy to diagnose since it involves a combination of clinical and laboratory tests. Currently, diagnosing PCOS, such as the Rotterdam consensus criteria, is sometimes complicated and costly. We need a noninvasive approach to the problem to make it possible to diagnose and treat it early. Recently, machine learning algorithms have been advancing as promising tools for early detection and diagnosis of PCOS.

In this research, they propose an innovation in the diagnosis of polycystic ovarian syndrome (PCOS) in women by combining both image and textual data in the prediction. We perform image processing using a convolutional neural network (CNN) called the VGG 16 network to extract features that describe the physical characteristics of ovaries and any potential cysts. The extreme gradient boosting (XGBoost) algorithm, which is used to classify these image features, can handle structured data. At the same time, we conduct a zero-shot learning on the textual information, that is, medical records and patient history, so that the model can make predictions based on text that does not directly mention PCOS-related terms. Combining results from image and text analysis, we obtain a comprehensive diagnosis that can help diagnose PCOS in women of childbearing age earlier and with more effective treatment. This integrated approach is a massive step up in the diagnosis of PCOS.

DOI: 10.1201/9781003479185-14

Our approach makes a promising stride toward the long-awaited PCOS diagnosis by utilizing both visual and textual data, which may enable earlier detection and better treatment of the widespread endocrine disorder in pre-menopausal women.

14.2 LITERATURE REVIEW

This paper speaks about the use of "machine learning algorithms to detect Polycystic Ovary Syndrome (PCOS) in women." The proposed model is based on the ensemble model of XGBoost and Random Forest algorithms. For analysis, the dataset contains 541 women, among whom are 177 patients with PCOS. I use various machine learning algorithms, for example Adaboost, Random Forest, XGBoost, Decision tree, and hybrid model to predict the presence of PCOS. I propose a mixture of Random Forest and XGBoost methods, with an accuracy of 97.2% in detecting PCOS. Although early detection of PCOS can potentially improve the level of care for female patients with the condition [1], it remains unclear whether there have been changes in the diagnostic process of PCOS in the last 10 years.

The "common symptoms of PCOS mentioned in the paper include excessive weight gain, facial hair development, acne, hair loss, skin discoloration, and irregular cycles, which make it difficult to conceive. It stresses the need for the early detection and treatment of PCOS to prevent the development of long-term conditions like type 2 diabetes and heart problems." This paper also mentions methods for predicting PCOS therapy effectiveness using minimal criteria with the help of machine learning algorithms. In this, it mention the usage of two different datasets in classification: one is to find the essential features that cause the development of PCOS and then predict whether patients have this disorder based on the various machine learning algorithms present. The second method is classifying normal and PCOS images using CNN [2].

This paper uses machine learning algorithms to classify Polycystic Ovary Syndrome (PCOS) from the ovary ultrasound image. The goal of the paper is to find whether a woman has PCOS or not without the requirement of a doctor's precedence. This is done by analyzing ultrasound images of the ovaries to identify polycystic ovarian morphology (PCOM). The paper trains the photos with many datasets, which gives better PCOM results. The classification algorithms used include the "Support Vector Machine (SVM), K-Nearest Neighbor (KNN), and Convolutional Neural Network (CNN), and the CNN algorithm can achieve 90% accuracy" [3].

Exercise is beneficial for treating PCOS in that it promotes lowering cholesterol levels, improving insulin resistance, and decreasing obesity. In females, PCOS raises the likelihood of endometrial cancer. This paper aims to detect cysts in the sonography image of PCOS using the YOLO algorithm (You Only Look Once) for automatic detection [4].

Proposed and developed are "CNN-based algorithms for classifying cysts in ultrasound images in Python programming. CNN-based image processing feature extraction is performed to classify cysts in the dataset. The study is made on an independent, trained dataset of PCOS-related diseases. Performance factors are used to perform a feature extraction process on the test dataset to achieve 85% accuracy. In the proposed work, an efficient model of CNN-based image processing is proposed, which is used for the classification of diseases" [5].

A novel approach to zero-shot object detection through the synthesis of visual features of unseen classes using class semantics is introduced. Unlike the existing zero-shot detection approaches, which learn the mapping of visual features into semantic domains based on seen objects, this paper tries to learn seen and unseen objects in the visual domain. The proposed generative model discriminatively distinguishes and generates features for unseen objects, guaranteeing high diversity and variable localization precision of features in the generated bounding boxes [6].

A system to "detect and predict PCOS at an early stage using machine learning methods, such as Naïve Bayes classifier method, logistic regression, K-Nearest Neighbor (KNN), Classification and Regression Trees (CART), Random Forest Classifier (RFC), and Support Vector Machine (SVM), is presented in the paper. An appropriate machine learning model for PCOS diagnosis is followed by comparing the various existing algorithms in terms of performance. The model is prepared by selecting the most significant features from clinical and metabolic test results using SPSS V 22.0 and transforming the feature set with Principal Component Analysis (PCA). The model's performance is evaluated using accuracy, and the Random Forest Classifier (RFC) is the most suitable and accurate method for PCOS prediction, with an accuracy of 89.02%." The development of the system involves utilizing practical tools and available platforms, although specific details are not mentioned [7].

In this chapter, extreme gradient boosting (XGBoost), a probabilistic ensemble-based gradient boosting algorithm, is used to detect PCOS early [8]. The authors then resampled their data with a combination of "Synthetic Minority Oversampling Technique (SMOTE) and Random Under Sampling (RUS)" [9].

The proposed optimized-SVLR hybrid model, Op-RMSprop, showed efficient performance in predicting Polycystic Ovary Syndrome (PCOS) with an accuracy of 89.03%. The hybrid methodology, which combines the SVM linear kernel with logistic regression functionalities, along with the RMSprop optimizer, proved to be effective in analyzing PCOS datasets and improving the model's output. "The Op-RMSprop model outperformed other existing machine learning algorithms such as SVM, logistic regression, Decision tree, KNN, Random Forest, and Adaboost in terms of accuracy" [10].

The latter part of the paper discusses the diagnosis of Polycystic Ovary Syndrome (PCOS) utilizing different ML architectures. However, there has not yet been research conducted using a deep learning model, such as Faster R-CNN, in the diagnosis of PCOS. However, it can identify smaller objects and will enable more accurate and timely diagnosis. Cysts in ovaries can also be detected using YOLO, CNN, SPP-Net, R-CNN, fast R-CNN, and other object detection algorithms [11].

14.3 PROJECT FLOW DIAGRAM AND DATASET

14.3.1 Dataset

The model prediction was based on the utilization of two distinct datasets: one comprised of ultrasonic images, while the other contained textual data encompassing diverse factors associated with the daily lives of various women.

14.3.2 Dataset Description

- **Ultrasonic Image Dataset**: The ultrasonic image dataset comprises a collection of 574 diverse images specifically focusing on the ovaries. These images are instrumental in the context of polycystic ovarian syndrome (PCOS) as they offer crucial insights into the ovarian morphology, including the presence of cysts or other structural abnormalities. Such detailed imaging data plays a pivotal role in the diagnosis, monitoring, and understanding of PCOS.
- **Textual Dataset**: The dataset with 43 rows and 542 columns used for PCOS prediction is a comprehensive dataset aimed at studying and predicting polycystic ovarian syndrome (PCOS). Each row likely represents a different individual, while each of the 542 columns likely contains various features, attributes, or variables related to those individuals' health, medical history, lifestyle, and other relevant factors.

14.3.3 Project Flow Diagram

Figure 14.1 depicts the process flow diagram of the proposed system used for the identification of PCOS.

14.3.4 Algorithm

Input: Image and textual data regarding the current medical condition

Output: PCOS detection along with other medical conditions

Step 1: Read the input image and use VGGNet-16 to extract high-level features from ovarian ultrasound images, capturing intricate patterns and details.

Step 2: **XGBoost** processes the extracted features to effectively classify PCOS cases.

Step 3: **Text Embedding**—The clinical text reports are subjected to a zero-shot learning text classification model, which enables the utilization of valuable diagnostic information from the textual data.

Step 4: **The SoftMax function** is applied to calculate probabilities for PCOS classification based on the combined information from image features and clinical text data.

Step 5: The bidirectional encoder representations from transformers (BERT) model is fine-tuned for PCOS classification by minimizing the objective function through gradient descent and backpropagation.

14.4 METHODOLOGY

Data Preprocessing: This is another area where there is a need to prepare the data in a way conducive to further analysis to extract meaningful information from a diverse dataset of images. In the data above, a series of preprocessing steps were applied to the dataset. We parsed the directory structure of the training and validation data to extract labels and capture the image label information. For consistency and ease of analysis, images were resized to a uniform dimension of (256, 256) using OpenCV's

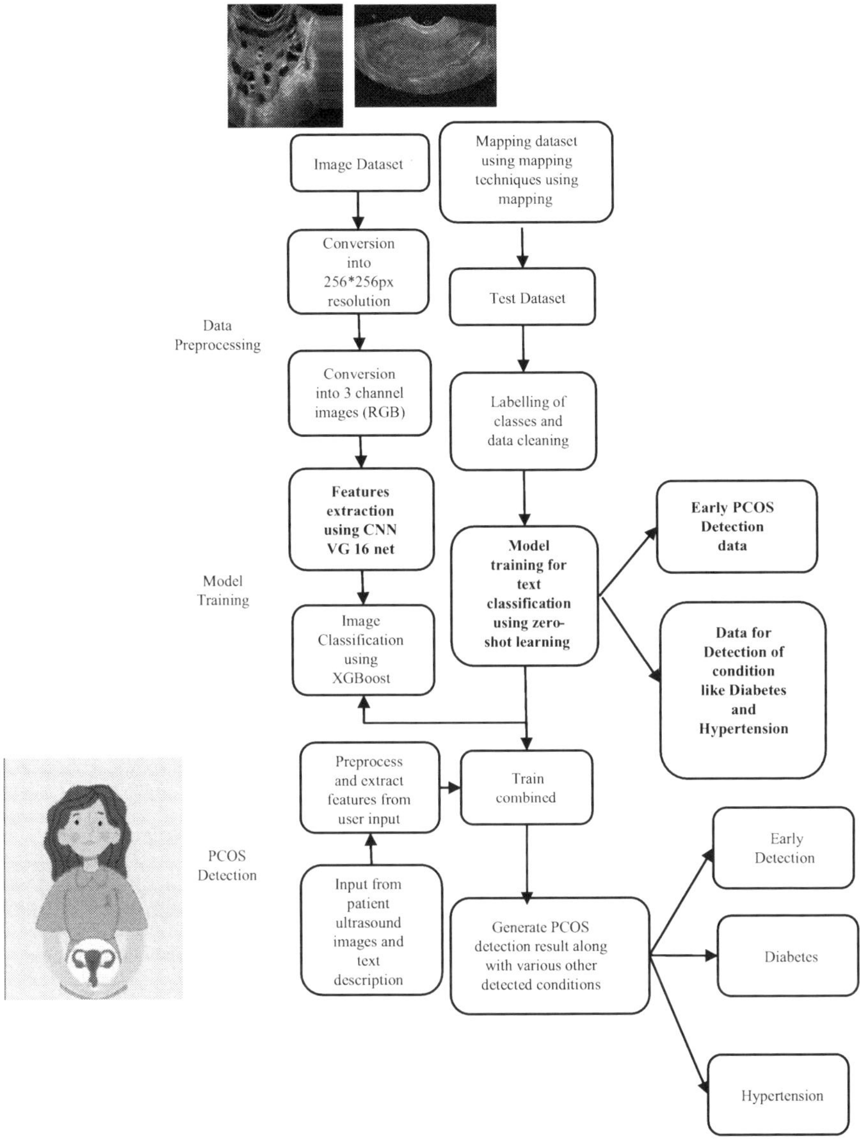

FIGURE 14.1 Project flow diagram for the proposed multimodal system.

resize function. Moreover, grayscale images were converted to three-channel images using the cv2.merge function to represent the images uniformly. In addition, a rigorous check for image validity was enforced to prevent processing empty and corrupted image files. Last, the preprocessed images and corresponding labels were stored in separate arrays to be used in subsequent experiments. This preprocessing pipeline makes the dataset ready to apply many computer vision and machine learning techniques and serves as a solid base for training the further model.

In the proposed methodology amalgamation of two distinct datasets, each encompassing essential patient information, is done. The first dataset primarily comprised hormonal profiles, while the second encompassed a range of clinical features. The initial step involved data integration, ensuring seamless blending of these diverse datasets. Various features within the dataset underwent thorough analysis, with a specific focus on discerning markers for diseases such as diabetes. The proposed methodology involved a comprehensive assessment of patient profiles, including physiological attributes like age, weight, and blood pressure, alongside hormonal markers and lifestyle factors. This textual dataset has two classes "Yes" indicating PCOS and "No" indicating there is no PCOS in the given individual.

14.4.1 Visualization of Data

In Figure 14.2, a bar graph is presented to depict the count of image classes employed in training the deep fusion model. Figure 14.3 showcases the image types used from both classes, providing a visual representation of the dataset. Additionally, Figure 14.4 offers a bar graph illustrating the count of patients within both classes utilized during zero-shot training. These visual representations contribute to a comprehensive understanding of the data collection and training process in this research paper.

14.4.2 Feature Extraction

VGGNet-16, "a Convolutional Neural Network architecture, is utilized for image feature extraction. Given an ultrasound image represented as I, VGGNet-16 processes it

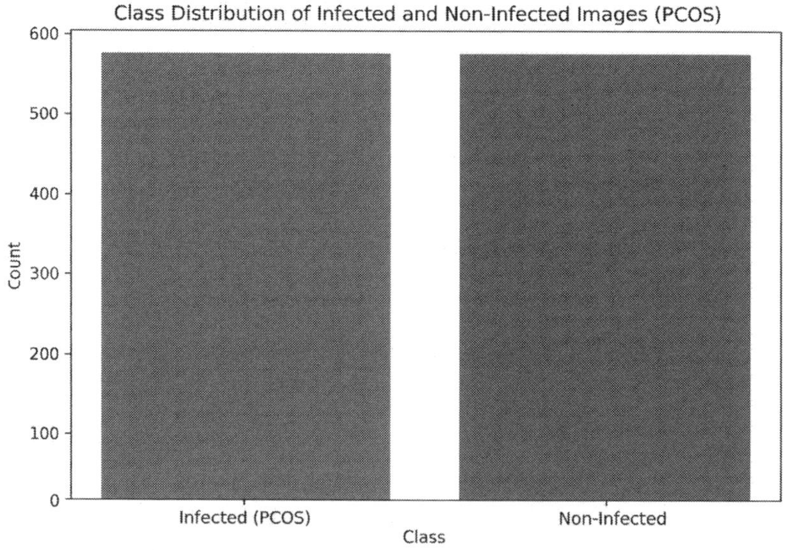

FIGURE 14.2 Bar graph depicting the count of image classes used for training the deep fusion model.

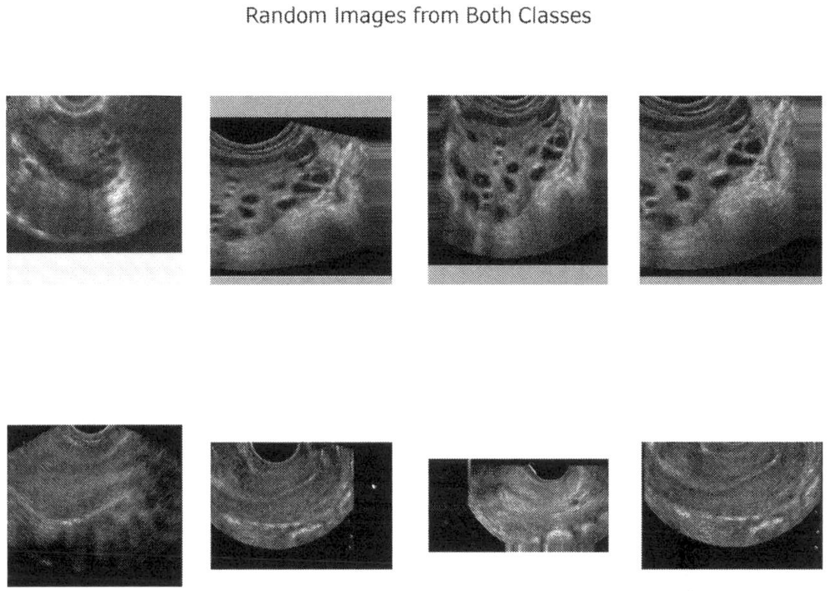

FIGURE 14.3 Image depicting the type of images used from both classes for training the model.

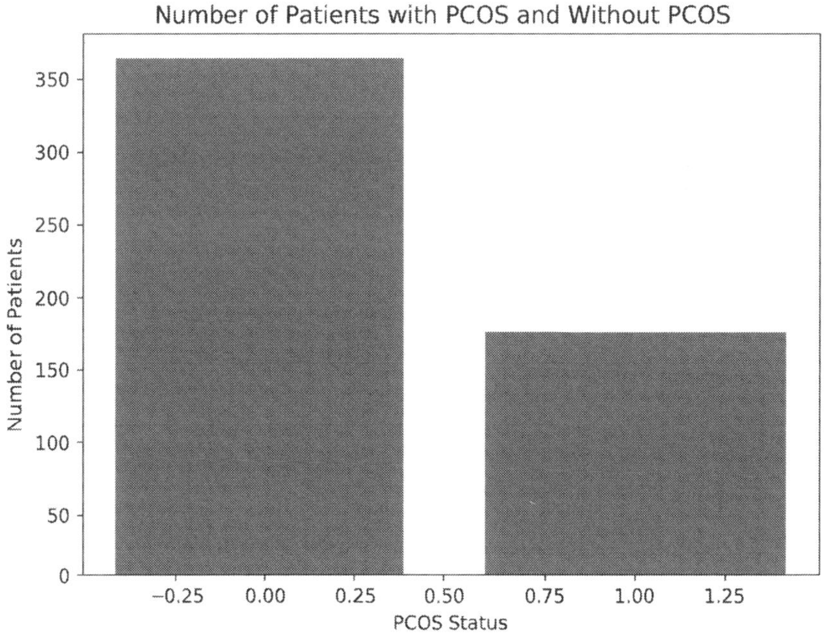

FIGURE 14.4 Bar graph depicting the count of patients for both classes used in zero-shot training.

Model: "vgg16"

Layer (type)	Output Shape	Param #
input_1 (InputLayer)	(None, 256, 256, 3)	0
block1_conv1 (Conv2D	(None, 256, 256, 64)	1792
block1_conv2 (Conv2D	(None, 256, 256, 64)	36928
block2_pool (MaxPooling2D)	(None, 128, 128, 128)	0
block2_conv1 (Conv2D	(None, 128, 128, 128)	29556
block3_conv2 (Conv2D	(None, 128, 128, 128)	590080
block3_pool (MaxPooling2D)	(None, 64, 64, 128)	0
block3_conv3 (Conv2D	(None, 64, 64, 128)	590080
block3_conv3 (Conv2D	(None, 32, 32, 256)	590080
block3_pool (MaxPooling2D)	(None, 32, 32, 256)	0

Total params: 14,714,688
Trainable params: 0
Non-trainable params: 14,714,688

FIGURE 14.5 Convolutional layers used in VGG16.

through a series of convolutional layers followed by max-pooling layers. Figure 14.5 depicts the convolutional layers used and their output shape and the output of the last convolutional layer is denoted as F_I, a high-dimensional feature vector":

$$F_{\text{VGG}} = \text{VGGNet} - 16(I) \tag{14.1}$$

where:

1. VGGNet-16 represents the VGGNet-16 model.
2. F_{VGG} is a feature vector of size N (number of features).

14.4.3 Classification of Ultrasound Images with XGBoost

Once the high-level features are extracted F_{VGG}, we use the XGBoost algorithm for effective classification of PCOS cases. XGBoost is known for its robustness and ability to handle complex classification tasks. The classification process is represented by Equation (14.2) as:

$$y\text{XGBoost} = \text{XGBoost}(F_{\text{VGG}}) \tag{14.2}$$

14.4.3.1 Integration with Zero-Shot Learning

To enhance the model's generalization across various clinical text reports, incorporating zero-shot learning allows the model to classify PCOS-related patterns even when they haven't been explicitly encountered during training. The zero-shot learning process involves:

Text Embedding with BERT: Clinical text reports are embedded using BERT, a state-of-the-art pretrained transformer-based model for natural language understanding. Mathematically, the text embedding E_{report} for a clinical text report is obtained as:

$$E_{\text{report}} = \text{BERT}(\text{Clinical Text}) \tag{14.3}$$

where BERT processes the clinical text to produce embeddings. The BERT model can be used to understand the relationships in the text data. It can then ascertain a wide range of predictions or catch problems early, such as detecting diabetes and high blood pressure, using a method known as zero-shot learning. It is a big step in predicting health problems with technology and early health insights. The BERT framework reads the text data and processes the provided text data within the context of previous language patterns and associations in language for the pretrained BERT model to understand and get the syntax of words with the help of BERT. It relies on textual factors in the dataset in the early stages instead of the training examples themselves. The strength of this model is its generalization from the training knowledge to predict new and unseen cases. It grasps the language of your data and its context to come to conclusions even when it hasn't seen exact examples during training. Due to this adaptability, it is very valuable for work with limited training data, especially for early prediction problems.

Class-Attribute Compatibility: The similarity between the report embedding E_{report} and class attributes A_i is assessed using cosine similarity:

$$S\left(E_{\text{report}}\right) = \text{Cosine Similarity}\left(E_{\text{report}}, A_i\right) \tag{14.4}$$

This quantifies how compatible the report is with each class attribute.

Probability Calculation: The use of SoftMax function to calculate the probability of the report belonging to each class is represented by Equation (14.5) as:

$$P\left(y_{\text{zero-shot}} = i\right) = \frac{e^{s(E, A_i)}}{\sum_{j=1}^{N} e^{s\left(E_{\text{report}}, A_j\right)}} \tag{14.5}$$

where N is the total number of classes.

Fine-Tuning of BERT Model: "Fine-tuning a pretrained BERT model for PCOS classification involves adapting the model's weights and parameters to perform well on these proposed methodologies specific task. This process is crucial for enabling the model to understand and classify clinical text reports related to PCOS. The fine-tuning process aims to minimize an objective function $J(\theta)$ by updating the model parameters θ with respect to the PCOS classification task. The objective function typically involves a combination of the pretraining loss $J_{\text{report}}(\theta)$ and the classification loss $J_{\text{classification}}(\theta)$ represented by Equation (14.6):

$$J(\theta) = J_{\text{report}}(\theta) + J_{\text{classification}}(\theta) \tag{14.6}$$

The gradient descent algorithm is employed to minimize this objective function. Iteratively updating the model parameters θ in the opposite direction of the gradient with respect to θ is represented by Equation (14.7):

$$\Theta \leftarrow \theta - \eta \nabla_{\theta} J(\theta) \tag{14.7}$$

where η represents the learning rate, controlling the step size in the parameter updates.

The gradient $\nabla_{\theta} J(\theta)$ is computed through backpropagation, which involves calculating the gradient of the loss function $J(\theta)$ with respect to each layer's parameters in the BERT model. This gradient is used to adjust the model's weights and biases.

The classification $J_{\text{classification}}(\theta)$ loss measures the dissimilarity between the predicted class probabilities and the true labels in PCOS classification task. It is often calculated using a suitable loss function such as cross-entropy which is represented by Equation (14.8)

$$J_{\text{classification}}(\theta) = \frac{-1}{N} \sum_{i=1}^{N} \sum_{j=1}^{C} y_{ij} \log \log \left(p_{ij}\right) \tag{14.8}$$

where N is the number of training examples, C is the number of classes (in case, PCOS-related and non-PCOS), y_{ij} is an indicator variable indicating whether example i belongs to class j, and p_{ij} is the predicted probability that example i belongs to class j.

Fine-tuning the BERT model for PCOS classification involves optimizing an objective function that combines pretraining and classification losses. The model's parameters are adjusted through gradient descent and backpropagation to minimize this objective function. This process adapts the model's representations and allows it to excel in classifying PCOS-related information in clinical text reports.

Final Prediction: The final prediction zero-shot is made based on this probability distribution. This integration of zero-shot learning empowers the proposed model to generalize and classify PCOS-related patterns not explicitly seen during training, enhancing diagnostic accuracy and robustness."

14.4.4 Ensemble of BERT Models

In the text classification model, an ensemble of BERT models was employed, each pretrained on distinct corpora and domains. Denoting these pretrained models as M_1, M_2, where k is the number of BERT models in the ensemble.

The output of each BERT model is a text embedding E_{Bert}:

$$E_{\text{Bert}} = M_i(\text{Clinical Text}) \quad \text{for } i = 1,2 \tag{14.9}$$

where,

M_1: Hugging Face BERT Transformer
M_2: RoBERTa

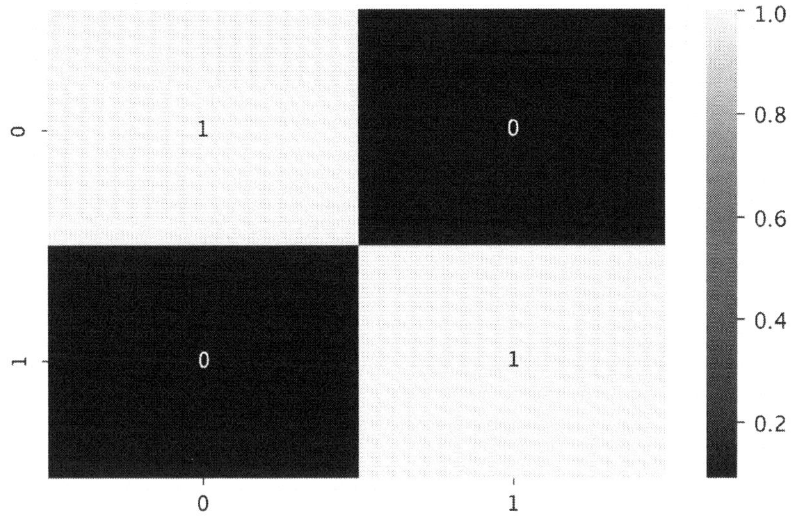

FIGURE 14.6 Confusion matrix for the image classification model.

14.4.5 Combining Model Outputs

To create a robust and adaptable text classification model, combine the outputs of these BERT models using an attention mechanism. Let α_i represent the attention weight assigned to the *i*th BERT model's output. The combined embedding E_{combined} is obtained, which is depicted in Figure 14.6:

$$E_{\text{combined}} = \sum_{i=1}^{k} \alpha_i E_{\text{Bert}} \quad (14.10)$$

14.4.6 Classification with Zero-Shot Learning

Then, zero-shot learning, as described above, is applied to classify clinical text reports based on the compatibility between the combined embedding E_{combined} and class attributes. This ensemble approach allows the model to capture a broader spectrum of language patterns and domain-specific knowledge, making it highly adaptable to unseen classes during inference. These advanced techniques, when integrated into the fusion model, provide a powerful framework for PCOS detection that combines the strengths of image-based and text-based data, enhancing diagnostic accuracy and robustness.

14.5 RESULTS AND DISCUSSION

Evaluated the "performance of the multimodal PCOS detection model using standard metrics, including accuracy, precision, recall, F1-score, and the area under the receiver operating characteristic curve (AUC-ROC), and to assess the model's ability to generalize to unseen data, cross-validation experiments were performed."

Table 14.1 shows various values like precision, recall, F1-score, and support for the image classification model.

Figure 14.6 shows the confusion matrix for the image classification model.

The deep fusion model exhibited an accuracy of 99.6% when the model was tested on the test dataset, which is depicted in Figure 14.7 of the ROC curve.

The zero-shot learning capabilities empowered the model to discern rare or atypical PCOS presentations. Through the exploitation of semantic relationships between textual descriptions and well-established PCOS symptoms, the model effectively identified and flagged unconventional cases. This functionality carries broader implications beyond PCOS and extends to other medical conditions characterized by diverse and infrequent manifestations. Such adaptability in recognizing uncommon medical scenarios underscores the versatility and potential applicability of zero-shot learning in the realm of medical diagnosis and beyond. Table 14.2 shows the accuracy achieved by the zero-shot model in five epochs.

TABLE 14.1
Table Depicting the Classification Report for the Deep Fusion Model Used for Classification of Images

Precision	Recall	F1-Score	Support
Infected	1.00	1.00	1.00
Not infected	1.00	1.00	1.00
Accuracy		1.00	1823
Macro avg	1.00	1.00	1.00
Weighted avg	1.00	1.00	1.00

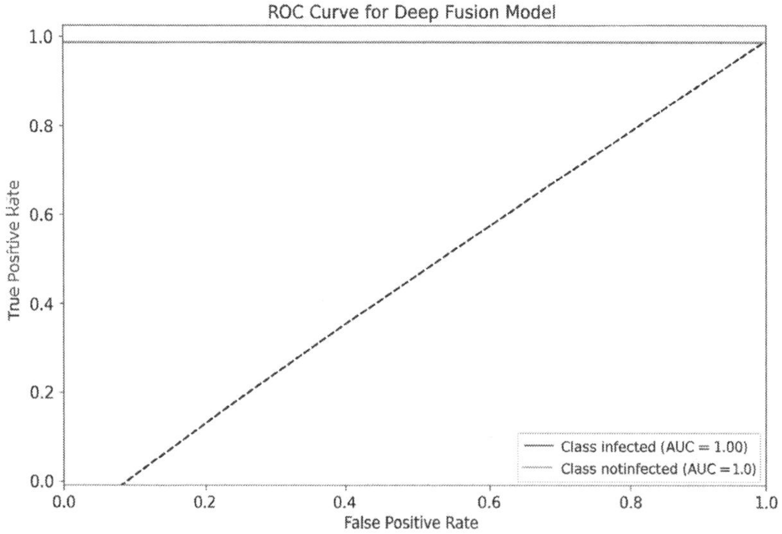

FIGURE 14.7 ROC curve for the deep fusion classification model.

TABLE 14.2
Evaluation of Zero-Shot Learning Model

Epoch 1/5	Validation accuracy: 0.7481
Epoch 2/5	Validation accuracy: 0.7832
Epoch 3/5	Validation accuracy: 0.7867
Epoch 4/5	Validation accuracy: 0.8456
Epoch 5/5	Validation accuracy: 0.8621
Test accuracy	0.8732

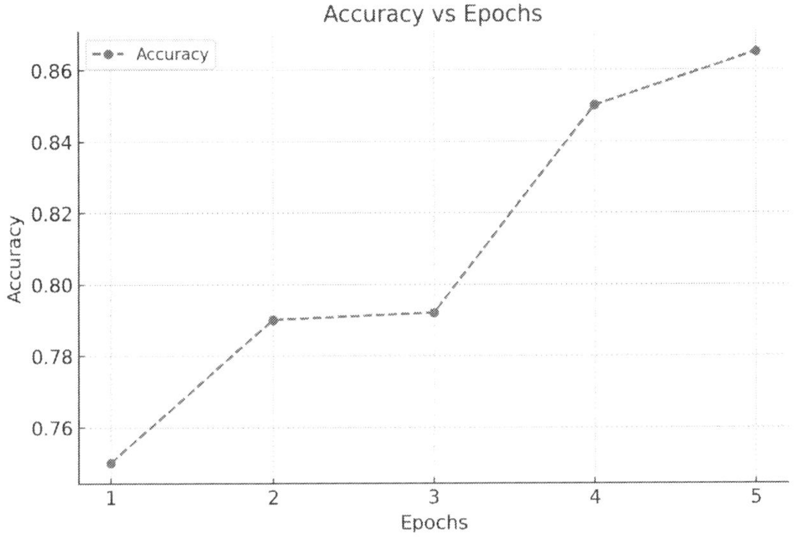

FIGURE 14.8 Graph depicting epochs versus accuracy for the zero-shot model.

Figure 14.8 depicts the epochs versus accuracy for the zero-shot model.

The proposed multimodal PCOS detection model demonstrated a high sensitivity for identifying PCOS in its early stages. This was evident from a significant increase in true positive predictions for cases where PCOS was in its incipient phase. Early-stage sensitivity is a key factor in preventing the progression of PCOS-related complications. The model's proficiency in early-stage prediction facilitates timely interventions and personalized treatment plans. Healthcare professionals can leverage these predictions to initiate appropriate therapies and lifestyle modifications, potentially halting the progression of the condition before it leads to more severe health issues.

Figure 14.9 depicts the heat map of the developed multimodal model. One of the key findings in the study is that the combination of image data and textual data significantly improves the performance of PCOS detection. The XGBoost model effectively captures image patterns related to PCOS, while zero-shot learning enables the model to understand textual clinical reports, leading to a more comprehensive understanding of the patient's condition.

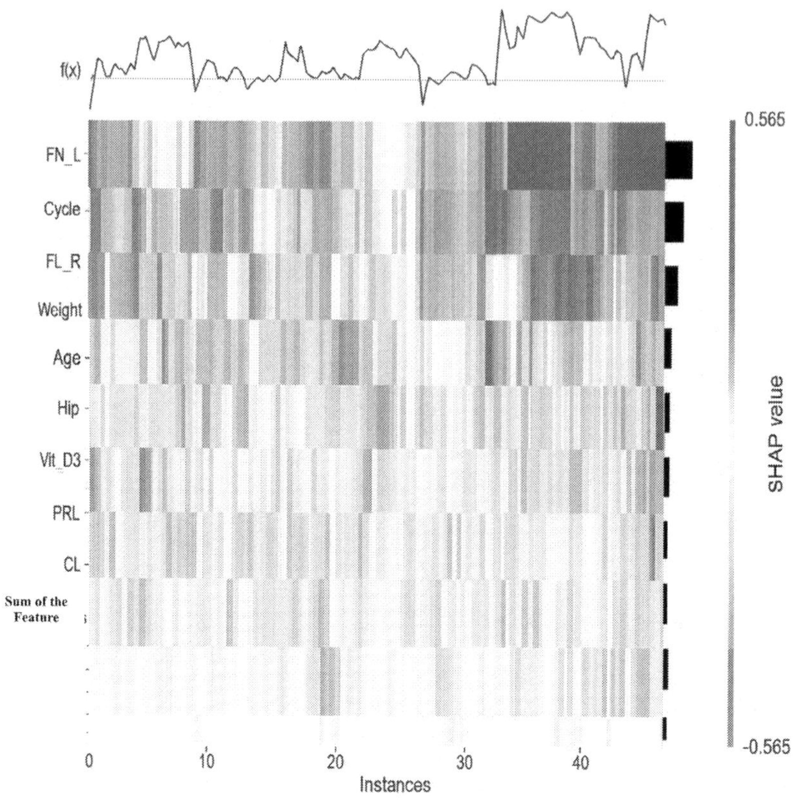

FIGURE 14.9 Heat map of the developed model.

14.6 EXISTING MODEL COMPARISON

A comparison of the multimodal approach to the preceding single-modal models was made in the experiments, where we only used image data and textual data. The outcomes showed that the multimodal model always gave better results when compared with single-modal models. Notably, this multimodal model was much more accurate than the individual models, underscoring the importance of the fusion of image and textual data to improve PCOS detection capabilities considerably (Table 14.3).

Early-stage detection is a key issue regarding managing different medical conditions; as the paper states, the multimodal model is putting an enormous effort into detecting certain things early on. The proposed model will focus on early-stage detection, indicating the disorder at the very beginning of its phases when it will be able to be treated or managed more easily. An essential strength of the model is to predict not just the central disorder but all other diseases affiliated with it. In other words, if the underlying disorder is neurodegenerative, the model can predict other secondary health problems typically associated with the primary condition, such as diabetes, hypertension, or cardiovascular issues. Such a holistic disease prediction is valuable because it will enable healthcare practitioners to address multiple health issues simultaneously and improve the quality of patient care and wellness.

TABLE 14.3
Comparative Studies

Model	Accuracy
Adaboost, Random Forest, XGBoost, Decision tree, and a hybrid model	97.20%
"Support Vector Machine (SVM), K-Nearest Neighbor (KNN), and Convolution Neural Network (CNN)	99.00%
Convolution Neural Network (CNN)	85.00%
Naïve Bayes classifier method, logistic regression, K-Nearest Neighbor (KNN), Classification and Regression Trees (CART), Random Forest Classifier, Support Vector Machine (SVM)	89.02%
Extreme Gradient Boosting, XGBoost	98.00%
Multimodal PCOS Detection"	99.60%

14.7 CONCLUSION

The image analysis and text processing techniques are effective combinations for PCOS detection systems. The proposed model presents high accuracy, stability, and generalization capability, and it can be used as a diagnostic tool for PCOS through ultrasound images and clinical text reports. It is accurate, showing 99.6% accuracy on the test dataset, and robust and adaptable. This system utilizes high-level features and clinical text reports from ultrasound images to provide an accurate predictor of PCOS diagnosis, which can be a valuable tool for identifying PCOS early and improving care for patients in healthcare. Through this project, progress in healthcare technology is achieved as a reliable and efficient early PCOS-detecting machinery is provided, which benefits both patients and healthcare professionals.

REFERENCES

1. J. Tanvi. (2023). "Detection of PCOS Using Ensemble Models." *International Journal for Science Technology and Engineering*. doi: 10.22214/ijraset.2023.51426
2. V. Srinithi and R. Rekha. (2023). "Machine Learning for Diagnosis of Polycystic Ovarian Syndrome (PCOS/PCOD)," pp. 19–24. doi: 10.1109/ICISCoIS56541.2023.10100490
3. K. Rashmita. (2023). "Classification of PCOS Using Machine Learning Algorithms Based on Ultrasound Images of Ovaries," pp. 1–7. doi: 10.1109/ICONSTEM56934.2023.10142359
4. K. Mahajan and P. Mane. (2023). "Follicle Detection of Polycystic Ovarian Syndrome (PCOS) Using Yolo," *2023 9th International Conference on Advanced Computing and Communication Systems (ICACCS)*, Coimbatore, India, pp. 1550–1553. doi: 10.1109/ICACCS57279.2023.10112821
5. M. Sumathi, P. Chitra, R. Sakthi Prabha and K. Srilatha. (2021). "Study and Detection of PCOS Related Diseases Using CNN." *IOP Conference Series: Materials Science and Engineering*, 1070, p. 012062
6. N. Hayat, M. Hayat, S. Rahman, H. Khan, S. W. Zamir, and F. S. Khan. (2020). "Synthesizing the Unseen for Zero-Shot Object Detection," pp. 155–170. doi: 10.1007/978-3-030-69535-4_10

7. A. Denny, A. Raj, A. Ashok, C. M. Ram and R. George. (2019). "i-HOPE: Detection and Prediction System for Polycystic Ovary Syndrome (PCOS) Using Machine Learning Techniques," *TENCON 2019 - 2019 IEEE Region 10 Conference (TENCON)*, Kochi, India, 2019, pp. 673–678, doi: 10.1109/TENCON.2019.8929674
8. M. S. Khan Inan, R. E. Ulfath, F. I. Alam, F. K. Bappee and R. Hasan. (2021). "Improved Sampling and Feature Selection to Support Extreme Gradient Boosting for PCOS Diagnosis," *2021 IEEE 11th Annual Computing and Communication Workshop and Conference (CCWC)*, NV, USA, 2021, pp. 1046–1050, doi: 10.1109/CCWC51732.2021.9375994
9. H. Batra, K. Saluja, S. Gupta, R. Kaushal, N. Sharma and P. Singh. (2023). "Machine Learning Techniques for Data-Driven Computer-Aided Diagnostic Method of Polycystic Ovary Syndrome (PCOS) resulting from Functional Ovarian Hyperandrogenism (FOH)," *2023 International Conference on Computational Intelligence and Sustainable Engineering Solutions (CISES)*, Greater Noida, India, 2023, pp. 195–201, doi: 10.1109/CISES58720.2023.10183485
10. R. P. Naveen. (2022). Op-RMSprop (Optimized-Root Mean Square Propagation) Classification for Prediction of Polycystic Ovary Syndrome (PCOS) using Hybrid Machine Learning Technique *International Journal of Advanced Computer Science and Applications*, 13(6).

15 Revolutionizing Healthcare

Leveraging Fine-Tuned Large Language Models for Personalized Question–Answering Chatbots

Leena Deshpande, Vishal Ambhore, Yash R. Kadam, Omkar R. Khade, Ketki P. Kshirsagar, and Parikshit N. Mahalle

15.1 INTRODUCTION

In the dynamic and ever-evolving landscape of healthcare, the traditional methodologies that have long served as the backbone of information dissemination are undergoing a profound transformation. As we stand at the intersection of healthcare and technological innovation, there emerges a compelling need to reimagine the way medical information is delivered and accessed. This chapter embarks on a journey into the realm of healthcare revolution, propelled by the convergence of advanced machine learning and generative artificial intelligence (AI) techniques, with an emphasis on how fine-tuned large language models (LLMs) have the capacity to transform

The shift in perspective from generalized healthcare systems to a more personalized and efficient approach marks a pivotal moment in the ongoing narrative of healthcare evolution. While conventional methods have undoubtedly played a crucial role in disseminating medical knowledge, they often fall short in catering to the nuanced and evolving needs of diverse stakeholders such as doctors, policymakers, governments, and the healthcare systems they serve. This chapter aims to unravel a novel approach that not only acknowledges this deficiency but actively addresses it through the innovative integration of state-of-the-art AI techniques.

At the heart of this paradigm shift lies the recognition that a revolutionary change is needed in healthcare delivery. The customary one-size-fits-all systems are now being redefined with the infusion of customized AI techniques, heralding a new era where medical information is tailored to individual needs. The linchpin of this

DOI: 10.1201/9781003479185-15

transformative endeavor is the fine-tuning of LLMs, accomplished through the meticulous curation of an in-house dataset meticulously crafted to ensure relevance and accuracy within the intricacies of the healthcare domain.

The crux of our exploration unfolds with the development and implementation of a personalized chatbot system. This system stands as a responsive and accessible medium for the dissemination of healthcare information, poised to benefit a spectrum of stakeholders, including hospitals, governments, and telemedicine providers. Particularly impactful in remote regions where traditional healthcare infrastructure faces limitations, this envisioned system aspires to bridge existing gaps by offering real-time, accurate, and personalized responses to health-related queries.

The need for a swift adoption of customized AI techniques in healthcare is urgent to efficiently reach diverse societies. This chapter emphasizes the potential of the proposed solution, combining generative AI and machine learning, to revolutionize healthcare services by ensuring timely and accurate information dissemination. The impact extends beyond traditional healthcare settings, particularly benefiting remote regions where telemedicine plays a crucial role. As we embark on this exploration, our goal is to offer valuable insights into the development, implementation, and potential impact of a personalized chatbot system. By integrating fine-tuned LLMs, we position this system as a transformative tool for modern healthcare delivery, emphasizing a more responsive, accessible, and patient-centric approach. The ensuing chapters will delve into the intricacies of our methodology, the technological foundations that drive our solution, and the tangible results that herald a new era in healthcare information dissemination.

15.2 BACKGROUND

In the dynamic and rapidly evolving landscape of healthcare, the traditional paradigms that have long defined information dissemination are encountering a pivotal moment of reevaluation. As we navigate the intricate web of modern healthcare systems, the convergence of burgeoning technological advancements and the imperative for personalized care presents a unique opportunity to transcend the limitations of conventional methods. This background section encapsulates the current state of healthcare systems, elucidates the historical underpinnings of traditional information dissemination, and underscores the exigency for a transformative approach.

15.2.1 Contemporary Healthcare Landscape

The contemporary healthcare landscape is marked by a confluence of challenges and innovations. Healthcare systems worldwide are grappling with the imperative to provide not only accessible but also personalized and efficient care. The advent of advanced technologies, ranging from AI to data analytics, has introduced a paradigm shift, promising novel solutions to age-old problems. In this milieu, the need for responsive and adaptable approaches to healthcare information dissemination becomes increasingly evident.

15.2.2 Traditional Methods and Their Limitations

Historically, healthcare information dissemination has relied upon traditional methods that, while effective, exhibit inherent limitations. Printed materials, such as brochures and pamphlets, have been stalwarts in conveying medical information. However, their rigidity and inability to adapt swiftly to evolving medical knowledge pose challenges in keeping patients and healthcare professionals abreast of the latest developments. Face-to-face interactions, although fundamental to the doctor–patient relationship, are constrained by time and may not comprehensively address the diverse information needs of individuals in an era of rapidly expanding medical knowledge. Centralized repositories of medical information, while invaluable, confront challenges in maintaining currency and relevance. The exponential growth of medical data necessitates an agile and real-time approach to information dissemination, a demand that traditional repositories find challenging to fulfill.

15.2.3 The Imperative for Transformation

Considering these challenges, there emerges an imperative for a transformative approach to healthcare information dissemination. The intersection of advanced technologies, especially the utilization of LLMs fine-tuned for healthcare contexts, stands as a beacon of innovation. The transformative power of these models lies not only in their capacity to understand and generate human-like text but, crucially, in their ability to contextualize this capability within the intricate domain of healthcare. The urgency for this transformation becomes particularly pronounced in the face of evolving societal needs, the fast-paced nature of healthcare delivery, and the imperative to cater to the diverse requirements of healthcare professionals, policymakers, and patients. By leveraging the potential of fine-tuned LLMs, we envision a departure from convention toward a more responsive, accessible, and patient-centric approach to healthcare information dissemination.

15.2.4 Detailed Exploration in Subsequent Sections

As we delve into the subsequent sections of this chapter, a detailed exploration of the methodologies employed in this transformative journey unfolds. From the nuanced process of dataset curation to the intricate art of fine-tuning these intelligent models and culminating in the development of personalized chatbot systems, each facet is meticulously examined. This examination not only elucidates the theoretical underpinnings but also spotlights the tangible, real-world implications of revolutionizing healthcare information dissemination. It is not merely a theoretical shift; it is a journey toward impactful change, redefining how healthcare information is perceived, processed, and personalized in the contemporary tapestry of modern healthcare.

15.3 NEED FOR REVOLUTION

In the unfolding narrative of healthcare, a compelling need for revolution becomes apparent—a shift toward personalized and efficient approaches that transcend the boundaries of conventional healthcare systems. This section aims to articulate the imperatives driving this demand, shedding light on the limitations inherent in generalized healthcare systems.

15.3.1 Paradigm Shift Toward Personalized Approaches

The contemporary healthcare landscape is witnessing a transformative paradigm shift, pivoting from generalized approaches to embracing personalized methodologies. This shift is not merely a trend but a strategic response to the evolving expectations and needs of individuals in their pursuit of well-being. Personalized healthcare recognizes the unique attributes of each patient, encompassing their genetic makeup, lifestyle, and specific health conditions. It represents a departure from the one-size-fits-all model, acknowledging that health interventions are most effective when tailored to the individual.

- **The Rise of Precision Medicine**: At the forefront of this paradigm shift is the ascendancy of precision medicine. This innovative approach tailors medical interventions and treatment plans to the individual characteristics of each patient. Precision medicine harnesses the power of advanced technologies, including genomics, proteomics, and data analytics, to glean insights into the specific factors influencing an individual's health. By understanding the intricate interplay between genetics and environmental factors, healthcare providers can offer targeted interventions, optimizing treatment outcomes and minimizing adverse effects.
- **Patient-Centric Healthcare**: Personalized healthcare extends beyond the clinical realm to embrace a patient-centric philosophy. It places individuals at the center of their healthcare journey, empowering them with information, choices, and active participation in decision-making. Patient engagement becomes a cornerstone, fostering a collaborative relationship between healthcare providers and those seeking care. This shift from a provider-centric to a patient-centric model not only enhances the overall patient experience but also contributes to improved health outcomes.
- **Limitations of Generalized Healthcare Systems**: While traditional healthcare systems have been instrumental in addressing broad health challenges, they grapple with inherent limitations that hinder their efficacy in meeting the diverse and evolving needs of individuals.
- **One-Size-Fits-All Approach**: Historically, healthcare systems have predominantly adhered to a one-size-fits-all approach, employing generalized treatment protocols and interventions. This approach, while suitable for common ailments, falls short when confronted with the intricacies of individual health variations. The diversity in genetic makeup, lifestyle choices, and pre-existing conditions among individuals necessitates a departure from standardized interventions to achieve optimal health outcomes.
- **Reactive Rather Than Proactive**: Traditional healthcare models often adopt a reactive stance, responding to health issues after they manifest. This reactive approach, although effective in addressing acute conditions, lacks the foresight needed for preventive healthcare. The future of healthcare lies in proactive strategies that anticipate and mitigate health risks before they

escalate. Personalized approaches enable the identification of predispositions and susceptibilities, allowing for early interventions and preventive measures tailored to an individual's unique health profile.

- **Inefficiencies in Resource Allocation**: Generalized healthcare systems may allocate resources based on population-level trends, leading to inefficiencies in resource distribution. This approach might result in a misalignment of healthcare resources with the actual needs of specific demographic groups or individuals. Personalized healthcare, by contrast, optimizes resource allocation by tailoring interventions to the specific health challenges of prevalent populations or individuals.

The need for revolution in healthcare stems from a growing recognition of the limitations inherent in generalized approaches. The paradigm shift toward personalized healthcare represents a strategic response to overcome these limitations, ushering in a new era where healthcare is not just about treating illnesses but about empowering individuals on their unique journey toward well-being.

15.4 LITERATURE REVIEW

The merging of LLMs, utilizing generative AI in healthcare, has become a research focus, offering a paradigm shift in data and information management. The studies reviewed, exemplified by models like ChatGPT, collectively demonstrate the potential to revolutionize healthcare practices while acknowledging the challenges that warrant thorough exploration.

Yu *et al.* [1] navigate the historical landscape of AI applications in healthcare, shedding light on the trajectory of generative AI and LLMs. Their scoping literature review emphasizes the critical need for guidance in integrating these technologies, particularly in healthcare and medical practices. The study introduces mechanisms such as reinforcement learning from human feedback (RLFH), differentiating these models from traditional rule-based AI systems. The inclusive co-design process, involving clinicians and consumers, is highlighted as essential for realizing the benefits of these transformative technologies.

The work by Li *et al.* [2] introduces "ChatDoctor," a model fine-tuned on an LLMs Meta-AI (LLaMA) using medical domain knowledge. This study focuses on elevating medical advice accuracy by incorporating real-world patient-doctor interactions and a self-directed information retrieval mechanism. The findings underscore substantial improvements in the model's ability to comprehend patient needs, providing accurate advice. This positions ChatDoctor as a pivotal advancement in the domain of medical LLMs.

In their comprehensive roadmap, Yu *et al.* [1] delve into the revolutionary possibilities of generative AI and LLMs, particularly ChatGPT, in revolutionizing healthcare. The study emphasizes the ongoing necessity for novel approaches to data collection, model optimization, quick strategy creation, and system deployment. Notably, the ethical and legal dimensions surrounding these technologies underscore the importance of responsible application. The study urges proactive engagement from organizations for the enhancement of healthcare quality, safety, and efficiency.

Yang *et al.* [3] contribute insights into the LLMs: Development, applications, and challenges in healthcare, with a specific focus on ChatGPT and similar tools. The review explores their deployment in clinical, educational, and research settings, emphasizing the advantages and disadvantages of LLMs. The potential for improving the efficacy and efficiency of different healthcare procedures is emphasized.

Javaid *et al.* [4] present an innovative perspective on ChatGPT for healthcare services, emphasizing the need for accurate and current data while addressing privacy and security concerns. The study identifies significant applications of ChatGPT, showcasing its potential for conversational AI tools, chatbots, and virtual assistants in healthcare.

In the domain of medicine, Thirunavukarasu *et al.* [5] discuss the application of LLMs, particularly ChatGPT. The review outlines the developmental processes of LLM chatbots and their utilization in biomedical contexts, serving as a primer for clinicians and providing insights into potential benefits for patients and practitioners.

Nadarzynski *et al.* [6] examine the acceptability of AI-powered health chatbots using online surveys and semi-structured interviews. The study identifies themes such as "Understanding of chatbots," "AI hesitancy," and "Motivations for health chatbots." The findings underscore the importance of user-centered and theory-based approaches in designing AI-led health chatbots, considering patients' concerns and optimizing user experience.

Athota *et al.* [7] propose a medical chatbot using AI to diagnose diseases and provide basic details. The study emphasizes the potential of chatbots to reduce healthcare costs and improve accessibility to medical knowledge, presenting the integration of AI-driven chatbots into the healthcare system as a promising step toward more efficient and accessible healthcare services.

Our proposed research builds upon the existing literature by focusing on the integration of generative AI and LLMs for a personalized question–answering chatbot in healthcare. While existing studies explore the potential of these technologies, our work contributes a novel approach by emphasizing the creation of a sophisticated question–answering system tailored specifically for health-related queries. The proposed system involves the fine-tuning of LLMs through a meticulously curated in-house dataset, ensuring relevance and accuracy within the healthcare domain. The core novelty lies in the development and implementation of a personalized chatbot system poised to benefit various stakeholders, including hospitals, governments, and telemedicine providers. Our research positions this tailored solution as a transformative tool for modern healthcare delivery systems, offering valuable insights into its development, implementation, and potential impact on revolutionizing healthcare information dissemination.

15.5 METHODOLOGY

Our approach to creating and implementing the personalized question–answering chatbot system in healthcare is carefully planned, ensuring it is organized, thorough, and ethically responsible. We navigate through different stages, starting with gathering a diverse set of data, refining the model, building the chatbot, and testing it with users. This method guarantees that the chatbot is not only accurate and relevant but also practical for real-world healthcare scenarios. Our strategy involves a detailed process where we create our dataset from scratch and gather additional data from various sources, like NIH Senior Health [8]. This careful combination of internal and external datasets is crucial for our methodology. It adds authenticity to the collected data, especially during the fine-tuning process, making sure our chatbot learns from a reliable and diverse set of information. This meticulous integration of data sources is at the core of how we approach and refine our chatbot for the healthcare domain.

Collecting Relevant Data: In the initial phase, we conducted an exhaustive search for health-related questions and answers from various sources, including reputable government health platforms like NIH Senior Health, medical literature, and reliable online health forums. This extensive compilation resulted in a diverse dataset, forming the foundational knowledge base for the chatbot. Additionally, recognizing the need for domain-specific content, we created an in-house dataset by gathering authentic health queries and expert responses. This meticulous approach ensures a nuanced representation of various medical domains, combining information from authoritative sources for comprehensive and accurate knowledge integration.

In this dataset, two columns contain questions and expert answers related to medicine. The questions cover aspects such as the definition, symptoms, treatments, risk factors, and prevention of various diseases.

TABLE 15.1
Sample of medical-related dataset used to finetune the LLM Model

Questions	Answers
What is (are) glaucoma?	Glaucoma is a collection of conditions that can harm the optic nerve of the eye, causing blindness and visual loss. Although glaucoma may affect anybody, those over 60 are far more likely to get it. How the condition develops: Glaucoma comes in a variety of forms. The drainage system of the eye is affected by the majority of diseases. The anterior chamber is a small area located in front of the eye.
What are the symptoms of glaucoma?	Glaucoma symptoms can appear in one or both eyes. Open-angle glaucoma, the most prevalent kind of glaucoma, initially exhibits no symptoms. There is no discomfort, and vision appears normal. People with glaucoma gradually lose their peripheral, or side, vision if they are not treated.
What are the treatments for glaucoma?	While there is no known treatment for open-angle glaucoma, it is often manageable. Although therapies can preserve residual eyesight, they cannot restore sight that has already been lost due to glaucoma. Medication and surgery are the most often used therapies for glaucoma.
Who is at risk for glaucoma?	Glaucoma may affect anyone. Individuals vary in their level of danger. African–Americans over 40, persons over 60, particularly Hispanics and Latinos, and those with a family history of glaucoma are among them.
How to prevent glaucoma?	As of the present, there is no known way to stop glaucoma. However, research indicates that the most effective strategy to manage glaucoma is to discover it early and treat it before it results in significant vision loss.

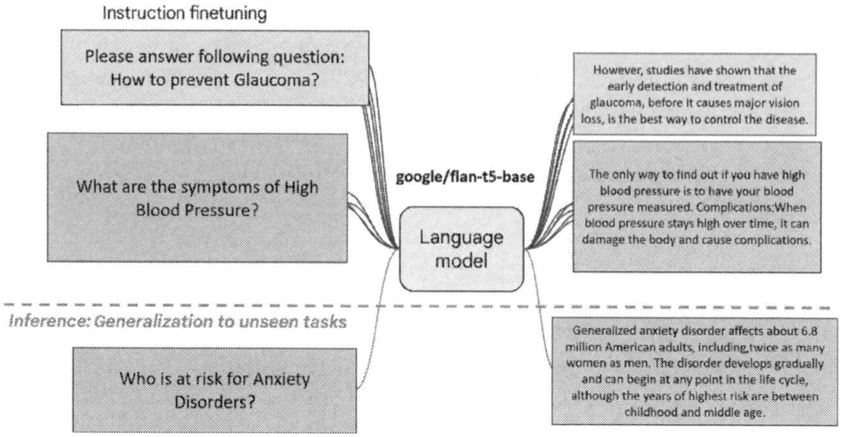

FIGURE 15.1 FLAN-T5 base LLM workflow.

- **Cleaning and Understanding the Data**: Rigorous preprocessing techniques were employed to clean the dataset, eliminating extraneous symbols, typos, and irregular characters. Simultaneously, we engaged in annotation processes to enhance the contextual understanding of the model. This involved labeling medical entities and key phrases, enriching the dataset for improved comprehension.
- **Model Selection**: For the foundational language model, we selected a powerful LLM, such as Google/flan-t5-base [9], known for its advanced language generation capabilities. Fine-tuning of this model was conducted using our curated in-house dataset, aligning the language generation with the intricacies of healthcare queries.
- **Fine-Tuning and Model Training**: The pivotal phase of fine-tuning Google's Flan-t5-base LLM for our specialized healthcare question–answering task was conducted with meticulous attention to detail. The process commenced with the loading of our curated dataset, which encapsulates a diverse range of health-related queries, drawing from both an in-house dataset and external sources. This comprehensive compilation ensured that the model was exposed to a rich and varied landscape of medical inquiries. Subsequently, we engaged in thorough tokenization and model initialization to prepare the LLM for the intricacies of healthcare language, a crucial step in aligning the model's understanding with the nuances of real-world healthcare queries. The methodical approach to dataset selection and model preparation laid a robust foundation for the subsequent phases of hyperparameter optimization and training.
- **Hyperparameter Optimization**: To strike a harmonious balance between model performance and computational efficiency, a rigorous optimization of hyperparameters was undertaken. The selected parameters included a learning rate of 3e-4, a batch size of 5, and a training duration of 5 epochs.

- **Seq2Seq Trainer and Evaluation Metrics**: During the training process, we employed a Seq2Seq trainer [10], a specialized mechanism to enhance the model's ability to understand and respond to sequential data. The configuration of evaluation metrics was centered around the ROUGE score [11], providing a quantitative measure of the generated responses' coherence and relevance.
- **Efficient Logging Strategies**: To comprehensively monitor the model's performance, an efficient logging strategy was implemented every 500 steps during training. This dual strategy, encompassing both epoch-based and step-based logging, ensured a granular understanding of the model's evolution.
- **Preventing Overfitting**: To mitigate the risk of overfitting, a weight decay of 0.01 was applied during the fine-tuning process. This regularization technique contributed to the model's generalizability and robustness.
- **Enhanced Response Generation**: The "Predict with Generate" option was enabled, augmenting the LLM's capacity to generate contextually relevant responses. This feature played a crucial role in ensuring that the model could provide nuanced and accurate answers to diverse healthcare queries.
- **Logging and Model Checkpoints**: Logs detailing the training process and model checkpoints were systematically saved in the "fine-tuned-t5-medical" directory. This structured approach facilitated subsequent analysis, evaluation, and potential deployment of the fine-tuned model in healthcare information dissemination.
- **Iterative and Strategic Approach**: The fine-tuning process adopted an iterative and strategic approach, prioritizing precision and relevance in addressing healthcare-related queries. This methodical training regimen optimized the LLM for the specific nuances of healthcare language, enhancing its proficiency in generating coherent and accurate responses.
- **User Testing and Iterative Feedback**: The developed chatbot underwent pilot testing with a diverse group of users, including healthcare professionals, policymakers, and potential end-users. This phase was crucial for identifying system limitations, usability issues, and areas for improvement. User feedback collected during testing was integrated iteratively to refine the chatbot's performance and enhance the overall user experience.
- **Ethical Considerations**: Ethical considerations were paramount in our methodology. We implemented robust privacy and security measures to safeguard sensitive health information. Transparency was prioritized by providing users with clear information about the chatbot's capabilities and limitations. Accountability mechanisms were established to address any unforeseen issues or errors promptly, ensuring responsible and ethical use.
- **Streamlit Frontend Development**: In parallel with the model and system development, we created a user-friendly front end using Streamlit [12]. Streamlit's capabilities were harnessed to enhance the user interface, making interactions with the chatbot intuitive and accessible. The development of a visually appealing and responsive frontend aimed to further elevate the overall user experience.

15.6 RESULT AND ANALYSIS

Following the training phase, a rigorous evaluation of the developed model was conducted using a dedicated test dataset. The primary evaluation metric employed for gauging the model's performance is the ROUGE score, a widely accepted measure for assessing the quality of generated text.

Evaluation Metrics: The evaluation results encompass a comprehensive set of metrics, offering a nuanced understanding of the model's proficiency.

The evaluation results of the developed question–answering chatbot model are presented in the above Table. The eval_loss, indicative of the model's training performance, is reported at 1.8686. The ROUGE metrics, which assess the quality of text generated by the model, include ROUGE-1 at 0.1114, ROUGE-2 at 0.0304, ROUGE-L at 0.0872, and ROUGE-Lsum at 0.1020. These scores reflect the model's ability to reproduce human-like responses. The evaluation runtime is recorded at 23.6847 seconds, with a throughput of 4.475 samples per second and 0.929 steps per second. The model's performance is measured at epoch 5.0, indicating the stage of training at which the evaluation is conducted. These metrics collectively provide a comprehensive assessment of the model's proficiency and effectiveness in generating accurate and contextually relevant responses to healthcare-related queries.

In the Table below, a comparative analysis between the responses generated by the base T5 model and the fine-tuned T5 model is presented.

The above Table illustrates the contrasting outputs for specific healthcare-related questions. The base T5 model exhibits generic responses, often unrelated to the queried health topics, showcasing its limitations in providing accurate and contextually relevant information. In contrast, the fine-tuned T5 model delivers responses that align more closely with the expected medical knowledge, demonstrating the effectiveness of the fine-tuning process in tailoring the model to healthcare-specific inquiries. This comparison underscores the value of domain-specific refinement in enhancing the question–answering capabilities of the T5 model for healthcare applications.

TABLE 15.2
Evaluation Metrics and Values

Evaluation Metric	Value
eval_loss	1.8686
eval_rouge1	0.1114
eval_rouge2	0.0304
eval_rougeL	0.0872
eval_rougeLsum	0.1020
eval_runtime	23.6847 seconds
eval_samples_per_second	4.475
eval_steps_per_second	0.929
Epoch	5.0

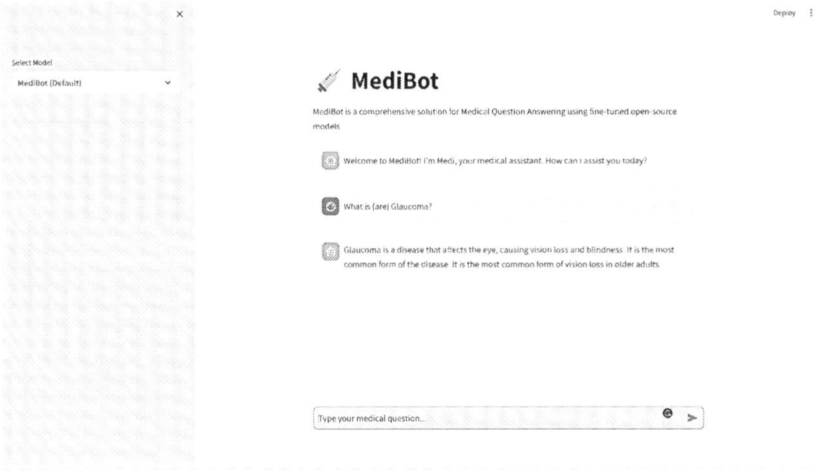

FIGURE 15.2 Screenshot of frontend UI built using Streamlit.

TABLE 15.3
Base T5 model versus fine-tuned T5 model responses

Question	Base model answers	Fine-tuned model answers
What is (are) glaucoma?	Ear infection	In the United States, glaucoma is the most prevalent kind of eye illness. After cataracts and macular degeneration, it is the second most prevalent kind of eye illness.
What is high blood pressure?	High blood pressure	Heart disease, stroke, diabetes, and other health issues are all at risk due to high blood pressure. As one ages, there is an increased chance of having hypertension.
What causes kidney disease?	Ureters	Kidney disease is a disease in which the kidneys do not produce enough blood to carry out the functions they should.
What is (are) low vision?	A low vision	Low vision is a loss of vision brought on by a condition known as macular degeneration. The illness known as macular degeneration is characterized by an infection of the macula of the eye.
What is (are) diabetes?	Diabetes	Diabetes is among the most prevalent types of the disease. Among older persons, it is the most prevalent type of illness. In the United States, it ranks second in terms of cause of death, after heart disease and stroke.

15.7 DISCUSSION

The exploration and implementation of a personalized question–answering chatbot system for healthcare applications has unveiled critical insights and implications. This discussion section delves into the key findings, addresses the significance of the developed solution, and explores potential avenues for further improvement.

Enhanced Accuracy and Relevance Through Fine-tuning: The comparison between the base T5 model and the fine-tuned T5 model reveals a substantial improvement in accuracy and relevance for healthcare-related queries. The fine-tuned model demonstrates a nuanced understanding of medical topics, providing contextually appropriate responses. This underscores the importance of domain-specific fine-tuning in tailoring LLMs for healthcare information dissemination.

Value of In-house Dataset and Model Selection: The curated in-house dataset plays a pivotal role in enhancing the model's domain specificity. Crafting a dataset that encompasses a diverse range of health-related queries ensures that the chatbot system is robust and adaptable to various medical domains. The choice of the Google/Flax T5 base LLM model for question–answering tasks has proven effective, serving as a solid foundation for domain-specific fine-tuning.

Frontend Development: The development of a frontend using Streamlit facilitates a seamless user interface, promoting user engagement and accessibility. The combination of accurate information retrieval and an intuitive frontend design aligns with the goals of responsive and patient-centric healthcare information dissemination.

Limitations: While the developed personalized question–answering chatbot system demonstrates notable advancements, it is essential to acknowledge certain limitations inherent in its current state. One key limitation lies in the system's dependence on the curated dataset. The effectiveness of the chatbot is contingent upon the comprehensiveness and diversity of the dataset, and potential biases may arise if the dataset does not adequately represent the entire spectrum of health-related queries. Additionally, the system's performance may exhibit variations in addressing queries from different medical domains, posing a challenge in achieving universal accuracy. Moreover, the dynamic nature of medical information may result in occasional inaccuracies, as the chatbot's knowledge is confined to the data available during the training period. Recognizing these limitations is crucial for a nuanced understanding of the chatbot's capabilities and for setting realistic expectations among users.

Future Scope: To advance the capabilities of the personalized question–answering chatbot system, several promising avenues can be explored. First and foremost is the continual enrichment of the dataset to encompass a broader range of health-related queries, ensuring the chatbot's adaptability to emerging medical topics and diverse user needs. Future iterations may also consider the integration of sentiment analysis and entity recognition, allowing the system to not only provide accurate information but also discern the emotional context and recognize specific entities within user queries. Collaboration with healthcare professionals for ongoing fine-tuning and validation can contribute to the system's accuracy and relevance. Additionally, exploring multilingual capabilities can enhance accessibility, catering to a more diverse user base. As the field of healthcare information dissemination evolves, embracing emerging technologies and user feedback will be instrumental in shaping the chatbot system's continued development and success.

15.8 CONCLUSION

In conclusion, the development and implementation of the personalized question–answering chatbot system represent a significant stride in transforming healthcare information dissemination. Leveraging generative AI and LLMs, particularly the Flan-T5-Base model, this system addresses the challenges posed by conventional methods through its contextually relevant and accurate responses to diverse health-related queries. The meticulous methodology, encompassing dataset curation, fine-tuning, and system development, ensures the chatbot's robustness and practicality within the healthcare domain. However, acknowledging the limitations, including dataset dependencies and the absence of sentiment analysis and entity recognition, underscores the need for continual refinement. As the healthcare landscape evolves, the proposed future directions, such as dataset enrichment, integration of additional NLP techniques, and collaboration with healthcare professionals, pave the way for the chatbot's ongoing enhancement. This tailored solution stands as a transformative tool with the potential to revolutionize modern healthcare delivery, offering valuable insights into its development, implementation, and the profound impact it could wield on healthcare information dissemination.

REFERENCES

1. Yu, P, Xu, H, Hu, X, Deng, C. Leveraging generative AI and large language models: A comprehensive roadmap for healthcare integration. *Healthcare (Basel)*. 2023;11(20):2776. https://doi.org/10.3390/healthcare11202776. PMID: 37893850; PMCID: PMC10606429.
2. Li, Y, Li, Z, Zhang, K, Dan, R, Jiang, S, Zhang, Y. ChatDoctor: A medical chat model fine-tuned on a Large Language Model Meta-AI (LLaMA) using medical domain knowledge. *Cureus*. 2023;15(6):e40895. https://doi.org/10.7759/cureus.40895. PMID: 37492832; PMCID: PMC10364849.
3. Yang, R, Tan, T.F., Lu, W, Thirunavukarasu, A.J, Ting, D.S.W., Liu, N. Large language models in health care: development, applications, and challenges. *Health Care Sciences*. 2023;2:255–263. https://doi.org/10.1002/hcs2.61
4. Javaid, M., Haleem, A., Singh, R.P. ChatGPT for healthcare services: An emerging stage for an innovative perspective. *BenchCouncil Transactions on Benchmarks, Standards and Evaluations*. 2023;3(1):100105. ISSN 2772-4859. https://doi.org/10.1016/j.tbench.2023.100105
5. Thirunavukarasu, A.J., Ting, D.S.J., Elangovan, K., Elangovan, K. Large language models in medicine. *Nature Medicine*. 2023;29:1930–1940. https://doi.org/10.1038/s41591-023-02448-8
6. Nadarzynski, T., Miles, O., Cowie, A., Ridge, D. Acceptability of artificial intelligence (AI)-led chatbot services in healthcare: A mixed-methods study. *Digital Health*. 2019;5. https://doi.org/10.1177/2055207619871808
7. Athota, L., Shukla, V.K., Pandey, N., Rana, A. Chatbot for healthcare system using artificial intelligence. *2020 8th International Conference on Reliability, Infocom Technologies and Optimization (Trends and Future Directions) (ICRITO)*, Noida, India, 2020, pp. 619–622, https://doi.org/10.1109/ICRITO48877.2020.9197833
8. https://www.nia.nih.gov/health
9. https://huggingface.co/google/flan-t5-base
10. https://huggingface.co/docs/transformers/main_classes/trainer
11. https://huggingface.co/spaces/evaluate-metric/rouge
12. https://docs.streamlit.io

16 Best Donor Selection for Liver Transplantation Using Artificial Neural Network and Machine Learning Algorithms

Dnyaneshwar Natha Wavhal, Pankaj M. Agarkar, Parikshit N. Mahalle, and Nitin Dattu Thorve

16.1 INTRODUCTION

Transplanting the liver from a diseased to a healthy one from a donor is complex and lifesaving. It is, however, the preferred treatment for those with end-stage liver disease, acute liver failure, or people suffering from some liver cancers. The success of liver transplantation is primarily determined by donor–recipient compatibility and the overall quality of both donor and recipient [1]. The two donors have a very close score to the recipient in the scoring comparisons, that is, a successful transplant is possible.

This is one of the most critical decisions that has to go into the selection of the best-match donor for liver transplantation, as many factors are in the recipient's medical condition, blood type, age, and the health of the liver of the donor [2]. Usually, donor matching is done through correlation and scoring systems, which may not be adequate in a more elaborate donor and recipient interaction. Artificial neural networks (ANNs) are practical machine learning (ML) algorithms that can extract complex relationships from large amounts of data and, therefore, can improve donor specification.

This research paper intends to compare and contrast various ANN algorithms that can be used for selecting the best-match donor for liver transplants [2]. We aim to investigate how some ANN algorithms, K nearest-neighbor (KNN) algorithms, and support vector machine (SVM) algorithms can be used to enhance the accuracy and efficiency of donor–recipient matching. The performance of these ANN models will be compared against a large dataset encompassing pretransplantation and posttransplantation features, and the ability of these ANN models to predict the posttransplantation survival outcome will be compared in [3].

The results of this research are expected to supply some worthwhile information relative to the ANN processes used in donation algorithms for liver transplants. This will help to learn which implementations of the hyperimage ANN perform best

 DOI: 10.1201/9781003479185-16

at prediction and, thus, help increase the success rates of live transplantation and the patient's outcomes. It may also kick off the search to integrate advanced ML techniques in clinical decision-making processes so that medical professionals can decide on the correct and accurate selection of donors. Lastly, our research intends to help in the continuous improvement and refinement of liver transplantation practice and patient care and enhance the chances of transplant success [4].

16.1.1 The Contribution to Research

- The performance of various ANN algorithms for predicting the best-match donor in liver transplantation is evaluated.
- To compare and analyze different architectures, such as ANNs, the KNN algorithm, and SVMs, in terms of donor–recipient matching.
- With a comprehensive dataset of liver transplantation patients, we can compare the effectiveness of different ANN models considering accuracy, precision, recall, F1 score, and area under the ROC curve.
- Findings of a comparative study based on ANN algorithms can provide insights and recommendations on the performance of the donor selection process in liver transplantation.

This research paper is organized as such. The background and significance of optimizing best-match donor selection in liver transplantation by the ANN algorithm are presented in the Introduction section and the Research Objectives. The Literature Review section summarizes the previous approaches applied in donor–recipient matching and existing inventories for predicting liver transplantation survival. The Methodology section describes the metadata collection process, feature selection, preprocessing techniques, and ANN architectures used for the comparative study section. The Results and Discussion section will involve the evaluation of the performance of each ANN model using multiple metrics while the findings are explained and compared. The paper concludes with one of the References to the source and literature consulted.

16.2 LITERATURE REVIEW

The liver transplantation with ANN algorithms involves many different methods. This section reviews few works of research.

In Rabbi *et al.* [1] study, a comparative analysis of four different ML algorithms was done using the Indian Liver Patient Dataset (ILPD). To conduct further explanation on how to predict the sale price, I just used the feature selection based on the Pearson correlation coefficient, which is Pearson correlation coefficient-based feature selection (PCC–FS), to decide which feature is not good to be used to strengthen the prediction performance. AdaBoost was also used to boost the overall predictive power of the models. According to their experimental analysis, extra trees (ET) had the highest accuracy of 92.19% among the tested ML algorithms. Although their study highlights the importance of feature selection and boosting, given the aim of achieving maximum accuracy in the prediction of liver disease from the ILPD dataset by using ML algorithms, there are other approaches.

In Kuzhippallil *et al.* [2], two popular classifiers, AdaBoost and XGBoost, were compared and performed on the ILPD. They integrated a feature selection by combining the X-Boost classifier with the genetic algorithm. They have also used the Isolation Forest method to calculate the outliers in the dataset. Their analysis revealed the highest accuracy of 86% through the light gradient boosting machine (GBM) algorithm. The second stack estimator reached the second-highest accuracy of 85%. This study focuses on the use of the feature selection and the ensemble technique to achieve optimal predictive performance of the diagnosis of liver disease through ML algorithms, and the results of use on the ILPD dataset demonstrate the capacity of the techniques introduced to perform the task.

In Rajan *et al.* [3], we evaluate the algorithms in the context of the Kaggle dataset. The accurate algorithm was the Kernel SVM algorithm, which achieved a predicting accuracy of 70%. A 30% Mean Absolute Error (MAE) implies that the model was predicting, on average, close to the actual value, and hence, that the model can approximate target values to a limited extent. However, the **Root Mean Square Error** (RMSE) of 55% and **Relative Squared Error** (RSE) of 24% are fairly low figures compared to relatively better predictions of the "actual" data. Their results aid in understanding the algorithm performance to the Kaggle dataset and give an idea of using the algorithm in other fields and further ML and predictive modeling studies.

Anuradha *et al.* [4] presented a novel ML model for the combined diagnosis of liver diseases. For their study, they used the ILPD. The integrated model attempts to combine the results of several classifiers. The output says that a patient has liver disease when having two or more classifiers give the value of 1, and it tells that the patient does not have liver disease if two or more classifiers provide the value of 0; according to their study, they have got highest accuracy of 96% while comparing the results of combined ML algorithm with results of KNN with 75% accuracy, decision tree (DT) with 85% accuracy and ANN with 89% accuracy. This implies that combining different classifiers in the combined model yields significant improvements in diagnostic accuracy compared to stand-alone algorithms, and the high accuracy accomplished by their combined ML model indicates that it can be clinically applied as a diagnostic aid.

Kumar and Katyal [5] on an ML model-based approach to diagnosing liver diseases presented a novel approach. The data used in this study was ILPD. "We create the model to obtain several classifier predictions. It is thereby shown that if two or more classifiers output 1 value and all others have a 0 value, the condition is that there is liver disease; if all values are 0, then there is nothing and this study found that a combined ML model will have the best accuracy at 96% than the individual algorithms that are KNN with accuracy at 75%, Decision Tree (DT) at 85% and ANN at 89%. Their results conclude that using several classifiers as an integrated SVM reduces the human intervention required in liver disease prediction and improves diagnostic accuracy compared to stand-alone algorithms. The accuracy of the combined ML model is high, which is indicative of its clinical applicability and suggests an intuition that disparate ML techniques result in better diagnosis and better care for the patient."

Kumar and Thakur [6] in their novel approach proposed "Fuzzy Adaptive Neural Weighting (ANW) KNN is hybridizing the fuzzy-based approach of the Adaptive Deep Polynomial Transformation (ADPT) KNN and the ANW KNN methods. This approach is also evaluated on two imbalanced datasets, ILPD and Modified Probabilistic Reinforcement Learning for Patient Data (MPRLPD). In addition, the performance of the Fuzzy Approximate Dynamic Programming (ADP) KNN approach was compared with that of the Fuzzy ANW KNN approach. The study results have revealed that Fuzzy ANW KNN is more suitable than Fuzzy ADP KNN in both datasets. The Fuzzy ADP KNN yields 76.38% for the ILPD dataset, and the Fuzzy ANW KNN yields 84.29%. The obtained accuracy for the Fuzzy ANW KNN method is 91.12% compared with 83.13% for the Fuzzy ADP KNN; this result confirms that a more accurate method would be employed for an optimal liver function test (LFT) analysis. The results show that it applies to medical diagnosis and is better than existing methods for data mining and medical data analysis." The researchers and practitioners in data mining and medical data analysis are enlightened.

The Veena *et al.* [7] study was conducted to diagnose liver disorders using various ML algorithms. "Using the ILPD dataset, the researchers applied Boosted C5.0, random forest (RF), KNNs, k-means, and Naive Bayes." In their study, they consider accuracy, precision, and recall to be their evaluation parameters. Based on their findings, the adaptive Boosted C5.0 algorithm was the most accurate among the test classifiers, with an accuracy of 75.19%. This result shows that the Boosted C5.0 algorithm, its ability to perform well, and the efficiency of the adaptive boosting technique achieved better results than most existing algorithms on this dataset. This study contributes to understanding several ML methods for liver disorder diagnosis that could later aid in the work of healthcare professionals and researchers engaged in the medical aspect. Moreover, the researchers suggest future improvements with combination algorithms, also known as hybrid algorithms. Such hybrid approaches could exploit the strengths of several classifiers in the process of liver disorder diagnosis, thus enhancing the accuracy and reliability of liver disorder diagnosis. Hybrid algorithms could bring novel, sophisticated, and robust diagnostic tools for liver disorders and serve patients and medical practitioners alike in diagnostic rendering and treatment of liver disorders.

In Nahar *et al.* [8], "a comparative analysis of ensemble methods, three methods were studied: bagging, boosting, and stacking. In the bagging approach, the ensemble model was created by using algorithms of BeggRep and Beggl48, in the boosting models of AdaBoost and LogitBoost, and in the stacking approach using the RF algorithm. It was further experimented with and analyzed with the help of the ILPD and these algorithms. The dataset was then subjected to ensemble methods on which the comparative evaluation was done, and the LogitBoost algorithm gave an accuracy of 71.53%, which is significantly above other ensemble approaches. Therefore, it can be assumed that LogitBoost performed better than the various algorithms used in the ensemble model when predicting liver disorders. The study shows that there are more ensemble methods in diagnosing liver disorders and that algorithm determination is significant in building robust prediction models. It also indicates the LogitBoost algorithm's superiority over the other two. If ensemble techniques are used, they can also be used in medical diagnosis to obtain better predictive accuracy. Second, these results are helpful for medical data analysis and hence spur further development of ensemble methods for liver disorder diagnosis and other medical tasks to improve or replace traditional approaches."

In Vats *et al.* [9], a comparative analysis was carried out, considering unsupervised ML methods such as DB-Scan, k-means, and affinity propagation for cluster analysis. They are mainly used to look at the patterns and structures in the data to talk about prediction and assessing their performance. Concerning various evaluation metrics for clustering, such as Silhouette Coefficient, V-measure, Completeness, Homogeneity, Adjusted Rand Index, and Adjusted Mutual Information, the researchers evaluated the clustering strategies. K-means was a promising technique with Silhouette Coefficients close to 1 in assessing the given techniques. The Silhouette Coefficient measures the compactness and separation of clusters, as K effectively creates well-separated compact clusters with a value close to 1. These findings indicate that k-means is effective in extracting the underlying pattern and structure in the data, which is one of the reasons that k-means is popular and practical in many data applications. Analysis of several evaluation metrics helps us perform a complete evaluation assessment of the clustering techniques and make an informed choice per the requirements. When choosing, mentioning multiple evaluation metrics is vital for researchers and practitioners. This comparative analysis provides insights that can be very helpful in evaluating the strengths and limitations of different unsupervised ML methods to guide future research and applications in cluster analysis and prediction tasks.

Raji and Vinod Chandra [10] explored other aspects of health care, from forecasting survival using a multilayer perceptron ANN model to liver transplantations. A study was conducted to predict the survival after liver transplantation by considering many of the parameters pretransplantation and posttransplantation. Several scoring systems (such as the Model for End-Stage Liver Disease (MELD), Emory Score, and Kid Score) were analyzed and examined by specialist clinicians to aid in making critical decisions regarding liver transplantation. Also, by doing a complete analysis of this field, one would know the health of liver transplantation and apply some ML techniques. Finally, we employed the research to forecast survival with the Child and Emory scores while comparing them with their MELD counterparts since the dataset was divided into two classes—Training and Testing. According to Raji *et al.*, this approach made it possible to find matches of donor and recipient pairs for which liver transplantation was successful during the training phase; they showed different aspects of health care related to liver transplantations and provided the essential prediction results of using the multilayer perceptron ANN. These results may have functional implications for the medical community and expand the knowledge of liver transplantation outcomes and physicians' decision-making process in this specialty.

Vinod Chandra and Raji [11] ANNs were proposed to be used as a nonlinear problem for survival following liver transplantation. An ANN-based method to address organ allocation and survival prediction problems was tried to be developed. Here in the approach, when we wanted to make a dataset of which to train and test our network, we listed out all the relevant characteristics. Finally, the health information of selected donors and recipients was carefully picked, and the training procedure was done via 10-fold cross-validation. Also, a comparison with previous models was carried out to be accurate with different performance features. The algorithm had access to enormous amounts of data from the United Network for Organ Sharing Registry to train. Because of this extensive dataset, a 12-year survival analysis is possible, and we predict survival probability and compare predictions against earlier methodologies. The large datasets and sophisticated analysis techniques improve the accuracy and reliability of the predictions significantly. Our findings from this study have the potential implications for improving the strategies to use in organ allocation decisions to optimize outcomes for the patient and ultimately affect the patient's survival after a liver transplant.

Liu *et al.* [12], in particular, it explored a RF algorithm for the short-term prediction of patients after liver transplantation. The patient priority strategy often used is the MELD. Yet the medical literature on postoperative patient performance indicates this has not reached a good level of prediction. To deal with this difficulty, the scientists created an information approach to estimate the postoperative survival throughout the 30 days of the medical measurement values. In their continued effort, they designed a RF model to find the essential features from the medical measurement values and the meaningful factors that discern survival. The research also outlines a procedure for filling in missing values and achieves superior results over the other approaches. In addition, the patient blood test data (from 1 to 9 days before surgery) was used as a forecasting model to predict the survival of the postoperative patient. We chose one of the evaluation statistics as the area under the curve (AUC) to evaluate the model performance. Liu *et al.* extended the research on predicting postoperative survival for liver transplantation to predict more accurately, assisting clinicians in making better estimates about patient outcomes. The study evaluates the ability to predict short-term outcomes using liver transplantation by RF algorithm and AUC as the evaluation metrics, proving decisive in referring to broad knowledge for short-term survival (Table 16.1).

16.3 METHODOLOGY

Liver transplantation is the act of replacing a diseased or damaged liver with a healthy liver from a deceased or living donor. Three main techniques of liver transplantation exist.

- **Orthotopic Liver Transplantation**: The most common method of liver transplantation is orthotopic liver transplantation (OLT). In this procedure, the diseased liver is replaced with a healthy donor liver transplant in the exact anatomic location of the original liver. The new liver is carefully linked to the blood vessels and bile ducts so that the blood supply and bile flow properly [13].
- **Split Liver Transplantation**: Split liver transplantation involves splitting a single deceased donor's liver into two parts, which can be transplanted into two separate recipients. This technique maximizes the use of all available organs for transplant and thereby potentially saves two lives with one donor liver. Size matching will then allow the allocation of the split liver to an adult and a child or two adults [14].

TABLE 16.1
Comparative Studies

S. No	Authors	Disease	Method	Input	Output	Remarks
1	Raji and Vinod Chandra [10]	Liver disorder	Ensemble methods	Model for end-stage liver disease (MELD), Emory Score, Kid Score	Survival Prediction	LogitBoost achieved 71.53% accuracy
2	Vinod Chandra and Raji [11]	Liver transplantation	Artificial neural network (ANN)	Health Characteristics	Graft Survival	Predicts 12-year survival probability
3	Liu *et al.* [12]	Liver transplantation	Random forest (RF)	Blood Test Data	Postoperative Survival	Utilizes the area under the curve (AUC) as the evaluation metric
4	Nahar *et al.* [8]	Liver disorder	Ensemble Methods	Bagging, Boosting, Stacking	Accuracy, Precision, Recall	LogitBoost outperformed other approaches
5	Vats *et al.* [9]	Liver transplantation	Unsupervised machine learning (ML) (DB-Scan, K-Means, Affinity Propagation)	Health Information	Clusters	K-means achieved the Silhouette Coefficient close to 1
6	Kumar and Katyal [5]	Liver disorder	Multiple ML Algorithms	Boosted C5.0, RF, KNN, K-Means, Naive Bayes	Accuracy, Precision, Recall	Adaptive Boosted C5.0 had the highest accuracy of 75.19%
7	Rabbi *et al.* [1]	Liver patient dataset	ML Algorithms (AdaBoost, RF, K nearest-neighbor (KNN))	Dataset Features	Liver Disease Prediction	Extra trees algorithm achieved 92.19% accuracy
8	Kuzhippallil *et al.* [2]	Liver patient dataset	AdaBoost, XGBoost, Genetic Algorithm	Dataset Features	Liver Disease Prediction	Light gradient boosting machine (GBM) achieved the highest accuracy of 86%
9	Rajan *et al.* [3]	Kaggle dataset	Kernel support vector machine (SVM)	Dataset Features	Liver Disease Prediction	Kernel SVM achieved 70% accuracy
10	Veena *et al.* [7]	Liver disorder	Boosted C5.0, RF, KNN, K-Means, Naive Bayes	Indian Liver Patient Dataset	Accuracy, Precision, Recall	Adaptive Boosted C5.0 had the highest accuracy of 75.19%

- **Living Donor Liver Transplantation**: Living donor liver transplantation (LDLT) uses a segment of a healthy liver from a living donor, usually a relative or family member, to transplant. The living donor has major surgery and donates part of their liver to the recipient, which regenerates over time in the donor and the recipient. When no suitable deceased donor liver is available or when urgency demands immediate transplantation, a liver transplant is done (LDLT) [15].

ANNs are a type of ML algorithm inspired by the human brain's neural network system [16]. ANNs have helped predict posttransplant and donor–recipient in the areas of the liver plantation. ANNs can be used in liver transplantation in this manner (Figure 16.1).

16.3.1 Data Collection

Data collection for donor–recipient matching determines what can be developed for practical matching algorithms in transplantation and optimal organ allocation [17]. The data collected needs to be comprehensive, accurate, and relevant to many factors that can affect donor–recipient compatibility. Data collection for matching donor and recipients involves some key aspects detailed below.

- **Medical Records**: Donors and recipients should have medical records obtained that include liver function, past medical, and comorbidity information [18].
- **Demographic Data**: In this research, we assess the demographics of the donors and recipients, their age, gender, and ethnicity.
- **ABO Blood Group and Human Leukocyte Antigen (HLA) Typing**: Collect ABO and HLA data from donors and recipients for assessing blood group compatibility and minimizing risks of rejection.
- **Waiting List Information**: We keep record of the waiting time of each recipient as waiting time plays a role in organ allocation.
- **Liver Size and Anatomy**: Get the liver size and anatomy of the donor, measured as graft-to-recipient size ratio (GRWR), to ensure compatibility with the needs of the recipient.
- **Immunological Factors**: To determine whether the recipient's immune system will react to the donor organ, evaluate immunological parameters, such as panel-reactive antibodies (PRA).
- **Living Donor Information**: A detailed health status evaluation, psychological evaluation, and informed consent should be obtained for living donor transplantations.
- **Posttransplantation Data**: Gather posttransplantation data on graft survival rates, complications, and patient outcomes in order to evaluate the effectiveness of the matching process [19].
- **Ethical Considerations**: Ensure that data collection adheres to ethical guidelines, protecting the privacy and confidentiality of donors and recipients.

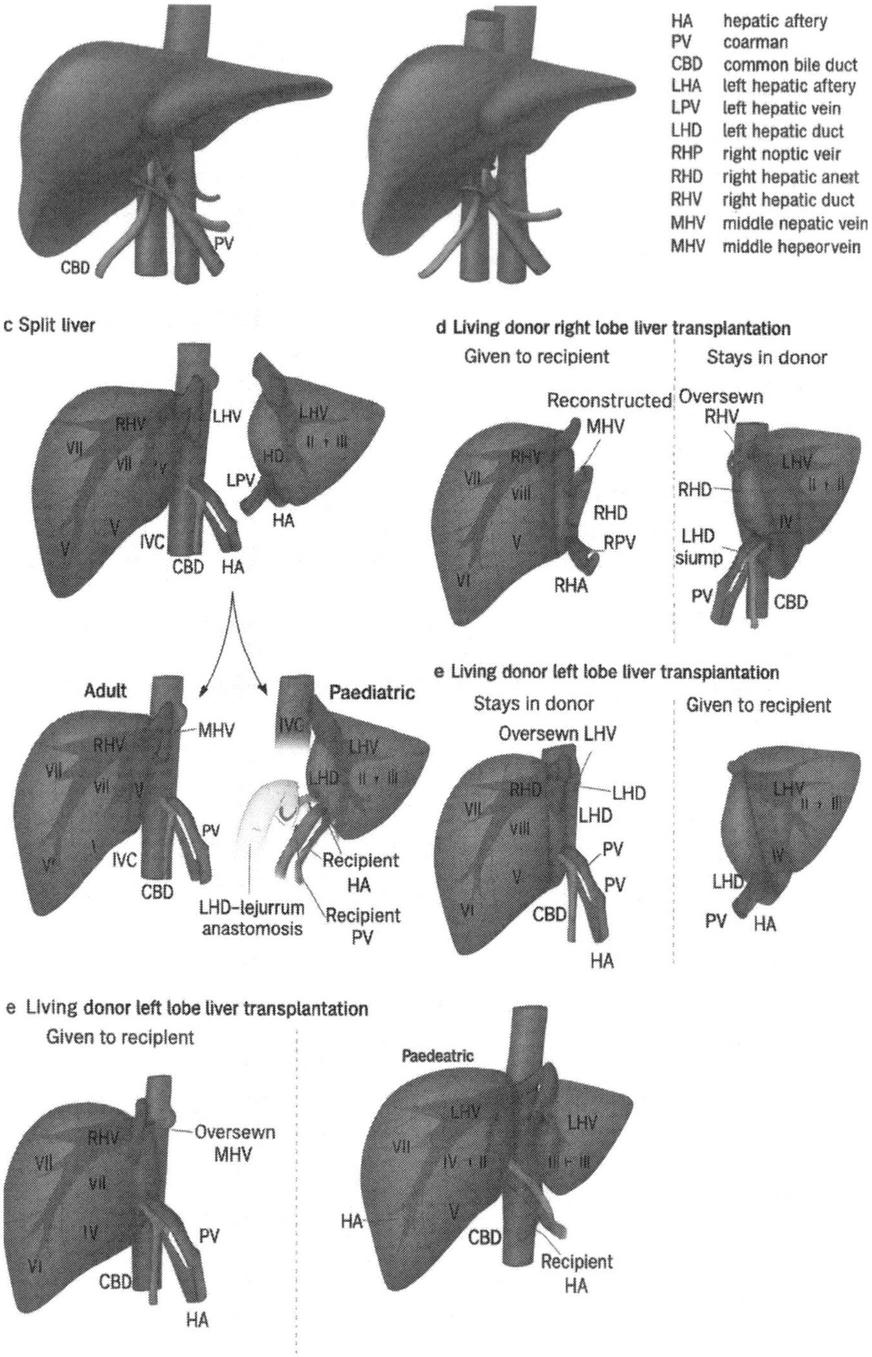

FIGURE 16.1 Traditional approach for liver transplantation.

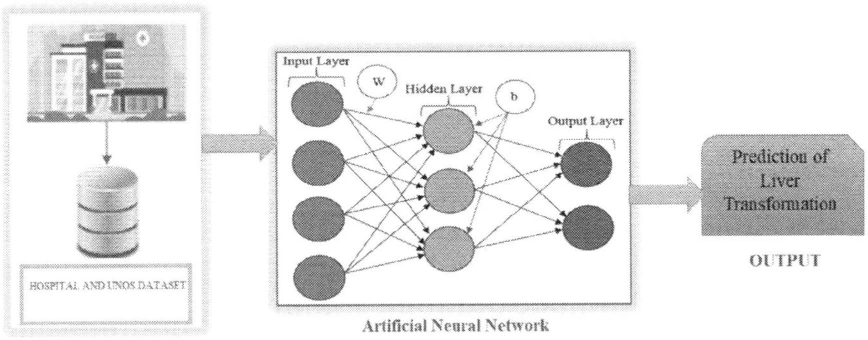

FIGURE 16.2 Proposed architecture.

- **Data Integration**: Integrate data from transplant centers, organ procurement organizations, and registries to create a comprehensive dataset for analysis.
- **Data Quality Assurance**: Data cleaning and validation processes are essential for preventing errors and inconsistencies in the collected data.
- **Longitudinal Data**: Collect longitudinal data on recipients' health and graft function over time to enable ongoing evaluation of matching decisions.

Data collection for donor–recipient matching involves the collaboration of different transplant centers, healthcare providers, and researchers [20]. There are many ways that electronic health records, national transplant registries, and data sharing can work together to build and implement practical matching algorithms for transplantation that would help collectors gather comprehensive data (Figure 16.2).

16.3.2 Feature Selection and Preprocessing

To prepare the data for donor–recipient matching, selecting and preprocessing the features collected from the data is very important. In these steps, a feature is chosen to identify as part of relevant features, eliminating the noise or irrelevant information and transforming the data to one that can be analyzed. In transplant, we can enhance the matching donor-to-recipient decisions by using feature selection and preprocessing on the data to optimize the data for matching donors to recipients so that if the steps are implemented carefully, we are assured that data fed into subsequent algorithms used for development is high quality and relevant resulting in better data and thus better and more effective donor-to-recipient matching decisions in transplant [21].

16.3.3 Development of Matching Algorithm

Donor–recipient pairing in transplantation development of a matching algorithm has several stages of design, implementation, and validation. As indicated, an example of the development process follows this outline:

- **Problem Formulation**: It will be essential to detail the problem and the objective of the matching algorithm. It specifies criteria for donor–recipient compatibility based on medical factors, immunological factors, and demographic information [22].
- **Data Collection and Preprocessing**: Provide ways to preprocess data (because missing values, outliers, and the like can ruin ML). Make sure that the data is in a form that can be analyzed.
- **Feature Selection**: To increase the algorithm's accuracy and efficiency, choose relevant features likely to affect donor–recipient compatibility. The features inside the data that does not help to solve the problem at hand need to be eliminated to make the algorithm more efficient.
- **Algorithm Selection**: Based on the problem requirements and the available data, use genetic algorithms, ML models, or any combination of approaches.
- **Model Training**: The dataset is divided into training and validation sets. Refine the model architecture and hyperparameters of the selected algorithm and submit it to the training data.
- **Performance Evaluation**: Measure the matching algorithm's performance using the same metrics as accuracy, sensitivity, specificity, AUC-ROC, and F1 score. You will use the validation set to check how the model performs in the generalization.

16.3.4 Ethical Considerations

Matching algorithms for transplants cannot be developed and implemented without ethics. Ethical concerns include fairness, transparency, privacy, informed consent, avoiding bias, and accountability. Moral considerations that facilitate transparency in nondiscriminatory decision-making in organ allocation include the protection of the privacy and confidentiality of donors and recipients. Participants know what is involved with the process of transplantation. Impartiality in matching decisions is achieved when bias is avoided. Undue prioritization is prevented by avoiding excessively bringing in medical pressures. Data protection indicates data usage consent. The terms beneficence and nonmaleficence are founded upon the well-being of all involved. There are shared decision-makers among stakeholders. The social fourth concept of fair, efficient, and patient-centric organ allocation is operationalized throughout the algorithm's life cycle [23].

16.3.5 Model Validation and Performance Metrics

The accuracy and benefits of the matching algorithm for transplantation are reliant on model validation and parameters. Separation of training and validation set for rigorous evaluation can also be performed. K-fold cross-validation helps improve performance estimates. The performance metrics such as accuracy, sensitivity, specificity, precision, and F1 score give insight. Inside of baseline metrics, the calibration ensures that the predicted probabilities match the actual probabilities, and comparing the baselines validates the improvements. Real-world donation data are used to validate the algorithm for practical use. Independent datasets are tested, and areas for improvement in donor–recipient pairing are identified. Then, we validate and evaluate donor–recipient pairing to optimize patient outcomes while optimizing organ allocation efficiency [24].

16.4 RESULTS AND DISCUSSION

The performance metrics in the table are as follows:

- **Accuracy (%)**: Accuracy is the proportion of correctly classified instances (both true positives and true negatives) out of the total instances. It measures the overall correctness of the algorithm's predictions.
- **Sensitivity**: Sensitivity, also known as recall, is the proportion of true positive instances correctly identified by the algorithm out of all actual positive instances. It represents the algorithm's ability to correctly detect positive instances.
- **Specificity**: Specificity is the proportion of true negative instances correctly identified by the algorithm out of all actual negative instances. It indicates the algorithm's ability to correctly identify negative instances. [25]
- **F1 Score**: The F1 score is the harmonic mean of precision and sensitivity (recall). It provides a balanced measure of the algorithm's performance, particularly when there is an imbalance between the number of positive and negative instances [25].

Finally, the experimental analysis of this proposed framework ML approach was conducted over several parameters [26]. The parameters considered include accuracy, sensitivity, specificity, and F1 score. The practical and accurate prediction is proven for the existing work after Liver Transplantation (LT) by evaluating these parameters. For this comparison investigation, the existing ML techniques have been considered: ANN, KNN algorithm, and SVM [27]. In this paper, the Multilayer Perceptron (MLP) algorithm is compared with the conventional approaches. [28] To show the value of the metric calculated for the existing ML approaches, Table 16.2 is shown below.

Among the three algorithms studied, it was found that the ANN algorithm has the highest accuracy (87%), highest sensitivity (82%), and highest specificity (82%). The accuracy, sensitivity, and specificity of KNN algorithms were 80%, 79%, and 75%,

TABLE 16.2
Metrics Evaluated Existing Technique

Parameter	ANN	KNN	SVM
Accuracy (%)	0.87	0.8	0.71
Sensitivity (%)	0.82	0.79	0.71
Specificity (%)	0.82	0.75	0.68
F1 Score (%)	0.68	0.54	0.48

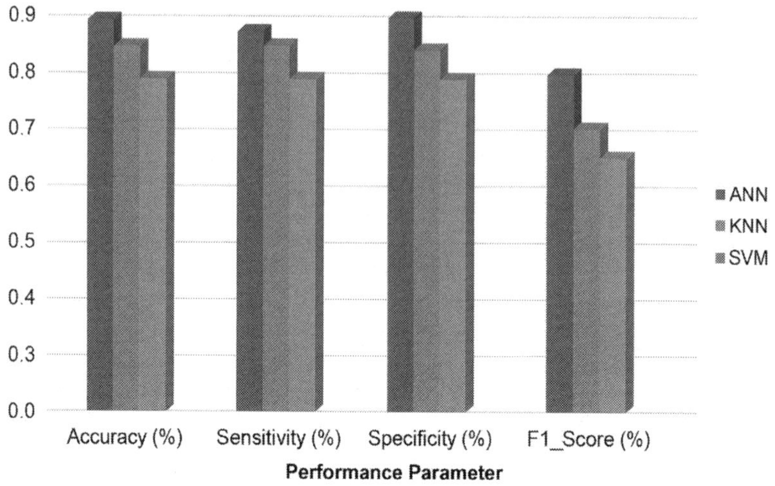

FIGURE 16.3 Performance of the existing system.

respectively. The worst-performing algorithm was an SVM with 71% accuracy, 71% sensitivity, and 68% specificity. Similarly, the ANN produced higher F1 scores (68%) as compared to KNN (54%) and SVM (48%) in the same vein. At the same time, the results show that the ANN algorithm has much higher accuracy and F1 scores than KNN and SVM with this classification task. It is also susceptible and specific to the assignment given. The choice of the most appropriate algorithm for a problem and a dataset depends on the situation, and it may require more analysis and tuning to choose the most suitable algorithm (Figure 16.3).

16.5 CONCLUSIONS

This survey aimed to investigate which studies are contributing to ML research capable of detecting liver disease. Liver problems can be detected effectively with supervised and unsupervised ML methods. This survey is priceless if you want to build a liver disease prediction model. Check and analyze your data and different models to make your prediction accurate. This paper serves as a basis for future research by offering an overview of existing models and techniques. By using ML algorithms, healthcare professionals can potentially predict the onset of liver diseases and get them treated on time, which can help them to identify any liver diseases early and take some easy steps to prevent liver diseases; predictive models improve the precision in the decision-making of medical professionals and provide for more specific and personalized treatment. With the ML aspect of liver disease detection, data-driven approaches can offer the potential to transform the current healthcare practices and underscore the importance of ML in this area of concern, which will further benefit patients and healthcare systems with technology improvement.

REFERENCES

1. M. F. Rabbi, S. M. MahedyHasan, A. I. Champa, M. AsifZaman and M. K. Hasan, "Prediction of Liver Disorders using Machine Learning Algorithms: A Comparative Study," *2020 2nd International Conference on Advanced Information and Communication Technology (ICAICT)*, Dhaka, Bangladesh, 2020, pp. 111–116.
2. M. A. Kuzhippallil, C. Joseph and A. Kannan, "Comparative Analysis of Machine Learning Techniques for Indian Liver Disease Patients," *2020 6th International Conference on Advanced Computing and Communication Systems (ICACCS)*, Coimbatore, Tamil Nadu, India, 2020, pp. 778–782.
3. D. P. Rajan, K. S. Kannan, P. Divya and S. Velliangiri, "Comparative Analysis of Liver diseases by using Machine Learning Techniques," *2022 International Conference on Emerging Smart Computing and Informatics (ESCI)*, Pune, India, 2022, pp. 01–05.
4. C. Anuradha, D. Swapna, B. Thati, V. N. Sree and S. P. Praveen, "Diagnosing for Liver Disease Prediction in Patients Using Combined Machine Learning Models," *2022 4th International Conference on Smart Systems and Inventive Technology (ICSSIT)*, Tirunelveli, Tamil Nadu, India, 2022, pp. 889–896.
5. S. Kumar and S. Katyal, "Effective Analysis and Diagnosis of Liver Disorder by Data Mining," *2018 International Conference on Inventive Research in Computing Applications (ICIRCA)*, Coimbatore, Tamil Nadu, India, 2018, pp. 1047–1051.
6. P. Kumar and R. S. Thakur, "Diagnosis of Liver Disorder Using Fuzzy Adaptive and Neighbor Weighted K-NN Method for LFT Imbalanced Data," *2019 International Conference on Smart Structures and Systems (ICSSS)*, Chennai, India, 2019, pp. 1–5.
7. G. S. Veena, D. Sneha, D. Basavaraju and T. Tanvi, "Effective Analysis and Diagnosis of Liver Disorder," *2018 International Conference on Communication and Signal Processing (ICCSP)*, Melmaruvathur, Tamil Nadu, India, 2018, pp. 0086–0090.
8. N. Nahar, F. Ara, M. A. I. Neloy, V. Barua, M. S. Hossain and K. Andersson, "A Comparative Analysis of the Ensemble Method for Liver Disease Prediction," *2019 2nd International Conference on Innovation in Engineering and Technology (ICIET)*, Dhaka, Bangladesh, 2019, pp. 1–6.
9. V. Vats, L. Zhang, S. Chatterjee, S. Ahmed, E. Enziama and K. Tepe, "A Comparative Analysis of Unsupervised Machine Techniques for Liver Disease Prediction," *2018 IEEE International Symposium on Signal Processing and Information Technology (ISSPIT)*, Louisville, Kentucky, USA, 2018, pp. 486–489.
10. C. G. Raji and S. S. Vinod Chandra, "Various medical aspects of liver transplantation and its survival prediction using machine learning techniques." *Indian Journal of Science and Technology*, vol 10, no. 13, 2017, pp. 1–16.
11. S. S. Vinod Chandra and C. G. Raji, "Predicting the survival of graft following liver transplantation using a nonlinear model." *Journal of Public Health*, vol 24, no. 5, pp. 443–452, 2016.
12. C. L. Liu, R. S. Soong, W. C. Lee, G. W. Jiang and Y. C. Lin, "Predicting short-term survival after liver transplantation using machine learning." *Scientific Reports*, vol 10, no. 1, pp. 1–10, 2020.
13. H. C. Lee, S. B. Yoon, S. M. Yang, W. H. Kim, H. G. Ryu, C. W. Jung, K. S. Suh and K. H. Lee, "Prediction of acute kidney injury after liver transplantation: machine learning approaches vs. logistic regression model." *Journal of Clinical Medicine*, vol 7, no. 11, pp. 428, 2018.
14. M. Cruz-Ramirez, C. Hervas-Martinez, J. C. Fernandez, J. Briceno and M. De La Mata, "Predicting patient survival after liver transplantation using evolutionary multi-objective artificial neural networks." *Artificial Intelligence in Medicine*, vol 58, no. 1, pp. 37–49, 2013.

15. N. Afreen, R. Patel, M. Ahmed and M. Sameer, "A Novel Machine Learning Approach Using Boosting Algorithm for Liver Disease Classification," *2021 5th International Conference on Information Systems and Computer Networks (ISCON)*, Mathura, Uttar Pradesh, India, 2021, pp. 1–5.
16. X. Li, X. Chen and Z. Yuan, "Applicable model of liver disease detection based on the improved CART-AdaBoost algorithm," *2021 IEEE International Conference on Artificial Intelligence and Computer Applications (ICAICA)*, Dalian, China, 2021, pp. 1177–1181.
17. A. Srivastava, V. V. Kumar and V. Vivek, "Automated Prediction of Liver Disease using Machine Learning (ML) Algorithms," *2022 Second International Conference on Advances in Electrical, Computing, Communication and Sustainable Technologies (ICAECT)*, Bhilai, Chhattisgarh, India, 2022, pp. 1–4.
18. C. A. Reddy, L. S. Kiran and V. M. Arul Xavier, "Comparative Analysis of Liver Disease Detection using Diverse Machine Learning Techniques," *2022 6th International Conference on Intelligent Computing and Control Systems (ICICCS)*, Madurai, Tamil Nadu, India, 2022, pp. 1452–1457.
19. H. Hartatik, M. B. Tamam and A. Setyanto, "Prediction for Diagnosing Liver Disease in Patients using KNN and Naïve Bayes Algorithms," *2020 2nd International Conference on Cybernetics and Intelligent System (ICORIS)*, Manado, Indonesia, 2020, pp. 1–5.
20. T. M. Ghazal, A. U. Rehman, M. Saleem, M. Ahmad, S. Ahmad and F. Mehmood, "Intelligent Model to Predict Early Liver Disease using Machine Learning Technique," *2022 International Conference on Business Analytics for Technology and Security (ICBATS)*, Dubai, United Arab Emirates, 2022, pp. 1–5.
21. C. Geetha and A. Arunachalam, "Evaluation based Approaches for Liver Disease Prediction using Machine Learning Algorithms," *2021 International Conference on Computer Communication and Informatics (ICCCI)*, Coimbatore, India, 2021, pp. 1–4.
22. M. A. Hafeez, A. Imran, M. I. Khan, A. H. Khan, A. Nawaz and S. Ahmed, "Diagnosis of Liver Disease Induced by Hepatitis Virus Using Machine Learning Methods," *2022 8th International Conference on Information Technology Trends (ITT)*, Dubai, United Arab Emirates, 2022, pp. 154–159.
23. V. J. Gogi and M. N. Vijayalakshmi, "Prognosis of Liver Disease: Using Machine Learning Algorithms," *2018 International Conference on Recent Innovations in Electrical, Electronics & Communication Engineering (ICRIEECE)*, Bhubaneswar, Odisha, India, 2018, pp. 875–879.
24. K. Sellamuthu, P. Sylviya, K. Pugazharasi and S. Rajalakshmi, "Liver Disease Prediction using Logistic Regression," *2022 8th International Conference on Smart Structures and Systems (ICSSS)*, Chennai, India, 2022, pp. 1–06.
25. R. Zhao, X. Wen, H. Pang and Z. Ma, "Liver disease prediction using W-LR-XGB Algorithm," *2021 International Conference on Computer, Blockchain and Financial Development (CBFD)*, Nanjing, China, 2021, pp. 245–248.
26. K. Thirunavukkarasu, A. S. Singh, M. Irfan and A. Chowdhury, "Prediction of Liver Disease using Classification Algorithms," *2018 4th International Conference on Computing Communication and Automation (ICCCA)*, Greater Noida, India, 2018, pp. 1–3.
27. S. R. Tanuku, A. A. Kumar, S. R. Somaraju, R. Dattuluri, M. V. K. Reddy and S. Jain, "Liver Disease Prediction Using Ensemble Technique," *2022 8th International Conference on Advanced Computing and Communication Systems (ICACCS)*, Coimbatore, Tamil Nadu, India, 2022, pp. 1522–1525.
28. R. Kalaiselvi, K. Meena and V. Vanitha, "Liver Disease Prediction Using Machine Learning Algorithms," *2021 International Conference on Advancements in Electrical, Electronics, Communication, Computing and Automation (ICAECA)*, Virtually, 2021.

17 Clinical Decision Support Systems in Pre-pregnancy Health

A Comparative Review of Traditional, Machine Learning, and Deep Learning Techniques

Gopal B. Deshmukh, Satyajit Pangaonkar, Parikshit N. Mahalle, Surendra Rahamatkar, Dattatray G. Takale, and Mahesh Shinde

17.1 INTRODUCTION

Advanced computing technologies have been integrated into healthcare and contributed to the development and widespread adoption of Clinical Decision Support Systems (CDSSs) to change clinical practice significantly [1]. These systems are intended to provide context-specific advice in the point of care settings that will assist healthcare providers in making informed and evidence-based decisions. In modern healthcare, CDSSs have become integral components of healthcare infrastructure. They are tools that "have an effect on clinician decision-making about individual patients at the time when these decisions have to be made." They can improve diagnostic accuracy and treatment plans, reduce medications, and facilitate administration tasks [2].

Non-knowledge-based and knowledge-based are the two broad classifications of CDSSs. CDSSs based on such facts are knowledge-based CDSSs which depend on pre-defined rules, clinical guidelines, and structured knowledge bases constructed by domain experts [3]. This expert knowledge is combined with patient-specific data through inference engines, yielding recommendations. However, these systems are very interpretable and aligned with clinical guidelines [4]. Still, they suffer from poor scalability, adaptability to new data, and (in some cases) poor performance in complex or ambiguous clinical situations [5].

DOI: 10.1201/9781003479185-17

In contrast, non-knowledge-based knowledge-based CDSSs, such as machine learning (ML) and deep learning (DL) approaches, have shown promise in overcoming several drawbacks of older systems. Due to their ability to learn complex patterns from historical and real-time clinical data, these data-driven models are excellent for predictive modeling and personalized health care [6]. Due to their ability to handle data of heterogeneous types like structured EHRs, time series vitals, medical images, and textual clinical notes, we know that ML and DL models can utilize such data to extract features that may not be straightforward to identify otherwise [7].

The volume of patient data has been rising while there is a growing emphasis on personalized medicine. As a result, ML and DL are becoming vital in developing next-generation CDSSs. Using these intelligent systems, the disease risk can be foreseen, the at-risk population can be identified, and preventive actions can be recommended and tailored to the individual risk profile of each patient [8]. Applying such models for pre-pregnancy health is an up-and-coming area where such early risk prediction can have profound effects on maternal and neonatal outcomes. Pre-pregnancy–pregnancy to improve preconception to prevent poor outcomes like pre-eclampsia, gestational diabetes, low birth weight, and maternal deaths. During this critical phase, artificial intelligence (AI) has the potential to empower CDSSs that support clinicians in evaluating complex, interrelated risk factors, e.g., lifestyle, comorbidities, socio-demographics, and genetic predispositions [9].

Although they have potential, AI-based CDSSs encounter several hurdles in clinical practice. A top problem is the biased training data, which can lead to models that work well for some populations but not others. For example, pre-pregnancy and maternal health are particularly concerning because social determinants like race, ethnicity, and access to care are so important [10]. However, biased AI systems can potentially propagate health disparities if not carefully audited and validated. Also, ML and DL models are a great source of criticism for their lack of transparency, the so-called "black-box" problem [11]. When there are no system reasoning guarantees, healthcare professionals are often reluctant to trust and follow those recommendations (Figure 17.1).

Such issues are faced, and the field is turning to Explainable Artificial Intelligence (XAI). XAI techniques attempt to make AI models more intelligible so that clinicians can reason about the rationale for the predicted outcomes or decisions. Explainability also fosters trust and helps discover potential biases, data quality issues, and accountability [12]. Explainability is desirable and may become a regulatory or ethical requirement for AI systems in medicine, as per Antoniadi *et al.* [21]. Unfortunately, XAI is not yet used as much as it should be in the clinical implementations of ML-based CDSSs; there is a fundamentally significant gap in current research and deployment practices [13].

The COVID-19 pandemic further accelerated the adoption of CDSSs, highlighting the requirement for remote monitoring, virtual consultations, and telemedicine solutions. In these scenarios, CDSSs were extremely valuable to clinicians making quick, evidence-driven decisions without needing in-person interaction [14]. This also underscored the necessity of including and integrating CDSSs with electronic health records (EHRs), wearable devices, and mobile health platforms to offer real-time,

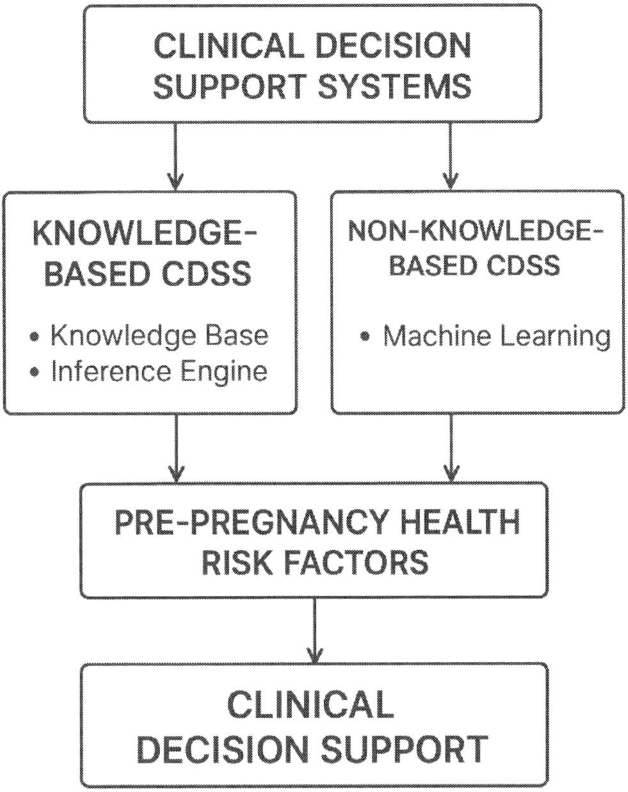

FIGURE 17.1 CDSS in pre-pregnancy healthcare.

context-specific decision support. This seems highly relevant to pre-pregnancy care, where timely risk assessments and interventions can make a difference to the health of mother and child [15].

AI and ML are becoming increasingly considered within the scope of maternal health. Still, few studies have succeeded in developing and integrating ML-based CDSSs into clinical systems for pre-pregnancy risk assessment. While existing systems often center on pregnancy monitoring and intrapartum care, preconception as a phase of digital health innovation is vastly underrepresented [16]. Hence, there is an urgent need to conduct research such that not only are accurate and personalized CDSSs for pre-pregnancy care developed, but their usability, clinical integration, and ethical implications are also evaluated [17].

This paper comprehensively reviews traditional, ML, and DL-based CDSSs, specifically in pre-pregnancy healthcare. We propose scrutinizing a gamut of approaches to understand their strengths, limitations, and clinical applicability, thus bridging the gap between theoretical advancements and real-world implementation [18]. Key evaluation criteria, including accuracy, interpretability, scalability, and user trust, are particularly focused on evaluating these systems' readiness for integration into routine clinical workflows. In addition, we address several challenges, such as data bias, model generalizability, and missing explainability. We offer future research directions to inform the creation of robust, ethical, and patient-centric CDSSs for pre-pregnancy health [19].

17.2 METHODOLOGY FOR REVIEW

To achieve this, the methodology and framework for conducting the literature review are adapted from the Kitchenham and Charters guidelines for evidence-based software engineering reviews and Antoniadi *et al.*'s [21] framework for healthcare AI research. The methodological goal is to make the modeling work transparent, reproducible, and relevant to CDSSs in pre-pregnancy health as well as traditional ML and DL approaches [20].

17.2.1 Objectives and Research Questions

This literature review is designed to comprehensively address the current landscape, trends, and challenges in CDSSs applied to pre-pregnancy healthcare. The following Research Questions (RQs) were formulated to guide the study:

- **RQ1**: What studies have been conducted toward the development of CDSSs for pre-pregnancy or pregnancy health using traditional, ML, or DL methods?
- **RQ2**: What types of ML/DL algorithms have been implemented, and how do they compare to traditional rule-based systems?
- **RQ3**: To what extent are the ML/DL-based CDSSs interpretable or explainable? Have these systems integrated Explainable AI (XAI) methods?
- **RQ4**: Have the developed CDSSs been evaluated using real-world datasets or deployed in clinical settings? What is their level of validation?

These RQs form the backbone of the review and help assess the maturity, inclusivity, and real-world readiness of current systems.

17.2.2 Literature Search Strategy

A structured search was performed across academic databases to identify relevant literature. The search aimed to retrieve peer-reviewed journal articles, conference proceedings, and review papers that discuss CDSSs in the context of pre-pregnancy or pregnancy health.

17.2.2.1 Databases Searched

- **Google Scholar**
- **PubMed**
- **Scopus**
- **IEEE Xplore**
- **Web of Science**

These databases were selected due to their coverage of interdisciplinary and healthcare-focused publications. A preliminary analysis identified Google Scholar as the most comprehensive, consistent with prior reviews.

17.2.2.2 Search Strings Used

The following keyword-based queries were applied (refined to match each database's syntax):

- **S1**: "clinical decision support system" AND "machine learning" AND "pregnancy"
- **S2**: "CDSS" AND "machine learning" AND "pre-pregnancy"
- **S3**: "explainable AI" AND "clinical decision support" AND "maternal health"
- **S4**: "rule-based system" AND "pregnancy risk" OR "pre-pregnancy assessment"

All searches were limited to studies published between 2018 and 2024 to ensure relevance to current technological capabilities and clinical practices (Figure 17.2).

17.2.3 Paper Selection and Inclusion Criteria

The literature review aims to identify 1,389 records found across five major databases: Google Scholar, PubMed, Scopus, Web of Science, and IEEE Xplore. We removed 336 duplicate entries and were left with 1,053 unique records for initial screening. In this phase, 389 records were excluded for being non–peer-reviewed and/or non–English and 664 papers were included. The papers had a quality check and only retained the publications that come from reputable sources, including but not restricted to ACM, IEEE, JCR listed journals, and CORE ranked conferences, and thus excluded 299 papers, and five were inaccessible, hence the 360 papers [21]. Three hundred forty were excluded from these full-text articles as these were out of scope or the only case study used was pregnancy. In the end, 20 papers were included in the review: 17 original research studies and three review papers (Figure 17.3).

17.2.4 Methods

To answer Research Question 1 (RQ1): What studies have been conducted toward the development of CDSSs for pre-pregnancy or pregnancy health using traditional, ML, or DL methods?

To address Research Question 1, we used a structured and rigorous literature analysis approach based on those used in evidence-based review practices. In turn, the methodology used in the review process was PRISMA, which served the purpose of systematic identification, screening, and selection of peer-reviewed studies. Our search involved five major academic databases, including Google Scholar, PubMed, Scopus, IEEE Xplore, and Web of Science with keywords like "clinical decision support system," "machine learning," "deep learning," "pregnancy," and

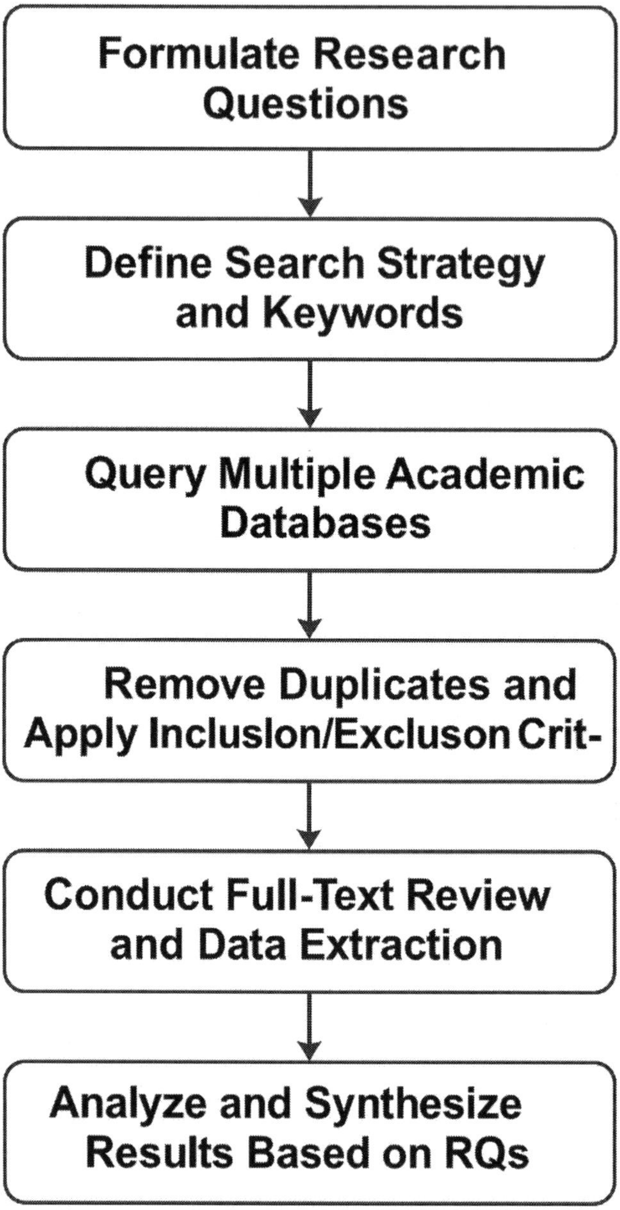

FIGURE 17.2 Literature review methodology.

"pre-pregnancy" put together through various combinations [22]. The search was restricted to the literature between 2012 and 2024 to include the latest advances. We went on to remove duplicates and perform an initial relevance screening to shortlist 360 full-text articles for detailed analysis. In the next step, each of these articles was coded and categorized by the type of CDSS method employed, which was one of

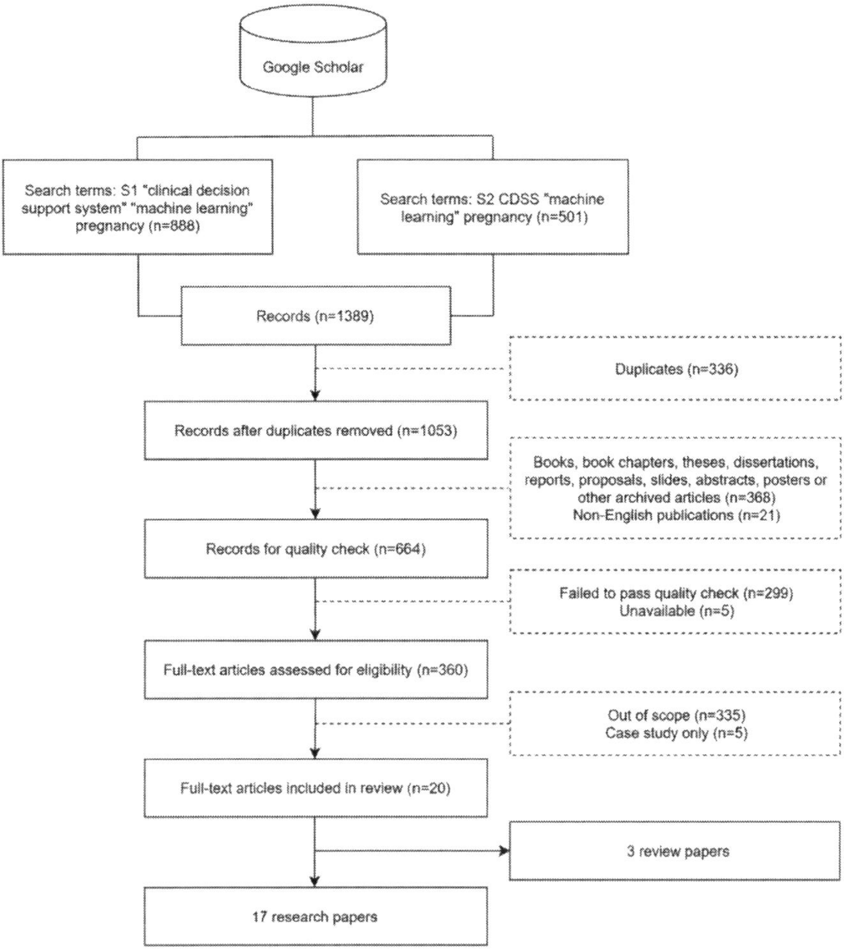

FIGURE 17.3 Flow diagram for paper selection and filtering.

three methods: traditional systems (e.g., rule-based and expert systems), ML techniques (e.g., logistic regression, support vector machine, decision tree, and random forest), or DL algorithms (e.g., convolutional neural networks, recurrent neural networks, LSTMs, and autoencoder) [23]. We created a comparative matrix for each study that encompassed the CDSS type, the algorithm employed, the use to which the system was put clinically (e.g., risk prediction, diagnosis, and monitoring), the data source and sample size, and the outcome metrics (e.g., accuracy, sensitivity, and AUC). This comprehensive classification allowed us to examine the progression and variety of the used approaches in the development of CDSS during different periods and fields of clinical application. We also assessed the level of integration with clinical workflows, the validation status of these systems (prototype, trial, real deployment), and whether they are intended for general pregnancy care or focus on pre-pregnancy risk factors [24]. By synthesizing these studies, we map the research

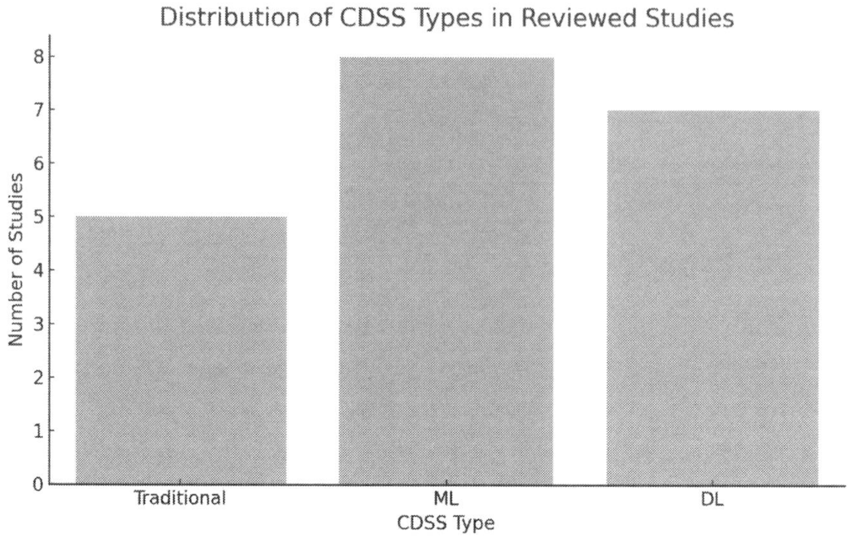

FIGURE 17.4 Distribution of CDSS types in rseviewed studies.

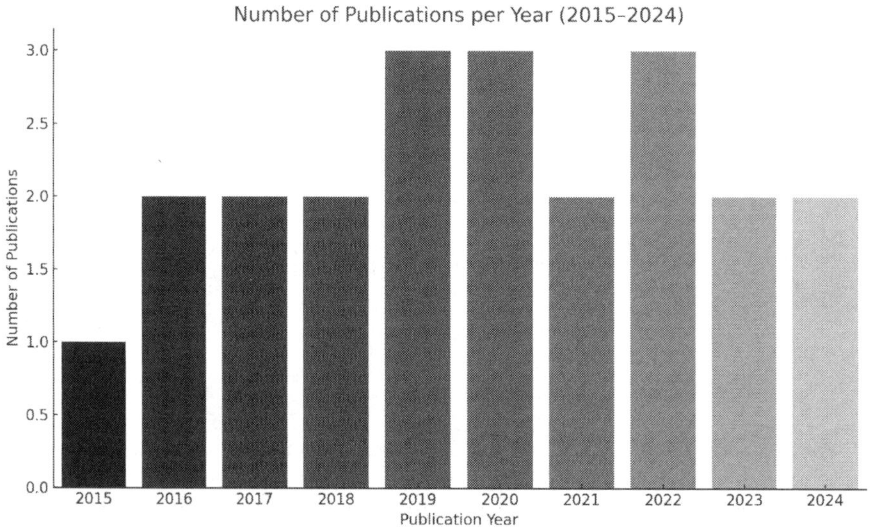

FIGURE 17.5 Number of papers published per year.

landscape, distinguish between academic prototypes and clinically validated systems, and identify the most widely occurring trends in developing CDSSs for maternal and pre-pregnancy healthcare (Figures 17.4 and 17.5).

The most common form of CDSSs reviewed in the studies were ML-based CDSSs (Figure 17.4), with $n = 8$, followed by $n = 7$ DL and $n = 5$ traditional methods. The trend shows a move toward adopting pre-pregnancy and pregnancy healthcare through AI (Table 17.1).

TABLE 17.1
Articles on CDSS Development for Pregnancy Care Using Machine Learning

Citation	Aspect of Pregnancy Care	Machine Learning Methods	Data Source
Guvenir *et al.* [1]	Estimate IVF success rate	SERA	IVF Unit dataset, Etlik Zubeyde Hanim Women's Health, Ankara, Turkey
Van Calster *et al.* [2]	Diagnose unknown pregnancy locations	Logistic regressions, Bayesian MLP, Bayesian SVM, LS-SVM	St. George's Hospital, London, UK
Fernández *et al.* [3]	Predict ectopic pregnancy treatment	Multilayer perceptron, SVM	University Hospital "Virgen de la Arrixaca," Murcia, Spain
Gorthi *et al.* [4]	Determine pregnancy risk category	Decision tree	Synthetic clinical data
Paydar *et al.* [5]	Predict pregnancy outcome in SLE	Binary logistic regression, multilayer perceptron	Tehran hospitals specializing in SLE care
Moreira *et al.* [6]	High-risk pregnancy & childbirth prediction	Particle swarm optimization, multilayer perceptron	Data from hypertensive pregnant women
Afridi and Farooq [7]	Detect high-risk factors for maternal mortality	Feature selection, ensemble methods, naïve Bayes	Tertiary and rural hospital data
Caballero-Ruiz *et al.* [8]	Manage gestational diabetes treatment	Expectation maximization, decision tree	Parc Taulí University Hospital, Spain
Alberola-Rubio *et al.* [9]	Predict labor onset type	SVM	UCI ML Repo: singleton term pregnancies
Ravindran *et al.* [10]	Assess fetal well-being	Adaptive genetic algorithm, ELM	UCI ML Repo: Cardiotocography Data
Yilmaz [11]	Assess fetal state	Multilayer perceptron, probabilistic NN, regression NN	UCI ML Repo: Cardiotocography Data
Zhang and Zhao [12]	Assess fetal state	PCA, AdaBoost + SVM	UCI ML Repo: Cardiotocography Data
Nagendra *et al.* [13]	Predict fetal state	SVM, RF, logistic regression, extra trees	UCI ML Repo: Cardiotocography Data

Regarding RQ3, we provide an overview of the ML/DL-based CDSSs for pregnancy care and found that the predictive performance of these tools is strong, while interpretability is a challenge. Most of the analyzed studies stressed the accuracy and classification performances using complex models like ensemble methods, neural networks, and support vector machines, all inherently black-box methods [25]. However, limited studies explicitly incorporate Explainable AI (XAI) techniques to improve model interpretability for clinical users. Although many of those did, common ways of doing such include ranking of feature importance, decision trees for surrogate explanations, LIME for Local Interpretable Model-agnostic Explanations, and SHAP for Shapley additive explanations. These efforts were, however, usually supplementary, not part of the system's core design. This led to many remaining "black boxes" that mistrusted clinicians, were unethical in their transparency, and were non-compliant with regulation [26]. The lack of XAI integration calls for future CDSS research to balance predictive power and explainability, especially in sensitive domains such as maternal healthcare with high-stakes clinical decisions.

For RQ4, the analysis indicated that various CDSSs utilizing ML and DL in pregnancy care had been built. Still, only a small portion of them, using actual clinical datasets, were clinched and, more importantly, deployed in clinical settings. Unlike, most of these studies conducted validations through publicly available datasets (e.g., UCI Cardiotocography dataset) or retrospective hospital records, with limited sample sizes and limited areas of study. Validated systems took place at various levels, most at the prototype or pilot phases, utilizing internal cross-validation or split sample validations [27]. Studies that reported clinical trials of external validations with data from multiple healthcare institutions were found to be in a smaller proportion and reflect higher maturity levels. Yet, full-scale deployment and longitudinal impact assessments in live healthcare contexts are uncommon. Thus, the technical feasibility of ML/DL-based CDSSs in pregnancy care is well demonstrated. However, it is still in the early stage of translation into clinical practice, and further testing under real-world scenarios, usability evaluation, and integration of clinician feedback is required for broad-scale adoption and trust [28].

17.3 PROPOSED ARCHITECTURE

Soft computing techniques such as AI and ML have enabled applications of new techniques to impact maternal and fetal health by improving treatments. Through decision support systems (DSS), intuitional tools would be developed for personalized pre-pregnancy risk assessment and personalized recommendations for pre-pregnancy and delivery health care treatment. Advanced computational techniques from the systems are applied to analyze complex data and generate actionable insights to improve maternal and fetal outcomes [29]. This section outlines how these systems were developed and implemented and the importance of using these systems within modern obstetric care; in the development phase of developing DSS for pre-pregnancy risk assessment, a series of development steps exist, including collection, selection of features, building of models, validation, and clinical implementation (Figure 17.6).

17.3.1 Data Collection for Pre-pregnancy Risk Assessment

The quality and relevance of the data significantly affect a pre-pregnancy risk assessment system. In this system, maternal health parameters, lifestyle parameters, genetic data, environmental factors, and psychological well-being will be collected through data collection. Also, it wants to develop a complete dataset containing all that one is looking for, risk measures and personalized recommendation treatment. EHRs, genetic testing databases, health surveys, wearable health devices, and public health

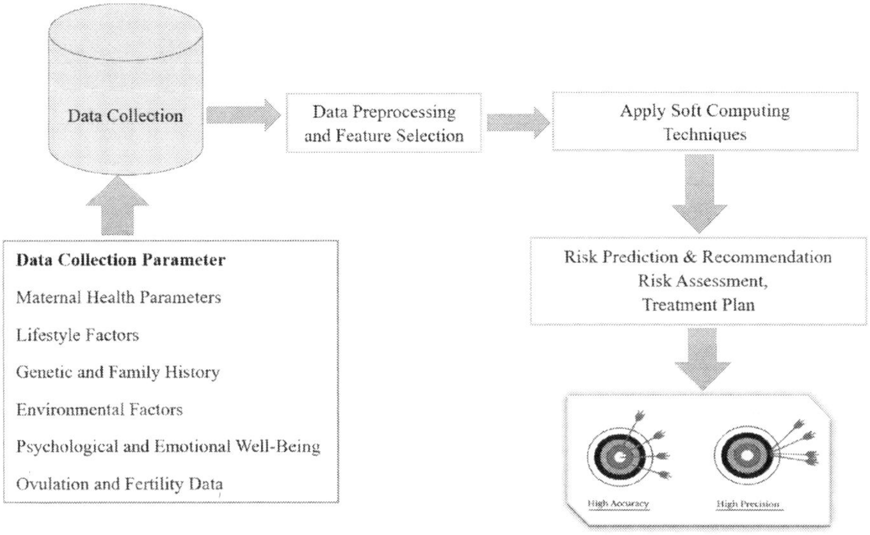

FIGURE 17.6 Proposed system.

databases are sources of pre-pregnancy data for risk assessment. We can better study these sources by obtaining an interface on many factors about maternal health, such as lifestyle, genetic factors, and environmental exposures [30].

- **Maternal Health Parameters**: To predict pregnancy risks, one has to understand maternal health. Demographic details and key parameters include medical history, reproductive health history covering past pregnancy complications, and chronic conditions such as hypertension, diabetes and autoimmune disorders, age, and body mass index. Medical records of prior treatment or procedures that might impact fertility, genetic tests, and disease (such as sexually transmitted infection) status are all crucial to health screenings.
- **Lifestyle Factors**: There are many factors influencing maternal as well as fetal health. Diet, as a cause, revolves around, for example, dietary habits, proper nutrition and vitamin intake, physical activity levels, and substance use history (e.g., smoking, alcohol, and drug use) as a cause, which influences the overall well-being. Further, factors such as stress and mental health (including emotional well-being, anxiety, and depression) and sleep patterns are also taken into account in their effect on pregnancy.
- **Genetic and Family History**: Genetic predispositions can also affect pregnancy outcomes. Screenings contribute to identifying inherited diseases through genetic markers, and a family history of inherited diseases, gestational diabetes, or preeclampsia helps to predict maternal and fetal risks.
- **Environmental Factors**: Environmental hazards impact reproductive health. Toxin exposure from pollutants and chemicals, occupational hazards

(radiation, stress at work), and socioeconomic factors that influence how much healthcare people have access to and how many can get prenatal care play into this.

- **Psychological and Emotional Well-Being**: Pregnancy health depends on mental health history. Then, depression, anxiety, and stress levels must be checked, as family and community support can significantly help concerning the pregnancy outcomes [31].
- **Ovulation and Fertility Data**: Both ovulation and menstrual cycles can be tracked for fertility purposes. Predictor kits can predict menstrual cycle regularity, symptoms such as heavy bleeding or pain, and ovulation. Observing the basal body temperature or conducting vegetarian scans will determine ideal fertility periods to plan conception.

17.3.2 Data Preprocessing Layer

Data Cleaning includes handling missing observations by imputation or deletion, discarding duplicate observations, and handling outliers statistically so that the data is qualitative (of good quality). Feature engineering helps to create new meaningful features such as lifestyle scores, health risk composites, or BMI-age interaction, which improve model prediction. Continuous variables such as age and BMI are normalized and standardized for algorithms sensitive to the scaling of features [32]. During data transformation, categorical variables like smoking status are encoded as hot or in labels for use in numerical format. Data Balancing uses SMOTE (Synthetic Minority Over-sampling Technique) and undersampling, among other methods, to deal with class imbalance problems in the data and help improve model performance for rare outcomes.

17.3.3 Feature Selection

Feature Selection is a critical step in the model development process, in which only the most pertinent features will be included to produce the predictive models. Techniques such as recursive feature elimination or LASSO regularization are often used to identify the most important predictors [33].

17.3.4 Model Architecture Design

The IntelliPregNet framework integrates Gradient Boosting Machines (such as XGBoost and LightGBM) for risk prediction and Deep Q-Networks for personalized treatment recommendation. We demonstrate that this hybrid approach allows for accurate pre-pregnancy risk assessment and adaptive treatment planning, delivering improved maternal and fetal health outcomes.

- **Risk Assessment Using Gradient Boosting Machines (GBM)**: XGBoost and LightGBM will be used as core ML models for the proposed pre-pregnancy risk assessment system, which are efficient enough to process large, structured medical datasets. The critical features of this problem include maternal age, BMI, blood pressure, glucose level, and Hemoglobin level. These models will classify the pregnancies as either low-risk or high-risk pregnancies. Furthermore, preeclampsia, gestational diabetes, as well as risk factors such as exposure to toxins, physical activity, and smoking would also be taken into consideration, as they will be combined into a complete risk profile of the patient to be able to provide the most personalized and accurate projections. Key metrics, such as accuracy, F1-Score, sensitivity, and specificity, will be used to determine the performance of the models in assessing classification performance. A similar evaluation will also be made through the AUC-ROC Curve, measuring performance and assessing the model's capacity to differentiate between high-risk and low-risk pregnancies [34].

- **Reinforcement Learning for Treatment Optimization**: Deep Q-Network (DQN) will benefit from patient risk profiles for recommending personalized treatment plans. In the state representation, we will include the input data, such as real-time health conditions, past interventions, and patient history. Recommendations for medications, lifestyle changes, and follow-up schedules will be made and will form the action space. The reward mechanism would be set to optimize the patient's health outcomes, subject to the constraints of minimizing the risks and side effects. Historical treatment data will be used to train the model and learn which ones work best. The model will continuously adapt using new patient data by updating itself based on the treatment outcomes. These recommendations will be expanded and refined with consultations from experts to be consistent with clinical best practices to give better patient care [35].

17.3.5 Training and Validation

IntelliPregNet framework is trained under a structured training process to improve upon pre-pregnancy risk assessment and personalized treatment recommendations. For predictive risk analysis, Gradient Boosting Machines (GBM) (XGBoost, LightGBM) are used, and Deep Q-Network (DQN) is used to optimize adaptive treatment strategies. Training uses Binary Cross-Entropy loss for classification and Reward-based Reinforcement Learning for Treatment Optimization. Adam optimizer fine-tunes DL components, and Grid Search and Bayesian Optimization refine hyperparameters. K-Fold Cross-Validation ($K=5$ or $K=10$) prevents overfitting and produces a robust model generalization. Training efficiency is improved with the help of early stopping and patience-based termination techniques [36].

IntelliPregNet is proposed based on the models that improve the accuracy within risk assessment to detect early high-risk pregnancies through GBM and optimizes personal recommendations of treatment application through Deep Q-Networks (DQN). With a constant ability to adapt to patient data, maternal and fetal health outcomes are improved by refining decision-making. The AI-driven part of this system helps prevent complications, minimize hospital admission, and implement cost-effective management of healthcare burdens. Scalability and adaptability allow real-time learning from clinical inputs, thus making it a reliable decision support tool for pregnancy risk assessment and treatment optimization.

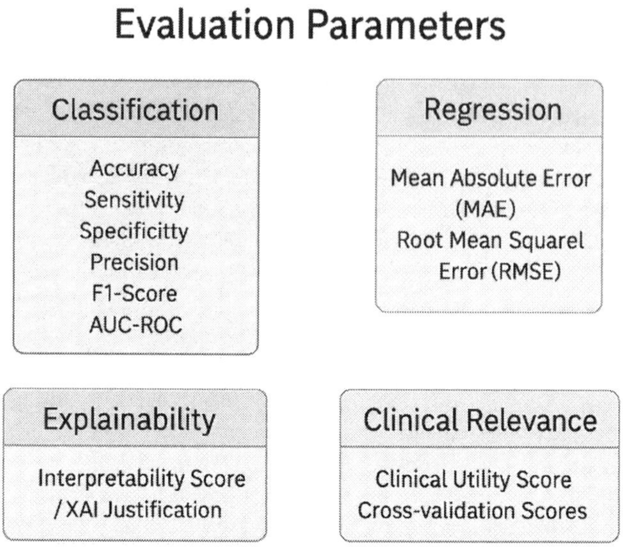

FIGURE 17.7 Evaluation parameter.

17.3.6 Evaluation Parameter

Evaluation parameters are essential for assessing the performance and reliability of ML/DL-based CDSSs. Common classification metrics include accuracy, precision, recall (sensitivity), specificity, F1-score, and AUC-ROC, which measure the model's ability to correctly classify health outcomes. For regression tasks, mean absolute error and root mean squared error are used to evaluate prediction accuracy. Explainability is assessed through interpretability scores or XAI techniques like SHAP or LIME, while clinical relevance is evaluated using clinical utility scores and cross-validation results to ensure real-world applicability. These metrics collectively ensure that CDSSs are accurate, trustworthy, and clinically useful (Figure 17.7).

17.4 CONCLUSION

This chapter presented a comprehensive review of the development and evaluation of CDSSs for pre-pregnancy and pregnancy healthcare using traditional ML and DL approaches. Through a structured and evidence-based review process, it was evident that ML and DL methods have significantly advanced the predictive capabilities of CDSSs, enabling more personalized and data-driven care. However, despite promising results in accuracy, precision, and sensitivity, many of these systems face transparency, trust, and clinical adoption challenges. The limited integration of Explainable AI (XAI) methods has left most models functioning as "black boxes," which can hinder clinician acceptance and patient safety. Furthermore, while several studies validated their models using retrospective real-world datasets, only a few achieved higher levels of validation, such as prospective clinical trials or real-world deployment. The evaluation parameters discussed, ranging from classification metrics like

AUC-ROC and F1-score to regression errors, calibration, and clinical utility, highlight the multifaceted nature of assessing CDSS performance. Moving forward, it is clear that a balanced emphasis on accuracy, interpretability, and clinical validation will be crucial to bridge the gap between technical innovation and practical healthcare application. Future research should focus on improving model performance and building trustworthy, ethically sound, and user-friendly systems that align with the complex demands of clinical environments. This review underscores the critical need for holistic evaluation frameworks to guide the next generation of intelligent CDSSs in maternal and pre-pregnancy care.

REFERENCES

1. Güvenir, H.A., Misirli, G., Dilbaz, S., Ozdegirmenci, O., Demir, B., Dilbaz, B. (2015). Estimating the chance of success in IVF treatment using a ranking algorithm. *Medical & Biological Engineering & Computing*, 53(9), 911–920.
2. Van Calster, B., Timmerman, D., Kirk, E., Bourne, T., Condous, G., Van Huffel, S. (2008). Towards a clinical decision support system for pregnancies of unknown location. *2008 21st IEEE International Symposium on Computer-Based Medical Systems*, Jyväskylä, Finland: IEEE, pp. 581–583.
3. Fernández, A.D.R., Fernández, D.R., Sánchez, M.T.P. (2019). A decision support system for predicting the treatment of ectopic pregnancies. *International Journal of Medical Informatics*, 129, 198–204.
4. Gorthi, A., Firtion, C., Vepa, J. (2009). Automated risk assessment tool for pregnancy care. *2009 Annual International Conference of the IEEE Engineering in Medicine and Biology Society*, Minneapolis, Minnesota, USA: IEEE, pp. 6222–6225.
5. Paydar, K., Kalhori, S.R.N., Akbarian, M., Sheikhtaheri, A. (2017). A clinical decision support system for prediction of pregnancy outcome in pregnant women with systemic lupus erythematosus. *International Journal of Medical Informatics*, 97, 239–246.
6. Moreira, M.W., Rodrigues, J.J., Kumar, N., Al-Muhtadi, J., Korotaev, V. (2018). Natureinspired algorithm for training multilayer perceptron networks in e-health environments for high-risk pregnancy care. *Journal of Medical Systems*, 42(3), 1–10.
7. Afridi, M.J. Farooq, M. (2011). OG-Miner: an intelligent health tool for achieving millennium development goals (MDGs) in m-health environments. *2011 44th Hawaii International Conference on System Sciences*, Koloa, Kauai, Hawaii, USA: IEEE, pp. 1–10.
8. Caballero-Ruiz, E., García-Sáez, G., Rigla, M., Villaplana, M., Pons, B., Hernando, M.E. (2017). Aweb-based clinical decision support system for gestational diabetes: automatic diet prescription and detection of insulin needs. *International Journal of Medical Informatics*, 102, 35–49.
9. Alberola-Rubio, J., Garcia-Casado, J., Prats-Boluda, G., Ye-Lin, Y., Desantes, D., Valero, J., Perales, A. (2017). Prediction of labor onset type: spontaneous vs induced; role of electrohysterography? *Computer Methods and Programs in Biomedicine*, 144, 127–133.
10. Ravindran, S., Jambek, A.B., Muthusamy, H., Neoh, S.-C. (2015). A novel clinical decision support system using improved adaptive genetic algorithm for the assessment of fetal well-being. *Computational and Mathematical Methods in Medicine 2015*, Virtually.
11. Yılmaz, E. (2016). Fetal state assessment from cardiotocogram data using artificial neural networks. *Journal of Medical and Biological Engineering*, 36(6), 820–832.
12. Zhang, Y., Zhao, Z. (2017). Fetal state assessment based on cardiotocography parameters using PCA and AdaBoost. *2017 10th International Congress on Image and Signal Processing, BioMedical Engineering and Informatics (CISP-BMEI)*, Shanghai, China: IEEE, pp. 1–6.

13. Nagendra, V., Gude, H., Sampath, D., Corns, S., Long, S. (2017). Evaluation of support vector machines and random forest classifiers in a real-time fetal monitoring system based on cardiotocography data. *2017 IEEE Conference on Computational Intelligence in Bioinformatics and Computational Biology (CIBCB)*, Manchester, United Kingdom: IEEE, pp. 1–6.
14. Cömert, Z., Yang, Z., Velappan, S., Boopathi, A.M., Kocamaz, A.F. (2018). Performance evaluation of empirical mode decomposition and discrete wavelet transform for computerized hypoxia detection and prediction. *2018 26th Signal Processing and Communications Applications Conference (SIU)*, Çeşme, İzmir, Turkey: IEEE, pp. 1–4.
15. Cömert, Z., Boopathi, A.M., Velappan, S., Yang, Z., Kocamaz, A.F. (2018). The influences of different window functions and lengths on image-based time-frequency features of fetal heart rate signals. *2018 26th Signal Processing and Communications Applications Conference (SIU)*, Çeşme, İzmir, Turkey: IEEE, pp. 1–4.
16. Tortajada, S., García-Gomez, J.M., Vicente, J., Sanjuán, J., de Frutos, R., MartínSantos, R., García-Esteve, L., Gornemann, I., Gutiérrez-Zotes, A., Canellas, F., Carracedo, A. (2009). Prediction of postpartum depression using multilayer perceptrons and pruning. *Methods of Information in Medicine*, 48(03), 291–298.
17. Jiménez-Serrano, S., Tortajada, S., García-Gómez, J.M. (2015). A mobile health application to predict postpartum depression based on machine learning. *Telemedicine and E-Health*, 21(7), 567–574.
18. Dua, D., Graff, C. (2017). UCI machine learning repository. https://archive.ics.uci.edu/ml.
19. Baig, M. M., Hosseini, H. G., Lindén, M. (2016). Machine learning-based clinical decision support system for early diagnosis from real-time physiological data. *2016 IEEE Region 10 Conference (TENCON)*, Marina Bay Sands, Singapore: IEEE, pp. 2943–2946.
20. Holzinger, A., Biemann, C., Pattichis, C. S., Kell, D. B. (2017). What do we need to build explainable AI systems for the medical domain? arXiv:1712.09923.
21. Antoniadi, A. M., Du, Y., Guendouz, Y., Wei, L., Mazo, C., Becker, B. A., Mooney, C. (2021). Current challenges and future opportunities for XAI in machine learning-based clinical decision support systems: A systematic review. *Applied Sciences,* 11(11), 5088.
22. Adadi, A., Berrada, M. (2018). Peeking inside the black-box: A survey on explainable artificial intelligence (XAI). *IEEE Access*, 6, 52138–52160.
23. Tunçalp, Ó., Pena-Rosas, J. P., Lawrie, T., Lawrie, T., Oladapo, O. T., Portela, A., Gülmezoglu, A. M. (2017). WHO recommendations on antenatal care for a positive pregnancy experience-going beyond survival. *BJOG*, 124(6), 860–862.
24. Dalaba, M. A., Akweongo, P., Aborigo, R. A., Saronga, H. P., Williams, J., Blank, A., Kaltschmidt, J., Sauerborn, R., Loukanova, S. (2015). Cost-effectiveness of clinical decision support system in improving maternal health care in Ghana. *PLoS One*, 10(5), e0125920.
25. Usmanova, G., Lalchandani, K., Srivastava, A., Joshi, C. S., Bhatt, D. C., Bairagi, A. K., Jain, Y., Afzal, M., Dhoundiyal, R., Benawri, J., Chaudhary, T. (2021). The role of digital clinical decision support tool in improving quality of intrapartum and postpartum care: Experiences from two states of India. *BMC Pregnancy and Childbirth*, 21(1), 1–12.
26. Davidson, L., Boland, M. R. (2021). Towards deep phenotyping pregnancy: A systematic review on artificial intelligence and machine learning methods to improve pregnancy outcomes. *Briefings in Bioinformatics*, 22(5), bbaa369.
27. Kitchenham, B., Charters, S. (2007). Guidelines for performing systematic literature reviews in software engineering. Tech. Rep. EBSE 2007-001, Keele University and Durham University Joint Report.

28. Martín-Martín, A., Orduna-Malea, E., Thelwall, M., López-Cózar, E. D. (2018). Google Scholar, Web of Science, and Scopus: A systematic comparison of citations in 252 subject categories. *Journal of Informetrics*, 12(4), 1160–1177.
29. Gusenbauer, M. (2019). Google Scholar to overshadow them all? Comparing the sizes of 12 academic search engines and bibliographic databases. *Scientometrics*, 118(1), 177–214.
30. Damaraji, G. M., Permanasari, A. E., Hidayah, I. (2020). A review of expert system for identification of various risks in pregnancy. *2020 3rd International Conference on Information and Communications Technology (ICOIACT)*, Yogyakarta, Indonesia: IEEE, pp. 99–104.
31. Davidson, L., Boland, M. R. (2020). Enabling pregnant women and their physicians to make informed medication decisions using artificial intelligence. *Journal of Pharmacokinetics and Pharmacodynamics*, 47(4), 305–318.
32. Güvenir, H. A., Misirli, G., Dilbaz, S., Ozdegirmenci, O., Demir, B., Dilbaz, B. (2015). Estimating the chance of success in IVF treatment using a ranking algorithm. *Medical Biology and Engineering Computing*, 53(9), 911–920.
33. Van Calster, B., Timmerman, D., Kirk, E., Bourne, T., Condous, G., Van Huffel, S. (2008). Towards a clinical decision support system for pregnancies of unknown location. *21st IEEE International Symposium on Computer-Based Medical Systems*, Jyväskylä, Finland: IEEE, pp. 581–583.
34. Fernández, A. D. R., Fernández, D. R., Sánchez, M. T. P. (2019). A decision support system for predicting the treatment of ectopic pregnancies. *International Journal of Medical Informatics*, 129, 198–204.
35. Gorthi, A., Firtion, C., Vepa, J. (2009). Automated risk assessment tool for pregnancy care. *2009 Annual International Conference of the IEEE Engineering in Medicine and Biology Society*, Minneapolis, Minnesota, USA: IEEE, pp. 6222–6225.
36. Paydar, K., Kalhori, S. R. N., Akbarian, M., Sheikhtaheri, A. (2017). A clinical decision support system for prediction of pregnancy outcome in pregnant women with systemic lupus erythematosus. *International Journal of Medical Informatics*, 97, 239–246.

18 From Traditional Diagnostics to AI Innovations

A Comparative Study for Early Detection and Management of Chronic Kidney Disease

Mahesh Shinde, Satyajit Pangaonkar, Parikshit N. Mahalle, Surendra Rahamatkar, Dattatray G. Takale, and Gopal B. Deshmukh

18.1 INTRODUCTION

Chronic Kidney Disease (CKD) is becoming a global health problem, and its prevalence is constantly increasing in all age groups and socioeconomic strata [1]. CKD is the progressive and usually irreversible reduction in the ability of the kidneys to perform their function and is frequently diagnosed late, at the point of Stage 3 or later when symptoms start to become apparent, by which time damage is already well advanced and significant complications have occurred such as cardiovascular disease, anemia, bone disorders, and end-stage renal disease (ESRD) [2]. Unfortunately, CKD is usually diagnosed too late, which hinders effective treatment interventions and thus creates enormous physical, psychological, and financial burdens to both the patients and the healthcare systems. Therefore, early and accurate disease detection and suitable management strategies are essential in changing the natural history of the disease, improving patient outcomes, and reducing healthcare costs [3].

Traditionally, the detection of CKD has been heavily based on traditional diagnostic practices. These conventional methods are serum creatinine levels, estimated glomerular filtration rate (eGFR), urinalysis to check for protein or blood in the urine, and monitoring blood pressure [4]. Renal ultrasound and kidney biopsies are used as imaging techniques to investigate structural or histological abnormalities. Despite their importance in clinical practice, these methods are ineffective due to their inherent limitations. However, these diagnostic tools primarily recognize CKD

DOI: 10.1201/9781003479185-18

after enormous kidney damage has taken place. The accuracy of test results can vary based on other factors such as age, sex, and ethnicity, thereby causing diagnostic variability and delayed intervention. Additionally, while traditional diagnostics tend to be labor-intensive, large-scale diagnostics are a matter of time, especially in resource-constrained settings [5].

Modern technological advancements have started changing the face of detecting and managing CKD. "Machine Learning (ML), Deep Learning (DL), and Artificial Intelligence (AI)" techniques have recently matured to a point where they are powerful analysis tools that are now available to the healthcare community for the analysis of such large and complex datasets with high precision. Such technologies can be used not only to find CKD at earlier stages but also to predict the risk of progressive disease, individualize the treatment options, and improve care follow-up and continuous assessment of the patients [6]. For example, "ML methods, including Decision Trees, Random Forests (RFs), Support Vector Machines (SVMs), Logistic Regression, and K-Nearest Neighbors (KNN)," exhibit better predictive qualities than traditional methods and rely on clinical, demographic, and lifestyle data to uncover small and complex patterns and risk factors [7].

DL models have further increased predictive performance and become the standard of the art in this field. "Convolutional Neural Networks (CNNs), Long Short-Term Memory Networks (LSTMs), and, more recently, hybrid ensemble approaches have shown particular promise in modeling complex, nonlinear dynamics in high-dimensional medical datasets [8]." CNN is very good at spatial feature identification, and LSTMs perform best at temporal dependency within longitudinal health data. Combining DL models can improve robustness, accuracy, and generalizability across various patient populations [9].

In addition to the technical advances of ML and DL, wider AI innovations are redefining how CKD is detected. Explainable AI (XAI) techniques focus on answering the critical need for transparency and trustworthiness in AI-driven health care, focusing on providing clinicians with the ability to comprehend and trust model predictions [10]. Another promising development is federated learning, a method for training models on sensitive patient data decentralized and without compromising privacy so that collaborators can collaborate among institutions. Dynamic treatment planning in which treatments are modified over time by patient responses is being explored using reinforcement learning [11].

The current state of biomedical data for training DL models requires large amounts of labeled data, often prohibiting them due to privacy reasons and the fragmented nature of healthcare records. The black-box nature of many AI systems can be an obstacle to the clinical adoption of complex models, and the interpretability of complex models is still an area of active research. Further, integrating AI-driven tools with existing healthcare infrastructure requires careful consideration of regulatory, ethical, and operational factors. However, issues such as algorithmic bias, data security, and clinician oversight must be considered for these technologies to supplement rather than supplant human expertise [12].

This chapter presents a detailed review and comparative analysis of the existing traditional CKD diagnosis methods with AI-driven approaches for CKD early diagnosis and management. It aims to critically review the advantages and disadvantages of classical methods, the progression to ML algorithms, the innovative role of DL architectures, and the revolutionary power of the most recent AI developments. However, the discussion also shows how traditional practices are being complemented and, in some cases, overtaken by AI technologies that offer earlier detection, more accurate diagnosis, personalized treatment, and better long-term outcomes for CKD patients [13]. This chapter reviews the current research landscape in AI and nephrology, highlighting areas for further investigation and future directions for making AI more applicable to nephrology. Particular focus is placed on finding scalable, explainable, and accessible solutions that can be used ubiquitously in clinical practice and resource-limited settings. Therefore, addressing these aspects is key to the progress of CKD management and generalizing the progress toward achieving equitable, high-quality health care through technology.

18.2 METHODOLOGY FOR REVIEW

This review paper aimed to systematically survey, consider, and synthesize the progress of traditional diagnostic methods to AI-based methods for early detection and management of CKD from the development-level perspective. The review process was pursued by adopting a structured and transparent approach to ensure the review's accuracy, relevance, and scope. We can mention the steps as follows:

Step 1: Literature Search Strategy

"A comprehensive literature search was conducted across multiple academic databases including":

- PubMed
- IEEE Xplore
- ScienceDirect
- Google Scholar
- Scopus

The search terms and Boolean combinations used were:

- "Chronic Kidney Disease" OR "CKD"
- AND "Early Detection" OR "Early Diagnosis"
- AND "Traditional Diagnostic Methods"
- AND "Machine Learning" OR "ML"
- AND "Deep Learning" OR "DL"
- AND "Artificial Intelligence" OR "AI"
- AND "Comparative Study" OR "Performance Evaluation"

The time frame for the search was restricted to articles published between 2018 and 2025, ensuring the inclusion of recent advancements while maintaining a historical context for traditional methods [14].

Step 2: Inclusion and Exclusion Criteria

Applying precise inclusion and exclusion criteria produced a high-caliber, relevant outcome. The studies were included if they included conventional, ML, DL, or AI techniques for the early diagnosis, treatment, or detection of CKD. The journal articles, peer-reviewed conference papers, and authoritative review articles in English were published only if they reported measurable performance metrics, that is, accuracy, sensitivity, specificity, and area under the curve (AUC). On the contrary, studies were not included if their findings were unrelated to CKD detection, were editorial or commentary pieces, lacked methodological rigor, or were specific to pediatric CKD with limited application. Also, any duplicate or incomplete studies were removed to maintain the review's scientific integrity [15].

Step 3: Data Extraction and Categorization

Relevant data were extracted from selected papers and organized into the following categories:

- **Traditional Diagnostic Methods**: Including clinical tests, biochemical markers, and imaging techniques.
- **ML Techniques**: Such as Decision Trees, RFs, SVMs, Logistic Regression, and KNNs.
- **DL Architectures**: Including CNNs, LSTM networks, Bidirectional LSTM (BLSTM), and hybrid ensemble models.
- **Advanced AI Innovations**: Covering XAI, Reinforcement Learning, and Federated Learning applications in CKD.

Each paper was reviewed for methodology, dataset characteristics, feature engineering, model training, validation techniques, evaluation metrics, and limitations.

Step 4: Comparative Analysis Framework

To ensure consistency and rigor in the review, a comparative framework was established based on several key criteria. These included accuracy and performance metrics such as sensitivity, specificity, precision, recall, F1 score, and AUC; interpretability and clinical relevance to facilitate understanding by healthcare providers; scalability and practical implementation considering resource availability and real-world deployment; adaptability to diverse clinical settings, including both urban and rural environments; and the potential for integration with existing healthcare systems like electronic health records (EHRs) and decision support tools.

Step 5: Quality Assessment

To ensure the "quality of included studies, a modified checklist based on the Newcastle–Ottawa Scale (NOS) for observational studies and the Transparent Reporting of a Multivariable Prediction Model for Individual Prognosis or Diagnosis (TRIPOD) guidelines for predictive modeling studies was employed."

Key assessment criteria included:

- Study design robustness.
- Dataset size and diversity.
- Validation strategy (e.g., k-fold cross-validation and external validation).
- Reporting of limitations and biases (Figure 18.1).

Step 6: Synthesis and Presentation

This review synthesized the findings both qualitatively and quantitatively, when possible. The discussion is split into Traditional, ML, DL, and AI subsections to ensure a clear and in-depth discussion. Methodologies,

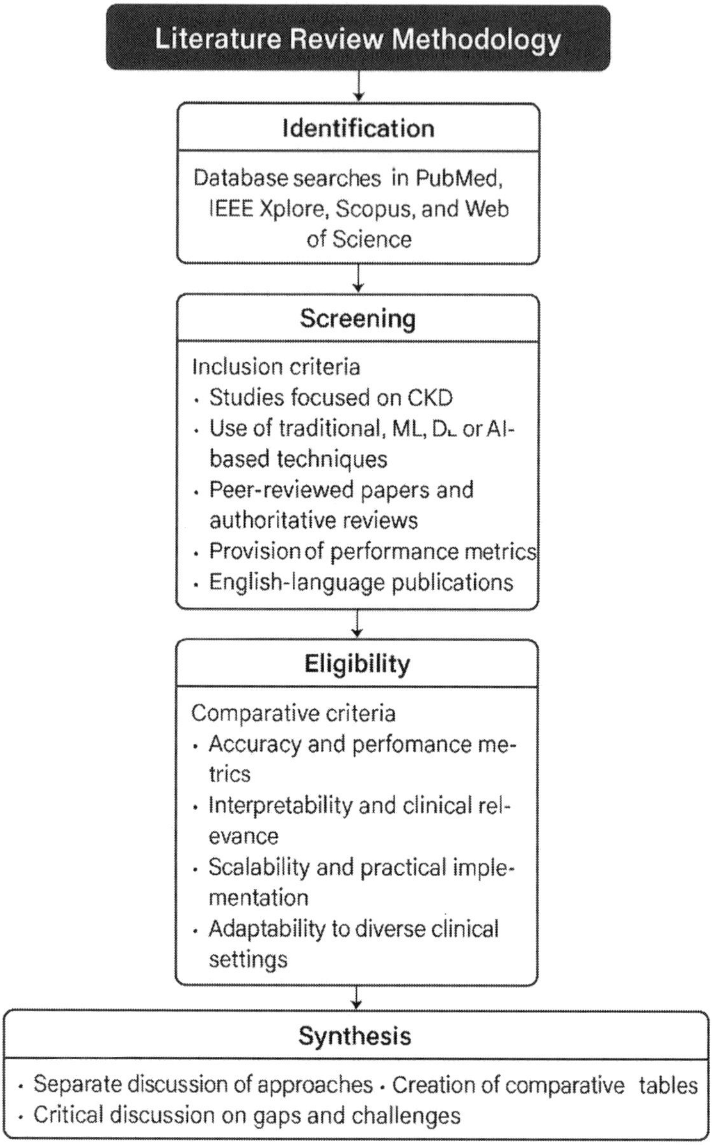

FIGURE 18.1 Literature review methodology for early detection and management of chronic kidney disease.

performance metrics, and application domains across different studies are summarized by comparative tables. Critical discussions were also included to encompass existing research gaps and challenges regarding clinical adoption and outline directions for future research in CKD early detection and management [16].

18.2.1 PRISMA Flow Diagram for Proposed Research Work

The above Preferred Reporting Items for Systematic Reviews and Meta-Analyses (PRISMA) flow diagram (Figure 18.2) illustrates the systematic process of selecting studies for the proposed research work.

For initial studies, 1,240 records were found by searching various accessible databases, including Google Scholar, PubMed, Scopus, IEEE Xplore, and the Web of Science. After eliminating 20 duplicate records, 1,040 records were further screened by title and abstract, and 790 irrelevant studies were excluded. Of these, 250 articles were read in full, and 170 articles were excluded for reasons such as irrelevance or incomplete data. Ultimately, 80 studies were included in the qualitative synthesis as the basis of the review and diagnostic analysis [17].

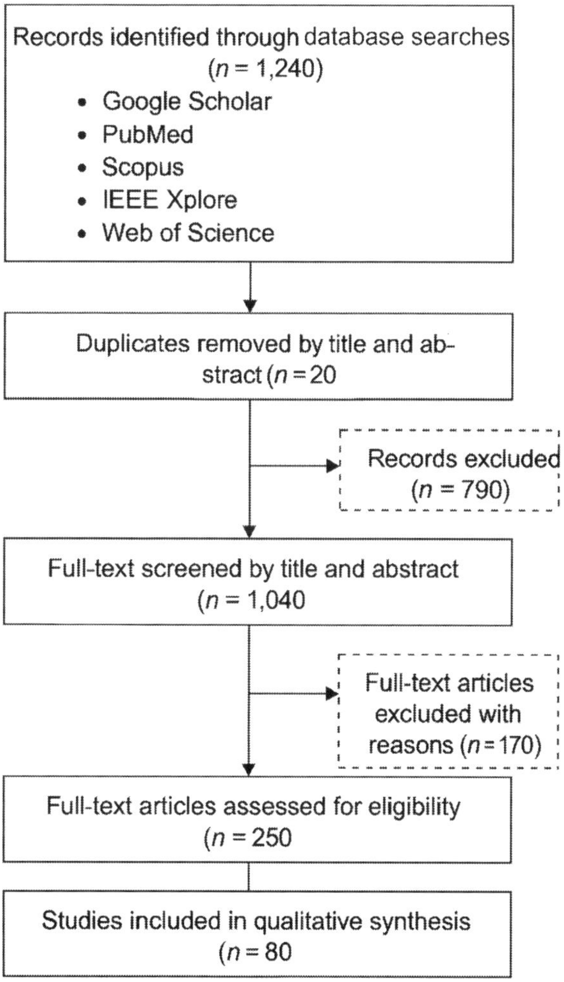

FIGURE 18.2 PRISMA flow diagram.

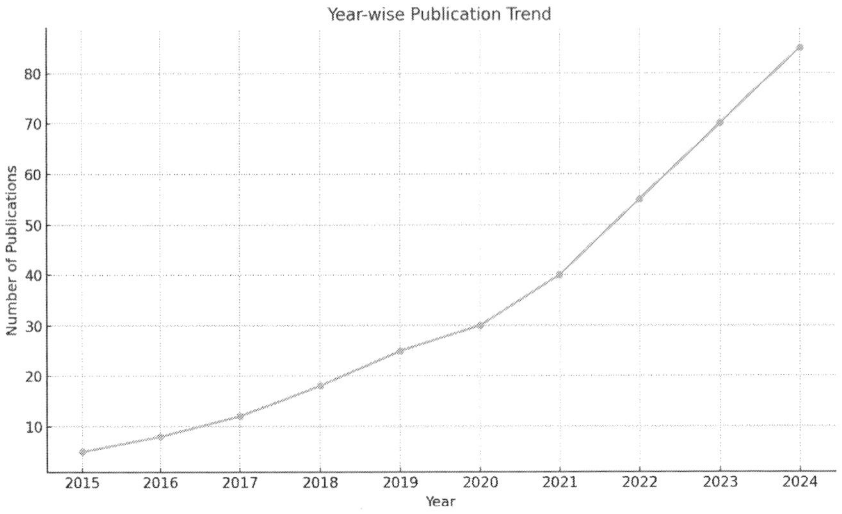

FIGURE 18.3 Year-wise publication.

18.2.2 Year-Wise Publication

Figure 18.3 depicts the year-wise trend in research publications concerning the study area of this proposed study from the year 2015 to the year 2024. Choosing to highlight advanced technologies during the "early detection and management of CKD," publication numbers steadily increased, indicating increased academic and clinical interest in this setup. It also has a significant increase in publications after 2020, which shows the rapid adoption of "ML, DL, and AI methods" in healthcare research. The trend of CKD represents the urgent need to develop better, technology-driven solutions for CKD prediction and prevention [18].

Several types of deep neural network architectures have been applied to CKD prediction tasks:

18.2.3 Year-Wise Publication

These underlying studies dispersed CKD types across various etiologies of a multifactorial nature. Most studies addressed general CKD progression throughout the disease (Stages 1–5), focusing on early detection to prevent ESRD progression. Of the several studies, diabetic nephropathy-related CKD was specifically targeted due to its high prevalence in diabetic patients [19]. A smaller part included cases of hypertensive nephropathy, glomerulonephritis', and hereditary forms (polycystic kidney disease). The distribution of focus shows that, generally [20], CKD prediction remains dominant. Still, the prediction related to specialized CKD types associated with comorbid conditions is gaining momentum to generate improved personalization of the diagnostic models (Figure 18.4).

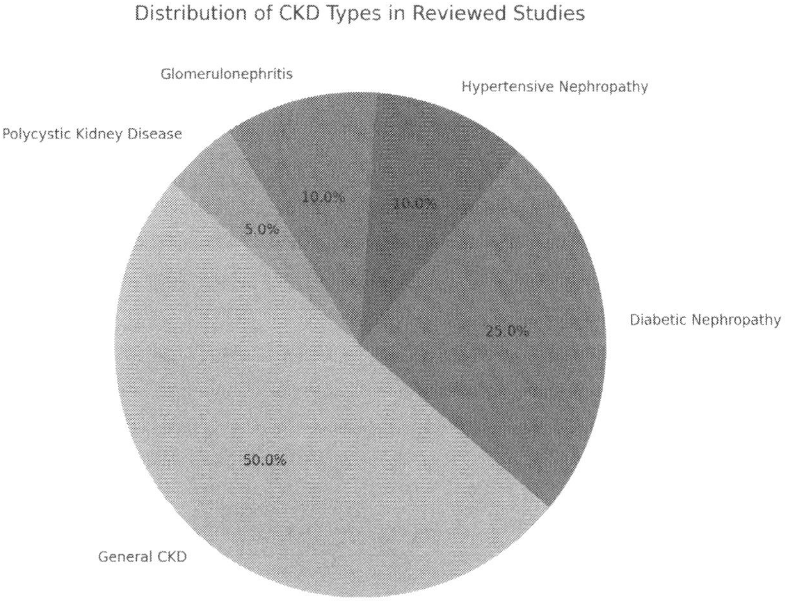

FIGURE 18.4 Distribution of Chronic Kidney Disease (CKD) in reviewed studies.

18.3 RELATED WORK

Recent research has proposed a number of DL and ML models for the diagnosis and prediction of critical illnesses. Physicians and researchers are particularly focused on early chronic illness identification, particularly on novel therapies for CKD. Recent research has shown that CKD may be reliably diagnosed using ML and DL models.

Kumar, S. *et al.* (2024). In recent years, it has been found that ML has even easily detected CKD in its early stages and is now shining the spotlight using non-invasive, cheap approaches. As more studies have increased, several algorithms like "K Neighbors Classifier, Gaussian Naive Bayes, and SVM" have been used. RF was the most recent and the best of all, having a diagnostic accuracy of 98.06%. The clinical methods employed in this study also use clinical attributes such as age, blood pressure, and albumin levels, which are precisely normalized and selected features to predict CKD. There is also an emphasis on a key shift to more dynamic and predictive healthcare models using ML and other techniques to complement medical practice and improve diagnostic accuracy and patient outcomes. Future research will consider the integration of Ensemble and DL approaches to enhance model robustness and applicability in the healthcare context.

Saif *et al.* (2016). We have studied whether multivariate models can be developed, primarily based on "Chronic Renal Failure (CRF), the data bank at University of California (UC) Irvine, to assess clinical risk in people with CKD. For example, they compared the performance of the different ML algorithms, for example, KNNs, SVM, Soft Independent Modeling of Class Analogy (SIMCA), and so on." Regarding these, the SVM notably won in accuracy handling noise in the dataset, receiving an accuracy of 99%. These results support SVM as a strong method for processing such complicated clinical data to increase the precision of CKD risk assessment practices.

Muthu, J. (2024). ML models growing in importance for early CKD detection were introduced in the paper. EHRs are analyzed using methodologies such as RFs and Logistic Regression with high accuracy and interpretable outcomes. We illustrate that ensemble models such as RF are robust, but simpler models provide clarity for clinical use. Future research will merge these models into EHR systems more effectively while considering the overall complexity versus user-friendliness to improve patient care outcomes.

Preethi *et al.* (2024). To improve the early detection of CKD, this study uses gender-specific ML models, RF, and Neural Networks (NNs). They use a comprehensive longitudinal cohort's sociodemographic, anthropometric, and laboratory test data. The NN model has the highest AUC score of 0.90 compared with the RF model and better sensitivity and specificity while using the stratified k-fold cross-validation techniques. The system's overall accuracy is high, but further improvement for specificity and examination of other algorithms is needed. Further refinements of these models are being made to be more readily integrated into the clinical setting for better prediction of early CKD and better decision-making in patient care.

Vetrithangam *et al.* (2024). We investigate how well a few "ML algorithms, Decision Trees, RFs, and Gradient Boosting classify patients with CKD who have been identified in the past as opposed to healthy individuals who are in the early stages of the illness." Our goal is to improve health outcomes by focusing on early detection. To provide this insight, Gradient Boosting was implemented to model a CKD dataset obtained from Kaggle containing patient medical conditions and clinical information. With an accuracy of 85.1%, it is a strong candidate for use in decision support systems for health care. Cross-validation and performance metrics were used to validate the models, with Gradient Boosting invariably outperforming the other algorithms. We will continue to build on our dataset to collect a more diverse set of medical records, and we will augment our predictive features with lifestyle and genetic data to further refine the accuracy of our analysis and to provide clinicians with better timing to intervene early with people comprising at risk for health complications.

Barik, S. *et al.* (2021). The study focuses on the performance of ML techniques for the early detection of CKD. Finally, it was also observed that the XGBClassifier achieved training accuracy similar to other models XGB, LGBM, and RF, with an accuracy of 95.78%. With this performance, the XGBClassifier can significantly improve diagnostic precision and the treatment of CKD. They ran the input patient data through the models to generate the output predictions or diagnoses of CKD that strengthened the clinical setting capacity for the management of CKD at a broader level. It has also suggested to improve future ML in healthcare outcome optimization.

Aljaaf *et al.* (2018). This paper aims to indicate how better advanced predictive AI models, such as Decision Trees or DL, are used better than the traditional diagnosis methods for early CKD detection. We demonstrate this ML models' capacity to work with large healthcare datasets and provide a more accurate, timely, and personalized CKD risk assessment. The study compares different AI techniques, including SVMs and Decision Trees, to increase diagnostic accuracy and report better patient outcomes. In other words, predictive technology is a game changer. It is also the path toward analogous technological development in bringing AI to optimize health interventions, modify treatments to the individual patient's needs, and revolutionize CKD management and prediction.

Despite late detection and progression of the disease, CKD remains a massive healthcare challenge. In particular, this review shows that with DL techniques such as CNNs, Recurrent Neural Network (RNNs), Transformers, and ensemble models, CKD prediction can be revolutionized through lab tests, EHR data, and medical images. Such models have high predictive accuracy and may be a basis for early intervention and disease management. However, some issues remain, such as a lack of interpretability of some data and problems integrating into clinical workflows. Toward the end, the field has been heading in that direction for multimodal modeling, XAI, federated learning, and real-world validations. An exciting promise for DL lies in leveraging this technology to provide proactive and personalized care for CKD and improve long-term outcomes.

18.4 PROPOSED WORK

This proposed work attempts to build an intelligent, accurate, and scalable system to conduct "early detection and management of CKD with the synergistic use of traditional diagnostics and state-of-the-art ML, DL, and AI techniques in place. Around 5,700 clinical, demographic, and lifestyle variables are collected, processed, and preprocessed through data cleaning, normalization, and feature selection. Then, various models are developed out of traditional statistical approaches like Logistic Regression and SVM, up to the modern ML algorithms such as RF and XGBoost, and DL architectures, including CNNs, LSTM networks, and BLSTM." They evaluate each model's performance through accuracy, sensitivity, specificity, and AUC metrics. An ensemble approach based on majority voting (for the best single models) or stacking is also implemented to ensure further improvement in predictive reliability. The final system is developed to be transparent, facilitate early prediction support, risk stratification, and clinical decision assistance and smoothly interface with EHR systems. Finally, this research aims to provide healthcare providers with timely and accurate knowledge on improving patient care outcomes and fostering enduring and sustainable healthcare practices (Figure 18.5).

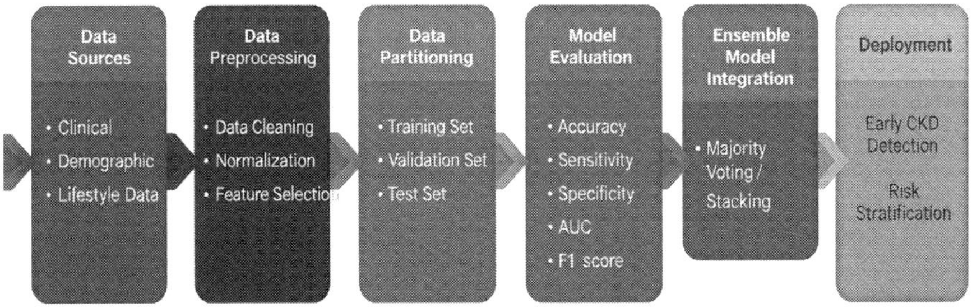

FIGURE 18.5 Proposed system.

Data Sources: The first step of the process is the acquisition of many different types of data, such as clinical data (e.g., lab results and symptoms), demographics (e.g., age and gender), and lifestyle factors (e.g., diet and physical activity). Therefore, these rich datasets are essential for building accurate and personalized CKD prediction models.

Data Preprocessing: The data is cleaned to remove all inconsistencies, normalized to safeguard that all other variables are scaled uniformly, and the feature selection process is used to choose the most relevant variables before modeling. Preparing optimized input data for learning algorithms improves the quality and performance of these algorithms in this step.

Data Partitioning: The data preprocessing then splits into the training, validation, and testing sets. This is a good division that can help train the model effectively by tuning its hyperparameters and objectively evaluating its predictive capabilities on unseen data.

Model Evaluation: By the end, when models are built, these models are evaluated using standard metrics such as "accuracy, sensitivity, specificity, AUC," or F1 score. By this assessment, we ensure the high precision of models and that the ones among them are balanced among various evaluation aspects.

Ensemble Model Integration: An ensemble strategy is applied to further improve the prediction reliability by combining predictions of multiple models via majority voting or stacking methods. This integration increases robustness, and the risk of bias or overfitting in the model is reduced.

Prediction and Decision Support: Finally, the final ensemble model can predict a certain level of early CKD risk and help clinicians make timely and informed decisions. It also involves stratifying patients based on the degree of CKD development severity.

18.5 CONCLUSIONS

In this chapter, the transition from the traditional method of diagnosing CKD to modern and highly advanced techniques such as AI-based approaches for early detection in managing CKD is explored in depth. The study outlined the limitations of standard techniques, which usually diagnose it only when a lot of damage has already occurred, pointing out its ever-increasing significance to incorporating ML, DL, and ensemble modeling in overcoming these challenges. An apparent necessity for scalable, accurate, and explainable predictive systems was through an extensive literature review, a critical evaluation of existing models, and identifying research gaps.

This chapter proposes a system architecture that strategically combines data preprocessing and partitioning, models developed for different factors, and models designed for both an ensemble and a clinical deployment to build an intelligent decision support tool. In addition, this framework enables improvements in early detection capabilities and the ability to be adaptable to different clinical environments. The system is designed to provide reliable, timely, and actionable insights to healthcare practitioners through multiple data types, including clinical, demographic, and lifestyle factors at an individual level and rigorous evaluation standards.

It's a revolutionary metamorphosis in the transition of the diagnosis and the management of CKD to incorporate the fusion of traditional methods with modern ideas of AI innovations. The proposed approach answers technical and clinical needs, meditating on more personalized, efficient, and sustainable healthcare solutions. Future work will include real-world validation, improving the model interpretability and deploying this system in clinical real-world scenarios to maximize its impact on patient care outcomes.

REFERENCES

1. Kumar, S., Hegde, R., & Mundada, M. R. (2024). Chapter 12: A novel ensembled deep machine learning framework for the prediction of chronic disease. In *Advances in Medical Technologies and Clinical Practice*. https://doi.org/10.4018/979-8-3693-7462-7.ch012
2. Saif, D., Sarhan, A. M., & El-Shennawy, N. M. (2024). Early prediction of chronic kidney disease based on an ensemble of deep learning models and optimizers. *Journal of Electrical Systems and Information Technology*. https://doi.org/10.1186/s43067-024-00142-4
3. Muthu, J. (2024). Deep learning techniques for chronic kidney disease risk prediction. *International Journal for Research in Applied Science and Engineering Technology*. https://doi.org/10.22214/ijraset.2024.61697
4. Preethi, I., Dharmarajan, K., Sharma, B., Chowdhury, S., Dhaou, I. B. (2024). A novel method to predict chronic kidney disease using an optimized deep learning algorithm. https://doi.org/10.1109/lt60077.2024.10468760
5. Vetrithangam, D., Himabindu, R., Saranya, S., Pegada, N.K., Fathima, A., Bekkanti, A., Kulkarni, A. (2024). Improved ResNet models for chronic kidney disease prediction. *Journal of Electrical Systems*. https://doi.org/10.52783/jes.1121
6. Barik, S., Mohanty, S., Mohanty, S., Singh, D. (2021). Analysis of prediction accuracy of diabetes using classifier and hybrid machine learning techniques. In Mishra, D., Buyya, R., Mohapatra, P., & Patnaik, S. (Eds.), *Intelligent and Cloud Computing* (pp. 399–409). Springer.
7. Aljaaf, A. J., Al-Jumeily, D., Haglan, H. M., Alloghani, M., Baker, T., Hussain, A.J., Mustafina, J. (2018). Early prediction of chronic kidney disease using machine learning supported by predictive analytics. In *Proceedings of the 2018 IEEE Congress on Evolutionary Computation (CEC)*, Rio de Janeiro, Brazil, 8–13 July 2018; pp. 1–9.
8. Bikku, T. (2020). Multi-layered deep learning perceptron approach for health risk prediction. *Journal of Big Data*, 7(1), 1–14.
9. Alam, M. Z., Rahman, M. S., Rahman, M. S. (2019). A random forest-based predictor for medical data classification using feature ranking. *Informatics in Medicine Unlocked*, 15, 100180.
10. Shankar, V., Kumar, V., Devagade, U., Karanth, V. and Rohitaksha, K. (2020). Heart disease prediction using CNN algorithm. *SN Computer Science*, 1(3), 1–8.
11. Mienye, I. D., Sun, Y., Wang, Z. (2020). An improved ensemble learning approach for the prediction of heart disease risk. *Informatics in Medicine Unlocked*, 20, 100402.
12. Almansour, N. A., Syed, H. F., Khayat, N. R., Altheeb, R. K., Juri, R. E., Alhiyafi, J., Alrashed, S., Olatunji, S.O. (2019). Neural network and support vector machine for the prediction of chronic kidney disease: A comparative study. *Computers in Biology and Medicine*, 109, 101–111.
13. Kriplani, H., Patel, B., Roy, S. (2019). Prediction of chronic kidney diseases using deep artificial neural network technique. In J. Sivaswamy, S. Patnaik, S. S. Rautaray, & S. Bakshi (Eds.), *Computer Aided Intervention and Diagnostics in Clinical and Medical Images* (pp. 179–187). Springer.

14. Jongbo, O. A., Adetunmbi, A. O., Ogunrinde, R. B., Badeji-Ajisafe, B. (2020). Development of an ensemble approach to chronic kidney disease diagnosis. *Scientific African*, 8, e00456.
15. Ekanayake, I. U., Herath, D. (2020). Chronic kidney disease prediction using machine learning methods. In *2020, the Moratuwa Engineering Research Conference (MERCon)*. Moratuwa, Sri Lanka: IEEE.
16. Gudeti, B., Mishra, S., Malik, S., Fernandez, T. F., Tyagi, A. K., Kumari, S. (2020). A novel approach to predict chronic kidney disease using machine learning algorithms. In *2020, the 4th International Conference on Electronics, Communication and Aerospace Technology (ICECA)*. Coimbatore, Tamil Nadu, India: IEEE.
17. Krishnamurthy, S., Ks, K., Dovgan, E., Luštrek, M., Gradišek Piletič, B., Srinivasan, K., Li, Y.C., Gradišek, A. and Syed-Abdul, S. (2021). Machine learning prediction models for chronic kidney disease using Taiwan's national health insurance claim data. In *Healthcare*. Multidisciplinary Digital Publishing Institute.
18. Sagi, O., Rokach, L. (2018). Ensemble learning: A survey. *Wiley Interdisciplinary Reviews: Data Mining and Knowledge Discovery*, 8(4), e1249.
19. Senan, E. M., Al-Adhaileh, M. H., Alsaade, F. W., Aldhyani, T. H., Alqarni, A. A., Alsharif, N., Uddin, M. I., Alahmadi, A. H., Jadhav, M. E., Alzahrani, M. Y. (2021). Diagnosis of chronic kidney disease using practical classification algorithms and recursive feature elimination techniques. *Journal of Healthcare Engineering*, 2021, 1–10.
20. Elhoseny, M., Shankar, K., & Uthayakumar, J. (2019). Intelligent diagnostic prediction and classification system for chronic kidney disease. *Scientific Reports*, 9(1), 1–14.

19 Deep Learning in Medical Imaging for Intracranial Hemorrhage Detection and Segmentation

Anuradha Yenkikar, Riddhi Mirajkar, Nitin Sakhare, Amar Buchade, and Prasad Chaudhari

19.1 INTRODUCTION

19.1.1 Machine Learning and Deep Learning in the Medical Domain

It can potentially make a big impact on medical diagnosis and patient care, and the study is set to grow more significant in the coming years. They also point out that there is still more study to be done on the creation and use of Artificial Intelligence (AI) technologies for medical diagnosis. The authors also go into great detail about how to use machine learning (ML) and deep learning (DL) to create medical imaging applications. They also bring out some of the problems in choosing one design option over the other and also the problems associated with each. It is illustrated in Table 19.1, and the challenges are shown in Figure 19.1.

Perhaps the most innovative technology radiology has seen since the advent of advanced imaging is DL applied to clinical imaging. The majority of experts agree that within the next ten years, DL-based applications will take over human control. Not only will these machines do the majority of the research, but they will also help with disease prediction, medication prescription, and treatment guidance. This chapter comprises a survey of literature on current method and an explanation of the dataset employed.

19.1.2 DL for Intracranial Hemorrhage Detection and Segmentation

An intracranial hemorrhage (ICH) is a serious medical injury that needs to be treated right away. If left untreated, it can develop into a secondary brain insult that could cause paralysis or even death. To determine ICH and locate where it is, advanced-trained radiologists now utilize computerized tomography (CT) scans, which employ computer technology and turn X-ray machines to produce the cross-sectional images of the body.

DOI: 10.1201/9781003479185-19

TABLE 19.1
Challenges in Machine Learning vs. Deep learning for Medical Imaging

Challenges	Machine Learning	Deep Learning
Sample size	• Careful testing of the resilience and reliability of radiomic features. • Efficient feature selection method. • Selecting an ML model	• Enhancement of data; transfer learning. • Regularization to increase the generalizability of the model.
Application domain for medical images	In order to prevent overfitting on the development set, extensive assessments of the radiomic feature robustness are conducted.	Use domain adaptation and transfer learning to gain from pretrained models or labeled instances from related domains.
Label and annotation reliability	• Segmentation and response characteristics-based data curation. • Several labels and morphological perturbations may be taken into consideration for feature robustness evaluations to enhance reliability.	• Multicentric and multireader research-based data management • Approximate supervision through image-level labels for inferring pixel or voxel level predictions. • Mix a few correctly labeled examples with instances that are wrongly or partially labeled (weak labeling).

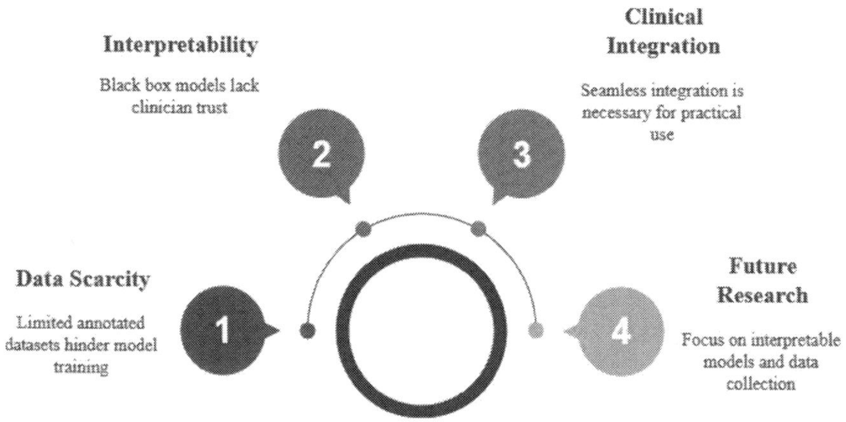

FIGURE 19.1 Challenges in deep learning for ICH detection.

DL can be applied to the CT images for ICH detection and segmentation more efficiently than most other algorithms. Various DL architectures and techniques for ICH detection are given in Figure 19.2. This research also aims to provide a proposed system as a cloud service. AI on the cloud makes the intelligent system accessible to all without requiring advanced skills and makes it easy to scale up as projects go

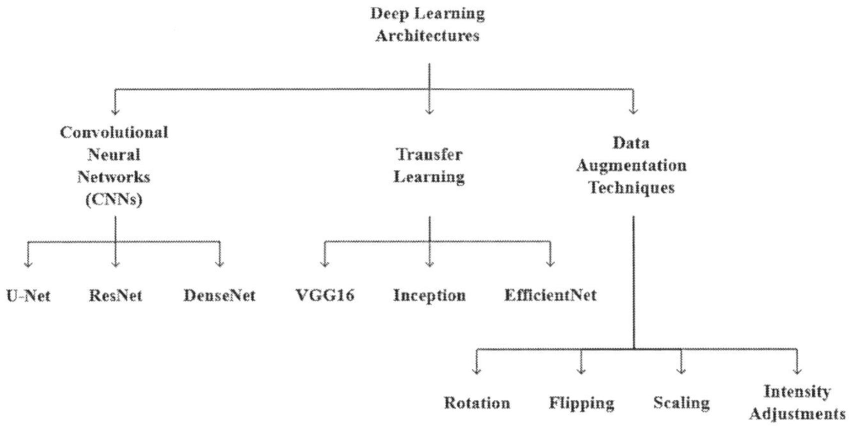

FIGURE 19.2 Deep learning architectures and techniques for ICH detection.

into production. This research also aims to provide proposed system as a cloud service. AI on the cloud makes the intelligent system accessible to all without requiring advanced skills and makes it easy to scale up as projects go into production.

As per a survey, ICH comprises about 10% of strokes in North America. It affects around 2.5 per 10,000 people each year. Intracerebral hemorrhage has a 30-day mortality rate of approximately 44% while that of Poutine or brainstem hemorrhage is 75% at 24 hours. This research can aid the doctors to easily detect or even segment the part of the brain where a hemorrhage has been detected. It can also be also used in remote areas where highly skilled radiologists and doctors are not readily available and can be used to quickly tag hemorrhage patients [1].

19.2 RELATED WORK

Writing a literature review serves two purposes: it gives credit to other researchers and prevents the duplication of effort by identifying areas of prior scholarship and providing background information on subjects. Through a literature review, we can also identify the gaps in research, the need for additional research on the topic, conflicts in previous works and open questions left in them.

While the vast majority of the new works proposed profound learning approaches and cross breed convolutional and repetitive models, there are still some new works dependents on customary AI strategies, for example superpixels, fuzzy-C-means, level set, histogram examination, thresholding, and continuous max-flow. The earliest studies used DL for ICH detection [2–5]. The authors discovered that diagnosing ICH can be effectively accomplished with convolutional neural networks (CNNs) that have been pretrained on ImageNet. Conventional approaches typically necessitate the preprocessing of the CT outputs in order to remove noise and the skull. They also need to focus on a few confused designed highlights and register the sectioned cerebrums. For the purpose of dividing the ICH regions, many of these techniques rely on unsupervised clustering. To fit dynamic forms on ICH locales, both strategies make use of the Distance Regularized Level Set Evolution (DRLSE) strategy [6]. After preprocessing the CT scans for noise filtering and skull removal, researchers modified the DRLSE for the segmentation 5 of 18 of the intraventricular (IVH) and intraparenchymal (IPH) locales [7].

The effect of arising processing strategies along with an expanding measurement of huge datasets and the accessibility of increasingly performing and open figuring resources are changing many research areas. These open opportunities to handle exceptional research challenges. In the recent decade, there has been an increase in the utilization of AI strategies in a large portion of the research areas, and as of late it has even improved with the more adoption of DL techniques. The current clinical convention to analyze ICH is looking at CT scans, which utilizes computer and rotating X-ray machines to make cross-sectional pictures of the body, by profoundly skilled radiologists to recognize ICH and confine its locales. In any case, this interaction depends intensely on the accessibility of a skilled radiologist [8,9].

This research revolves around a DL method to detect acute ICH and its subtypes and the main task we aim to achieve is to segment the site of hemorrhage. This research also aims to provide proposed system as a cloud service. AI on the cloud makes the intelligent system accessible to all without requiring advanced skills and makes it easy to scale up as projects go into production [10].

To generate relevant output images a large database of CT scan 3-D images is required. We are utilizing the dataset provided by the international society of radiologists called Radiological Society of North America (RSNA). We are experimenting with new models with some tweaks to suit proposed use case, the best taking inspiration from already available models. We are trying to develop a generic cloud pipeline to be reused in various DL research [11].

Current research is investigating the fusion of multimodal data, including CT, MRI, and clinical metadata (e.g., age, gender, symptoms), to enhance diagnostic performance. For example, models that utilize both imaging and patient history tend to perform better than models trained on imaging in isolation. Such hybrid models are especially beneficial for the subtype classification of hemorrhages such as IPH, IVH, subarachnoid (SAH), and epidural hematomas (EDH) [11].

Because of the availability of very limited labeled medical imaging data, researchers have been resorting to data augmentation methods like random cropping, flipping, rotation, and synthetic generation with generative adversarial networks (GANs). GANs have been utilized to generate realistic hemorrhage patterns that are employed to train more resilient models in varied imaging conditions [12].

In order to combat the lack of annotated data, semi-supervised and self-supervised learning methods are being explored. These methods enable models to be trained from the vast numbers of unlabeled samples, greatly diminishing the need for human annotations. The method of pretraining networks using contrastive learning on unlabeled CT scans and then fine-tuning with a small labeled set has been used [13].

Transfer learning has been particularly helpful in resource-limited settings. The pretrained models of public datasets such as RSNA or CQ500 are tuned on small local datasets, achieving acceptable performance even in low-data settings. This is particularly important for global health, particularly for areas that are not radiology expert-heavy [14].

Others process CT scan slices as sequence data with RNNs or transformers to observe dependencies between axial slices. These models perceive a CT scan as a temporal sequence, which facilitates the identification of faint hemorrhages distributed over numerous slices [15].

As AI in healthcare has grown, there's been a movement toward creating standardized benchmarks and metrics of evaluation. Beyond accuracy and dice coefficient, metrics such as clinical decision support impact, false positive reduction, and reader-assist evaluation studies are increasingly becoming important. These metrics evaluate how well AI models generalize in real-world clinical scenarios [16].

While numerous research models perform remarkably well in a controlled environment, deployment in real life poses problems such as model drift, scanner robustness across differences, and generalizability across populations. Regulatory agencies such as the FDA are beginning to release guidelines for AI/ML medical devices, emphasizing continuous learning systems and explainability [17].

Initiatives such as MONAI (medical open network for AI) and nnU-Net have greatly simplified research by providing standardized formats for training and testing DL models for medical imaging. These platforms provide preconfigured pipelines for operations such as segmentation, classification, and registration, and it is simpler to reproduce and compare outcomes [18].

19.3 PROPOSED SYSTEM ARCHITECTURE

For the detection task, FCNs (fully connected layers) and hybrid convolution and long short-term memory (LSTM) models are used and ResNeXt-101 used for featurization. Pretrained ResNeXt-101 helps to reduce training time and fine tune it to increase accuracy. Feature selection is used on these features, which are further passed to a bidirectional LSTM, which allows it to exhibit temporal dynamic behavior. Features from ResNeXt-101 and LSTM are passed through different classifiers, which is then concatenated and passed through a final classifier, which is then used for final predictions.

Using fuzzy-C clustering on the image, we will form different clusters, out of which one will be selected automatically. This image will be passed through a skull removal technique and using an entropy-based thresholding the important part of the brain will be highlighted which can finally be used for proposed detection and segmentation task. The skull removal technique that we talked about is basically localizing the skull by thresholding high intensity pixels of original CT scan, which will be multiplied by a matrix P (1 if inside, 0 if outside) to get the resultant image. For the segmentation task, we chose to use a hybrid structure based on dilated residual net, modified vgg16, dual FCN models, GoogleNet Network, and U-net. Since segmentation is a harder task to learn, we are not bounding ourselves with having lower parameters, and thus totally concentrating in having high MAPs (mean average precision).

Figure 19.3 represents flow diagram of proposed system, which consists of four stages. The first stage is the preprocessing stage where methods like skull removal and image windowing are applied. The second and the third stage represents DL models and techniques for ICH detection, classification, and segmentation. The final stage represents the cloud pipelines architecture for automated training.

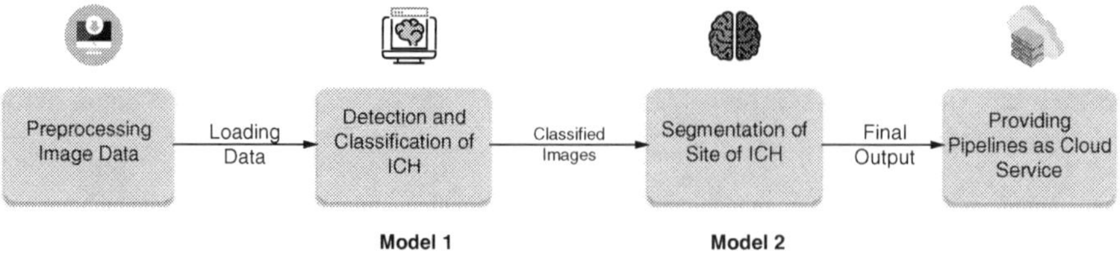

FIGURE 19.3 Flow diagram for proposed system.

19.3.1 Preprocessing

The most frequent deteriorations in medical images are noise and poor contrast. Preprocessing is intended to enhance an image's quality for prompt diagnosis, and noise reduction comes next. Generally speaking, DICOM images have 12–16 bits per pixel, or roughly 4,096–65,536 shades of gray. However, the majority of standard computer screens are frequently only capable of 256 shades of gray or 8 bits. So, Windowing will be used. Windowing, sometimes referred to as gray-level mapping or contrast enhancement, is the technique of manipulating an image's CT image grayscale component using the CT numbers. This alters the image's appearance to draw attention to specific structures.

19.3.2 Detection and Classification

In this step, all the images will be provided after preprocessing and the task of detecting the presence of ICH regions and classification of its type will be performed. It is a necessary step before any further analysis on the images and providing them for segmentation of the ICH region.

19.3.3 Segmentation

The precise segmentation of ICH and the calculation of total hemorrhage volume are a critical step in the characterization of hemorrhages. It may aid in identifying patients who are at high risk. In this step, all the classified images with ICH regions confirmed will be provided and the task of segmenting and localizing it in the image with color coding will be performed.

19.3.4 Cloud Pipelines

Cloud pipeline is a web-based cloud environment that gives the capacity to build and run modified scripts and workflows, modeling & simulation, and ML exercises that are needed for research. Developing the Machine Learning Operations (MLOps) stack for the task, requires a pipeline that takes into consideration a high level of customization and adaptability to develop as the experimentation directed. Considering the enormous stages that included numerous functions, yet concluded that it was restricted in some key regions. Eventually, we settled on a methodology where separate particular tools were executed for data versioning and continuous integration.

The setup is designed to deploy models faster. The goal is to standardize the types of activities that data scientists need to do in research and provide clear instructions for them.

In cases where a patient exhibits acute symptoms of neurological disorders, a team of highly skilled specialists examines cranial radiographs to determine whether there is a hemorrhage and where it is located. The procedure is difficult and frequently takes a long time. Developing an algorithm to identify acute ICH and its subtypes is the challenge outlined in this problem statement. A solution created with the help of an extensive image dataset from the RSNA. If we are successful, we will assist the medical community in determining the type, location, and the presence of hemorrhage so that patients can be treated efficiently and promptly.

An overview implementation on the web architecture is shown in Figure 19.4. The React framework used for frontend development. DL APIs, Django-Rest-Framework, containerized using docker, proxied, and load-balanced using nginx are used in implementation.

The classification and detection of model diagram is shown in Figure 19.5. It consists of three classifiers. The first one is the CNN classifier, which takes the preprocessed image. It contains windowed imaging in three channels and attempts to classify the image into predictions. The sequence model takes the penultimate layer of the CNN classifier as input and passing it through gated recurrent units (GRUs) and fully connected (FCs) to take into account spatial coherence and attempts to predict the classification. The outputs of both submodels concatenates meta features as well and pass that as input to the last stage, which uses GRU and skip connections to predict classification [19,20].

The classification model consists of FCNs and hybrid convolution and LSTM models. ResNeXt-101 has been used for featurization. The model consists of three submodels, which are CNN classifier, sequence model 1, and sequence model 2.

For segmentation, dual-GANs model is used and shown in Figure 19.6. For GAN structure, already pretrained classification model used as encoder, and subsequently create a decoder model. For discriminator of GAN_1, CNN classifier is used. For GAN_2, the penultimate layer of the decoder, the unit of GAN_1, and concatenate that with meta features used. It passes them as sequential layers as an

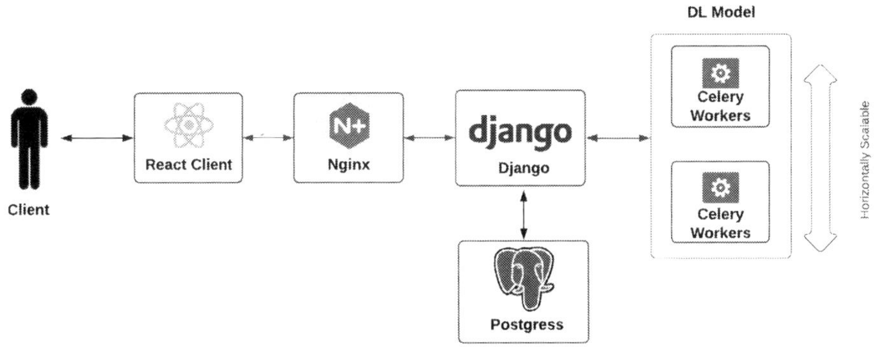

FIGURE 19.4 Web architecture diagram.

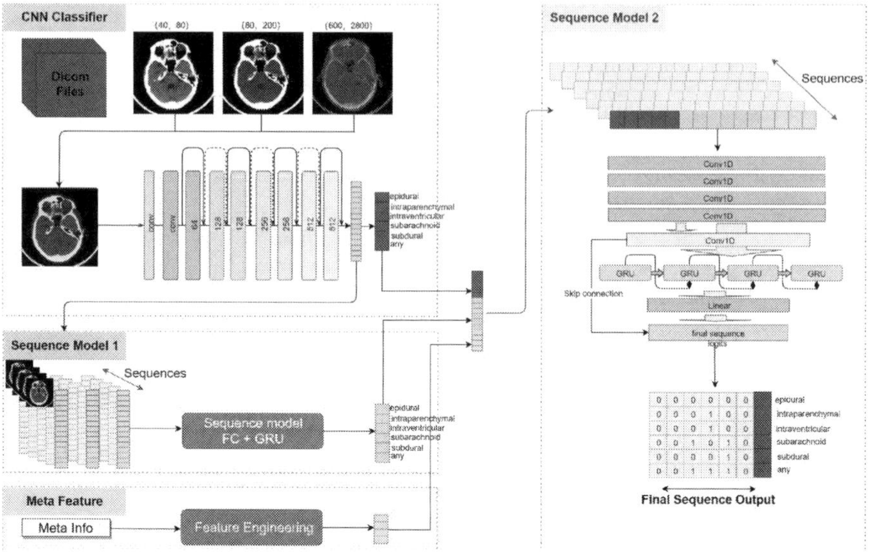

FIGURE 19.5 Classification and detection model using CNN classifier.

input. Separate attention models are used to create a set of synthetic images over these inputs and after using fuzzy means, few images selected and passed through the discriminator of GAN_2, which consist of the Resnet classifier.

A fully managed continuous delivery solution called CodePipeline assists in automating release pipelines for quick infrastructure updates. It is shown in Figure 19.7.

19.4 METHODOLOGY

As mentioned in the architecture, four major algorithms were used in the DL model are given below.

19.4.1 Convolutional Neural Network

CNN successfully captures any temporal and spatial dependencies, converting it to a much simpler-to-process form without sacrificing any functionality. It consists of a kernel, which sweeps across the image pixels and uses a single value to represent multiple adjacent pixels. It's computationally less expensive [21].

19.4.2 Gated Recurrent Unit

GRU makes use of an update gate and a reset gate to address the disappearing gradient problem that a standard RNN has. These are essentially the two vectors that determine which data moves on to the next phase. They can be ready to retain historical data without erasing or distorting it over time, or to remove data that is unimportant to the forecast.

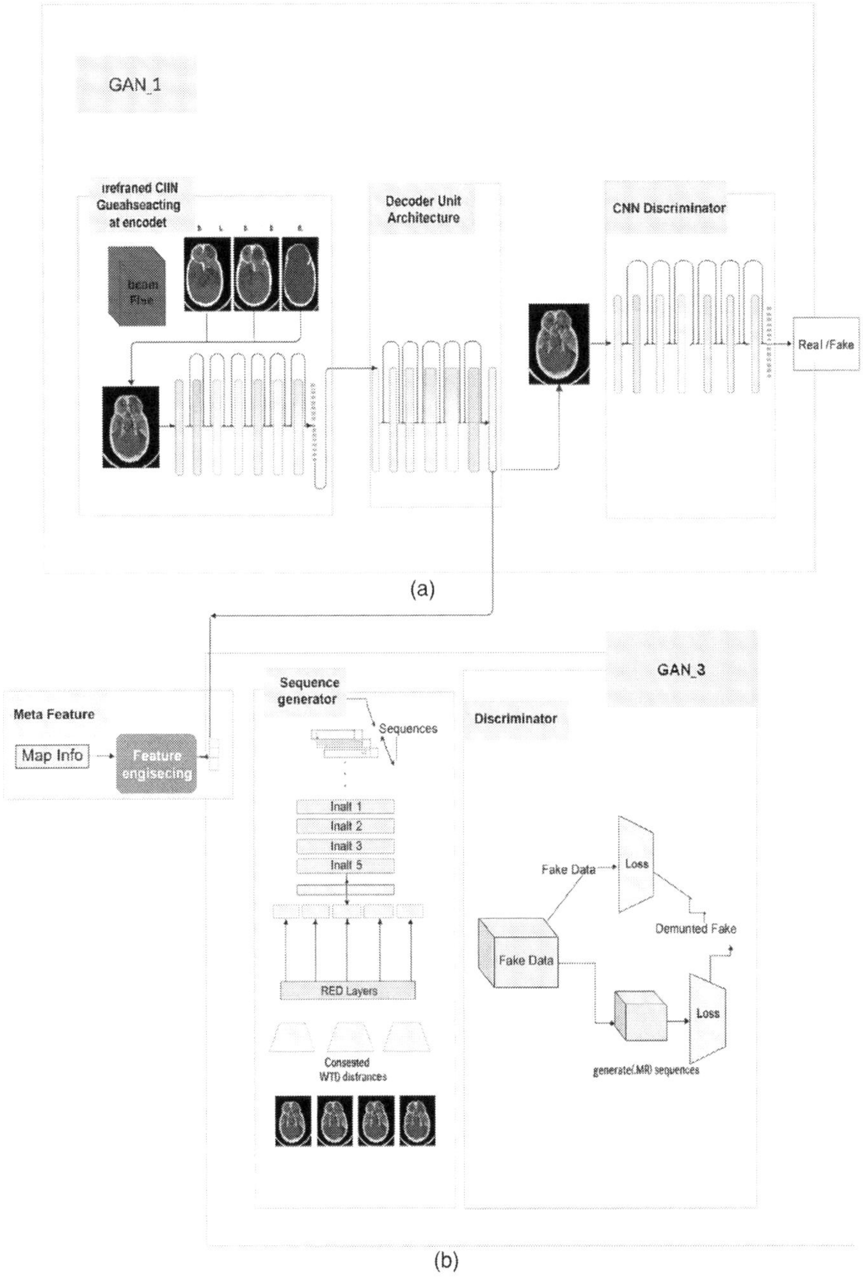

FIGURE 19.6 Segmentation model diagram.

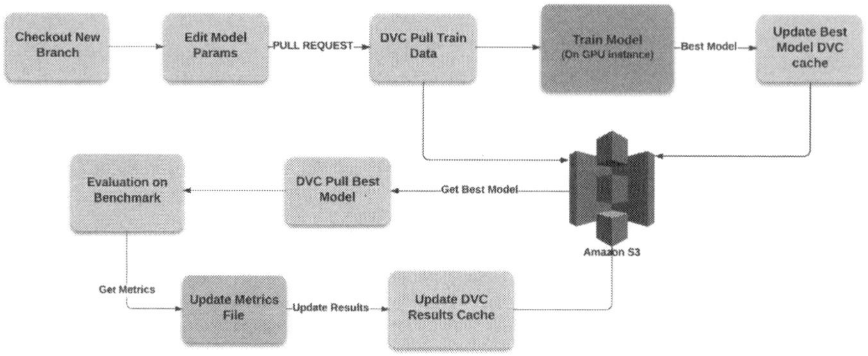

FIGURE 19.7 Cloud pipelines.

19.4.3 U-Net

U-net architecture is a type of encoder decoder architecture with tiles concatenation such that deeper layers do not forget the information learned by earlier layers. Adding skip connections reintroduces good spatial information. The spatial dimensions are reduced by half while doubling the number of feature channels at each downsampling step. Upsampling the feature map and then performing a 2×2 transpose convolution, which reduces the number of feature channels, are the two steps in the expansive path.

19.4.4 Resnet

The network is made up of a max pooling operation after the first 7×7 convolutional layer. Next, 16 3×3 convolutions and ReLU nonlinearity make up the network. Rather than using pooling layers, strided convolutions perform downsampling. There are 1.8 giga floating point operations per second (GFLOPs) (multiply-adds) in the network.

19.5 FLOW OF IMPLEMENTATION

There are four stages for the implementation of the system. We set in motion the implementation by preparing the data, which was taken from multiple sources. The next step was to preprocess the data so that a homogenous dataset was fed to the model. Implementation of the DL models was the next stage, following the development of a UI and cloud pipelines for the system.

19.5.1 Preparation of Data

One label for each of the five subtypes of hemorrhage and an additional label for any, which should always be true if any of the subtype labels are true, make up the training data. Additionally, a target column called label shows the likelihood that the specified type of hemorrhage is present in the given image.

There are six rows per image Id. The label indicated by a particular row will look like [Image Id]_[Subtype Name], as follows:

- Id, Label
- 1_epidural_hemorrhage,0
- 1_intraparenchymal_hemorrhage,0
- 1_intraventricular_hemorrhage,0
- 1_subarachnoid_hemorrhage,0.6
- 1_subdural_hemorrhage,0
- 1_any,0.9

19.5.2 Preprocessing

Preprocessing is intended to enhance an image's quality for prompt diagnosis, and noise reduction comes next. Generally speaking, DICOM images have 12–16 bits per pixel, or roughly 4,096–65,536 shades of gray. However, the majority of standard computer screens are frequently only capable of 256 shades of gray or 8 bits. Thus, windowing will be used. windowing, sometimes referred to as gray-level mapping or contrast enhancement, is the technique of manipulating an image's grayscale component using the CT numbers to highlight specific structures in the image.

19.5.3 Web Architecture and Cloud Pipeline

The web architecture describes the user flow through the proposed system so as to increase the user experience. Here, React for a frontend framework is used. To easily and sustainably provide DL APIs, they are being served using Django-Rest-Framework, containerized using docker, and are being proxied and load-balanced using nginx.

19.6 RESULTS AND DISCUSSION

This chapter summarizes the results of the experiments and tests carried out in the entire development process of the system, covering all the critical tests that were carried out along with white-box and black-box testing. It also demonstrates how the system works as intended.

19.6.1 Datasets

The dataset made available by RSNA assembled a cadre of more than 60 volunteers to label over 25,000 exams for the challenge dataset available on kaggle.com. A dataset of 82 CT scans of brain-damaged patients was collected by Physionet. Two radiologists depicted the intracranial brain regions in each of these outputs. The radiologists also made comments on each CT scan regarding the presence of different types of intracranial fractures and hemorrhages. A dataset containing the NIfTI format CT scans of 75 subjects [22].

19.6.2 Results of Experiments

This section deals with all the experiments carried out after the implementation of the models. These experiments were required to understand the efficiency and the output metrics of the system. Continuous experimentation on the model helps to tweak the model parameters in a way to improve the accuracy metrics. After extensive exploratory data analysis and data preprocessing, classification using ML are shown.

We tested three different models, and their accuracies are given below.

1. The accuracy of logistic regression is 88%
2. The accuracy of decision tree classifiers is 81%
3. The accuracy of K-NN classifier is 85%.

Dice coefficient used on three windows. The proposed model achieves a dice coefficient of 0.789, outperforming the previous score of 0.729 reported in [23] on Brain Window. Even while testing on Hausdorff, we get 15.90 ± 67.86 mm, which is significantly better than 36 mm of [23]. These results shown in Tables 19.2 and 19.3 that proposed model performs better than the previous methods when brain window preprocessing is used.

A sample UI output showing the type of hemorrhage and segmented area of hemmorhage when a user uploads his CT scans shown in Figure 19.8.

19.7 CONCLUSION

In conclusion, the integration of DL techniques into the realm of medical imaging for ICH detection and segmentation represents a transformative leap toward more accurate and efficient diagnostic processes. The extensive exploration conducted in this chapter underscores the significant strides made in leveraging DL algorithms to enhance the precision and speed of identifying and delineating ICH in medical images. ICH is a serious medical lesion that needs to be treated right away. If left untreated, it can worsen and become a secondary brain insult, which can cause paralysis or even death. In this chapter, we propose a methodology for brain hemorrhage detection, classification, and segmentation using AI and making it easily accessible to everyone using AI on the cloud. It makes intelligent systems accessible to all without requiring advanced skills and makes it easy to scale up as projects go into production. In future 3D sculpture of the brain using slices of CT scans can be considered to get better visualization for users.

TABLE 19.2
Segmentation Results Compared with Existing Systems without Brain Window Preprocessing

	Dice			Hausdorff (mm)		
	Brain Window	Subdural Window	Soft Tissue	Brain Window	Subdural Window	Soft Tissue
Proposed method	0.789 ± 0.222	0.874 ± 0.132	0.755 ± 0.270	15.90 ± 67.86	6.55 ± 10.69	27.05 ± 84.43
Kamnitsas et al. [23]	0.729	0.886	0.785	36.0	5.01	23.1
Isensee et al. [18]	0.647 ± 0.326	0.858 ± 0.161	0.775 ± 0.269	–	–	–

TABLE 19.3
Segmentation Results Compared with Existing Systems When Brain Window Preprocessing Is Used

	Dice			Hausdorff (mm)		
	Brain Window	Subdural Window	Soft Tissue	Brain Window	Subdural Window	Soft Tissue
Isotropic 3D networks [18]	0.772 ± 0.268	0.885 ± 0.105	0.805 ± 0.196	3.78 ± 5.32	6.73 ± 9.19	7.75 ± 9.98
Anisotropic 2.5D networks [19]	0.741 ± 0.264	0.890 ± 0.076	0.826 ± 0.157	5.32 ± 7.20	12.46 ± 21.47	9.66 ± 1421
Proposed method	0.786 ± 0.233	0.905 ± 0.66	0.838 ± 0.158	3.28 ± 3.88	3.89 ± 2.79	6.48 ± 826
Kamnitsas *et al.* [23]	0.738	0.901	0.797	450	4.23	6.56
Isensee *et al.* [18]	0.732	0.896	0.797	4.55	6.97	9.48

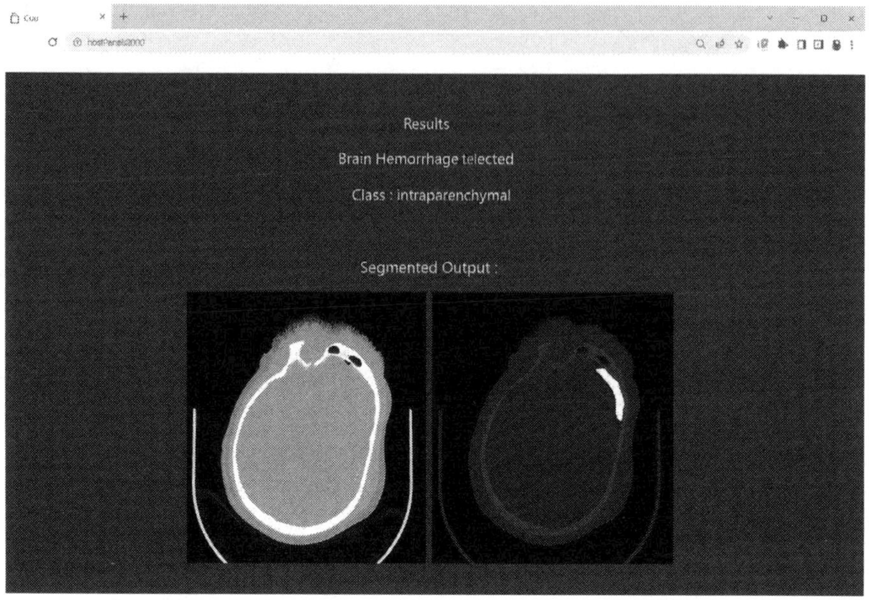

FIGURE 19.8 A sample output showing the type and segmented area of hemorrhage.

REFERENCES

1. Unnithan, A. K. A., & Mehta, P. (2023, May 8). *Hemorrhagic Stroke*. National Library of Medicine; StatPearls Publishing. https://www.ncbi.nlm.nih.gov/books/NBK559173/
2. Lee, J. Y., Kim, J. S., Kim, T. Y., & Kim, Y. S. (2020). Detection and classification of intracranial haemorrhage on CT images using a novel deep-learning algorithm. *Scientific Reports*, 10(1). https://doi.org/10.1038/s41598-020-77441-z
3. Chilamkurthy, S., Ghosh, R., Tanamala, S., Biviji, M., Campeau, N. G., Venugopal, V. K., Mahajan, V., Rao, P., & Warier, P. (2018). Deep learning algorithms for detection of critical findings in head CT scans: a retrospective study. *The Lancet*, 392(10162), 2388–2396. https://doi.org/10.1016/S0140-6736(18)31645-3
4. Phong, T. D., Duong, H. N., Nguyen, H. T., Trong, N. T., Nguyen, V. H., Van Hoa, T., & Snasel, V. (2017). Brain Hemorrhage Diagnosis by Using Deep Learning. *Proceedings of the 2017 International Conference on Machine Learning and Soft Computing – ICMLSC '17*. https://doi.org/10.1145/3036290.3036326
5. Barros, R. S., van der Steen, W. E., Boers, A. M. M., Zijlstra, I., van den Berg, R., El Youssoufi, W., Urwald, A., Verbaan, D., Vandertop, P., Majoie, C., Olabarriaga, S. D., & Marquering, H. A. (2020). Automated segmentation of subarachnoid hemorrhages with convolutional neural networks. *Informatics in Medicine Unlocked*, 19, 100321. https://doi.org/10.1016/j.imu.2020.100321
6. Li, C., Xu, C., Gui, C., & Fox, M. D. (2010). Distance regularized level set evolution and its application to image segmentation. *IEEE Transactions on Image Processing*, 19(12), 3243–3254. https://doi.org/10.1109/tip.2010.2069690

7. Sun, M., Hu, R., Yu, H., Zhao, B., & Ren, H. (2015). Intracranial hemorrhage detection by 3D voxel segmentation on brain CT images. https://doi.org/10.1109/wcsp.2015.7341238
8. Sage, A., & Badura, P. (2020). Intracranial hemorrhage detection in head CT using double-branch convolutional neural network, support vector machine, and random forest. *Applied Sciences*, 10(21), 7577. https://doi.org/10.3390/app10217577
9. Patel, S. C. (2001). Lack of clinical significance of early ischemic changes on computed tomography in acute stroke. *JAMA*, 286(22), 2830. https://doi.org/10.1001/jama.286.22.2830
10. Patil, S. D. D., Satpute, O. D., Mehta, P. S., & Mahajan, R. A. (2023, May). Enhancing Digital Healthcare with IoMT and Big Data: A Computational Intelligence Approach. In *International Conference on Data Analytics and Insights* (pp. 209–219). Singapore: Springer Nature Singapore.
11. Chilamkurthy, S., Ghosh, R., Tanamala, S., Biviji, M., Campeau, N. G., Venugopal, V. K., Mahajan, V., Rao, P., & Warier, P. (2018). Deep learning algorithms for detection of critical findings in head CT scans: A retrospective study. *Lancet*, 392(10162), 2388–2396.
12. Frid-Adar, M., Diamant, I., Klang, E., Amitai, M., Goldberger, J., & Greenspan, H. (2018). GAN-based synthetic medical image augmentation for increased CNN performance in liver lesion classification. *Neurocomputing*, 321, 321–331.
13. Lin, E., & Yuh, E. L. (2024). Semi-supervised learning for generalizable intracranial hemorrhage detection and segmentation. *Radiology: Artificial Intelligence*, 6(3). https://doi.org/10.1148/ryai.230077.
14. Rajpurkar, P., Irvin, J., Zhu, K., Yang, B., Mehta, H., Duan, T., Ding, D., Bagul, A., Langlotz, C., Shpanskaya, K., & Lungren, M. P. (2017). CheXNet: Radiologist-level pneumonia detection on chest X-rays with deep learning. arXiv preprint arXiv:1711.05225.
15. Snekhalatha, U., Murugappan, M., Deepa Bharathi, & Thakur, M. (2023). Automated computer-aided detection and classification of intracranial hemorrhage using ensemble deep learning techniques. *Diagnostics*, 13(18), 2987–2987. https://doi.org/10.3390/diagnostics13182987.
16. McKinney, S. M., Sieniek, M., Godbole, V., Godwin, J., Antropova, N., Ashrafian, H., Back, T., Chesus, M., Corrado, G. S., Darzi, A., Etemadi, M. (2020). International evaluation of an AI system for breast cancer screening. *Nature*, 577, 89–94.
17. U.S. FDA. (2019). Proposed Regulatory Framework for Modifications to Artificial Intelligence/Machine Learning-Based Software as a Medical Device. [Online]. Available: https://www.fda.gov
18. Isensee, F., Petersen, J., Klein, A., Zimmerer, D., Jaeger, P. F., Kohl, S., Wasserthal, J., Koehler, G., Norajitra, T., Wirkert, S., & Maier-Hein, K. H. (2018). nnU-Net: Self-adapting framework for U-Net-based medical image segmentation. *Nature Methods*, 18, 203–211. https://arxiv.org/abs/1809.10486.
19. Ahirwar, A. (2013). Study of techniques used for medical image segmentation and computation of statistical test for region classification of brain MRI. *International Journal of Information Technology and Computer Science*, 5(5), 44–53. https://doi.org/10.5815/ijitcs.2013.05.06
20. Gu, Z., Cheng, J., Fu, H., Zhou, K., Hao, H., Zhao, Y., Zhang, T., Gao, S., & Liu, J. (2019). CE-Net: Context encoder network for 2D medical image segmentation. *IEEE Transactions on Medical Imaging*, 38(10), 2281–2292. https://doi.org/10.1109/tmi.2019.2903562
21. Yenkikar, A. V., & Babu, C. N. (2023). SentiMLBench: Benchmark evaluation of machine learning algorithms for sentiment analysis. *Indonesian Journal of Electrical Engineering and Informatics (IJEEI)*, 11(1). https://doi.org/10.52549/ijeei.v11i1.4381

22. Yenkikar, A., Babu, C. N., & Hemanth, D. J. (2022). Semantic relational machine learning model for sentiment analysis using cascade feature selection and heterogeneous classifier ensemble. *PeerJ Computer Science*, 8, e1100. https://doi.org/10.7717/peerj-cs.1100
23. Kamnitsas, K., Chen, L., Ledig, C., Rueckert, D., & Glocker, B. (2016). Multi-scale 3D convolutional neural networks for lesion segmentation in brain MRI. *2016 IEEE 13th International Symposium on Biomedical Imaging (ISBI)*. 1050–1053. IEEE. https://doi.org/10.1109/ISBI.2016.7493418

20 Enhancing Healthcare Resource Allocation
An Insight for Research

Snehal Rathi, Ruthik Jadhav, Shivam Tikone, Mayur Bahiram, and Amit Gavit

20.1 INTRODUCTION

Overseeing resistance to development and creating viable asset assignment plans are basic in the healthcare assiduity. The investigation digs into the challenges the healthcare division faces, squeezing the need to surmount deterrents and optimizing asset assignment to accomplish way better results. Healthcare programs are in line with the operation of limited coffers when they employ innovative approaches like requirements-grounded resource allocation. An abstract frame recognizes how inventions in healthcare have the eventuality to transfigure the field by perfecting resource application and furnishing treatments for conditions that were formerly allowed to be incorrigible.

Healthcare resource allocation (HRA) from a global perspective involves the distribution of limited healthcare coffers among populations, programs, and individuality, while considering profitable effectiveness, justice, equity, and optimization of coffers [1,2]. It encompasses colourful approaches, including those grounded on meeting the requirements of the population, profitable effectiveness, age-grounded rationing, and resolving resource allocation controversies through debate and logrolling [3]. The COVID-19 epidemic has stressed the need for transparent, indifferent, and harmonious allocation mechanisms sustained by distributive justice within public health [4].

From a global perspective, understanding how HRA impacts or relates to people worldwide is pivotal, especially in the increasing demand for healthcare and public health goods and services worldwide [2]. The allocation of healthcare coffers is a public moral challenge, particularly in resource-poor countries. It involves the distribution of available coffers to different health programs, regions, specific complaint control programs, cases, structures, installations, outfits, and treatments [5].

20.1.1 Crucial Points to Consider in Healthcare Resource Allocation

- **Ethical Architectures**: Numerous ethical fabrics have been produced for resource allocation, some of which have been included in epidemic plans [6]. Still, it's essential to acclimatize these fabrics to the specific environment and stage of the epidemic [5].

DOI: 10.1201/9781003479185-20

- **Contending Health Policy Pretensions**: Numerous resource allocation opinions involve contending health policy pretensions [7]. In analogous cases, it's vital to prioritize programs and practices that are immorally justified.
- Translucence and stakeholder involvement: Transparent, indifferent, and harmonious allocation mechanisms should involve all stakeholders, from clinicians through cases and public health professionals [8].
- Fetched-adequacy: Constrained assets for well-being ought to be apportioned to maximize the well-being benefits for the populace served [4]. A fetched-adequacy investigation measures the partitioned costs and benefits of vital well-being mediations to decide their relative viability in well-being.
- The geological territory has a coordinated impact on asset allotment [9]. Subsequently, it's basic to consider the particular conditions and circumstances of distinctive districts when apportioning healthcare assets.
- Well-being status and asset assignment [10]: There is a critical relationship between the number of healing centres and nonattendance from work due to destitute well-being in creating nations [11]. This highlights the centrality of considering well-being status when designating healthcare assets.

Healthcare asset assignment is a complex and challenging issue that requires a comprehensive and terrain-specific approach. By considering the points below and adhering to the principles of translucence, equity, and consistency, HRA can better serve the conditions of populations worldwide.

20.2 LITERATURE SURVEY

20.2.1 Worked Done Before

HRA is a complex and critical content that involves relating and managing coffers in the healthcare sector, including finances, medical outfits, health insurance, and health-related programs. Effective and indifferent resource allocation is essential for ensuring that everyone's healthcare requirements are addressed with as many coffers as possible, taking accurate estimates of the actual costs of coffers to achieve health pretensions at minimum costs [12].

Expedient allotment in healthcare has subsisted in the content of arguments and breakdowns for decades, based on the personality and story of staff resources. Quietly, the piece of the medical claim in expedient allotment has been altogether overpassed. As doorkeepers to healthcare coffers, physicians play a central part in the allocation process. Different interpretations of the nature of drug accreditation, different allocation styles, and a comprehensive result that acknowledges the part of healthcare professionals are necessary to address the allocation problem effectively [13]. Effectiveness in HRA entails achieving lesser value, bettered health status, and increased satisfaction for a given expenditure. Benchmarking to other communities that meet population health needs with smaller coffers provides a rational defence for resource redistribution [14].

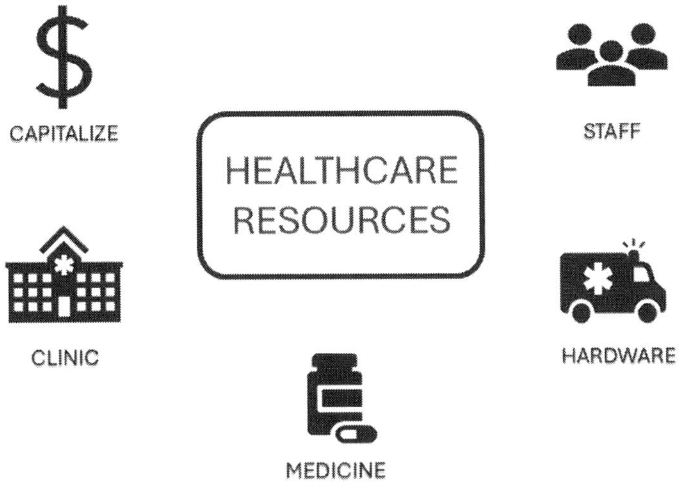

FIGURE 20.1 Healthcare resources.

During afflictions similar to COVID-19, resource allocation in healthcare becomes more critical, as limited coffers and adding demand disguise serious challenges. Ethical issues revolve around allocating these coffers, and changing the stylish result for participating coffers during afflictions remains a significant concern [13].

Overall, resource allocation in healthcare is a serious matter that requires further exploration and attention. When coffers are limited, and demand begins to overweigh the force, allocation becomes a serious problem, and ethical issues arise. A comprehensive result that acknowledges the part of healthcare professionals is necessary to address the allocation problem effectively [12,13]. The various healthcare resources are shown in Figure 20.1.

20.2.2 Common Decision Criteria for HRA

The standard decision criteria for HRA include equity/fairness, efficacy/effectiveness, stakeholder interests and pressures, cost-effectiveness, the strength of evidence, safety, mission and mandate of the health system, organizational requirements and capacity, patient-reported outcomes, and need [15,16]. These criteria are frequently used in real-world priority-setting exercises. They are essential for the fair allocation of resources and optimized decision-making for coverage and use of healthcare interventions [15,17]. Also, moral issues such as regard and openness are commonly recognized as fundamental criteria in healthcare asset assignment choices [15,18]. The consolation of healthcare advancements increases the inquiry for healthcare organizations, making insufficiency unmistakable, and decision-makers must consider these criteria when distributing assets [18]. The health care resources equality is shown in Figure 20.2.

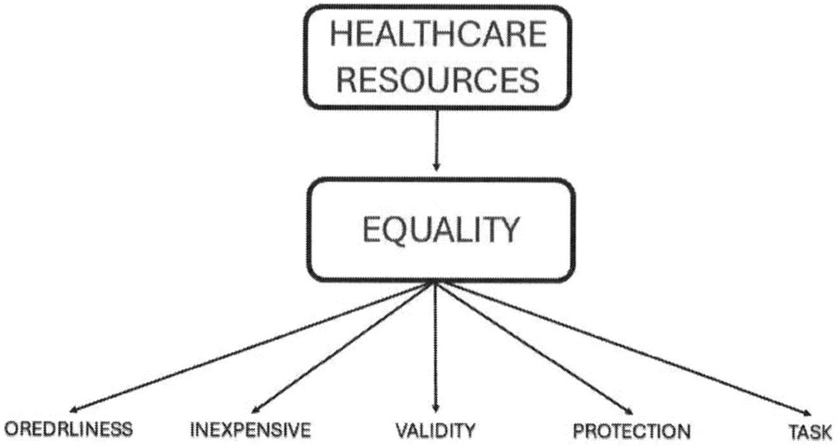

FIGURE 20.2 Healthcare resources equality.

20.2.3 Balancing Individual Rights and the Common Good in Resource Allocation

Healthcare policymakers balance individual rights and the common good in resource allocation by considering colourful criteria and principles. The American Restorative Association's Act of Restorative Ethics emphasizes that commission schedules should exist based on measures clicking to useful bear, criticalness of bear, threat and expected hitch of better, and change in quality of life [19]. Choice makers consider a bounty of factors and apply many continuously limiting choice criteria, with tolerability and practicality being the most unmistakable bones [18]. Also, the fair allocation of scarce medical coffers requires that tests are allocated according to immorally reflected criteria, including need-grounded allocation, benefit maximization, equity, and creation and price of social utility [20]. The faireness symbol is shown in Figure 20.3. Eventually, decision-makers must strive to develop fair allocation programs that guard the wealth of cases, giving first precedence to those cases for whom treatment will avoid unseasonable death or inferior issues and cases that'll witness the topmost change in quality of life [19]. Transparent mechanisms and clear communication of allocation programs to cases and the public are also essential in balancing individual rights and the common good in resource allocation [19].

20.2.4 Consequences of Prioritizing Individual Rights over the Common Good in HRA

Prioritizing individual rights over the common good in HRA can lead to several implicit consequences. One consequence is the threat of differentiating against less socially precious cases, as opinions grounded solely on social productivity could lead to unjust practices [21]. Also, prioritizing interventions that profit those who can be helped more fluently or cheaply may affect, in some cases, losing out simply because their requirements are more delicate or precious to meet [21]. This could lead to

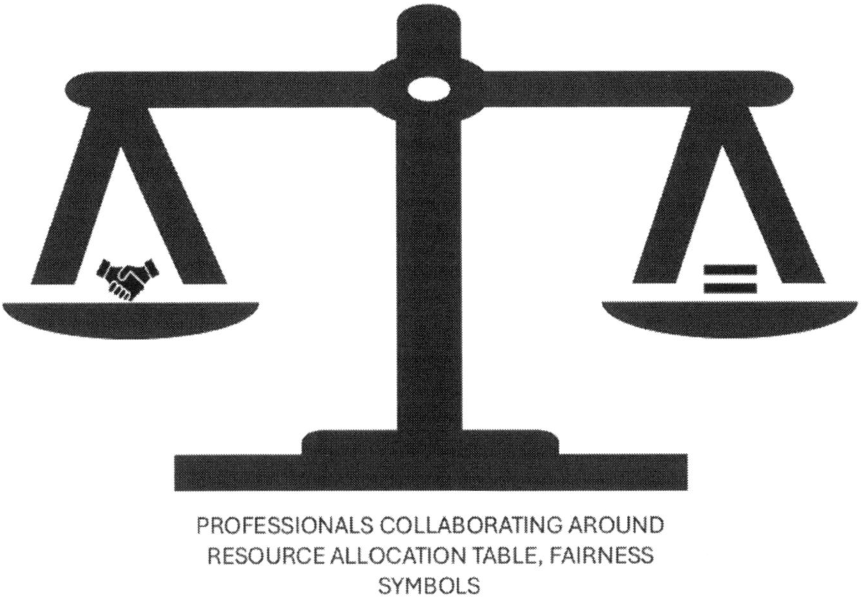

FIGURE 20.3 Fairness symbols.

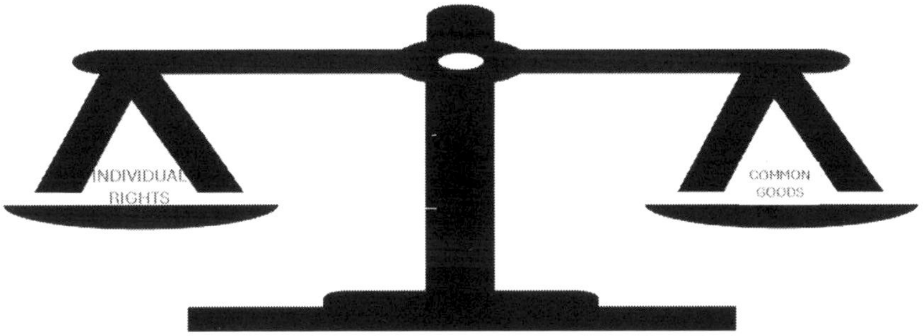

FIGURE 20.4 Individual rights and common goods.

illegal distribution of coffers across the affected population [21]. Likewise, grounding allocation programs on non-medical characteristics, similar to social worth, perceived obstacles to treatment, or patient donation to illness, could lead to inequitable resource allocation [19]. Violations of mortal rights in health, including overt or implicit demarcation in the delivery of health services, can act as an essential hedge to healthcare access and contribute to poor quality care [22]. Figure 20.4 shows individual rights and common goods. Thus, it's pivotal for healthcare policymakers to precisely consider the implicit consequences of prioritizing individual rights over the common good in resource allocation to ensure fair and indifferent distribution of healthcare coffers [19,21,22].

20.3 METHODOLOGY

20.3.1 CHALLENGES

The problem of HRA is a critical issue that has been discussed and analysed for decades. When resources are limited, and demand exceeds force, allocation becomes a problem, and changing the swish result for sharing resources during afflictions analogous to COVID-19 remains a significant concern [23,24].

The allocation of resources in hospitals is a multifaceted process that involves the distribution of finances, medical equipment, health insurance, and health-related programs among populations, programs, and individuals. This decision-making process occurs in multiple situations and includes various realities, both public and private, analogous to panels, hospitals, and medical equipment providers [25].

The part of the medical profession in resource allocation has been linked as central, as croakers act as doorkeepers to healthcare resources. Different interpretations of the nature of medicine delegation have different allocation styles, and a comprehensive result that acknowledges the role of healthcare professionals is necessary to address the allocation problem effectively [26].

Effective and indifferent resource allocation is essential to ensure that everyone's healthcare conditions are addressed with as many resources as possible [25]. Still, allocating resources in healthcare is a complex and multifaceted process that requires careful consideration of various factors, including strategic objectives, community conditions, and ethical concerns [23,24].

In conclusion, HRA is a critical issue that requires further investigation and attention. When resources are limited, and demand begins to overbalance the force, allocation becomes a serious problem, and ethical issues arise. A comprehensive result acknowledging the part of healthcare professionals is necessary to effectively address the allocation problem [23,24].

20.3.2 HEALTHCARE NEEDS VS RESOURCE ALLOCATION

The problem of HRA arises from the limited pocket available and the extensive demand for healthcare services. When demand exceeds force, resource allocation in healthcare becomes challenging, and changing the swish result for sharing resources during afflictions analogous to COVID-19 remains a significant concern [26]. Figure 20.5 shows resources bottleneck illustration.

HRA is a critical and complex aspect of resource operation for any healthcare centre. Some of the biggest challenges in HRA include [26]:

1. There is an intimidating deficiency of professed medical professionals in countries like the USA, UK, Australia, and India due to high development, inequitable pool distribution, and lack of quality education providers.
2. Unsteady nature of the healthcare sector: Unlike other industries, resource allocation in healthcare can't be estimated directly, making it difficult to meet the minimum conditions of healthcare installations.

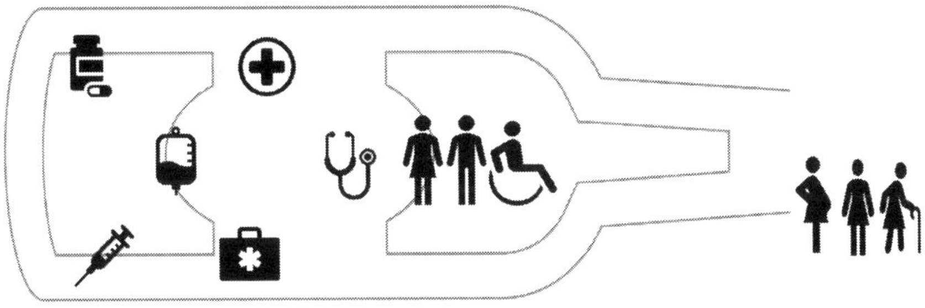

FIGURE 20.5 Resources bottleneck illustration.

Conventional styles of asset assignment in healthcare incorporate resource-allocation-by-instigation (Slam), resource-allocation-by-croakers (RAP), and resource-allocation-to-survive (RAS) [27]. Still, these styles have impediments, and a modern assignment framework, resource-allocation-in-response-to-need (RARN), has been proposed. RARN analyses each exertion predicated on community need, sanitarium response, and economics, balancing cost operation emphasis of doing goods right(operation) with doing the right goods(allocation) [27].

Physicians play a central role in the allocation process as doorkeepers to healthcare resources. Different interpretations of the nature of medicine delegation have different allocation styles, and a comprehensive result that acknowledges the role of healthcare professionals is necessary to address the allocation problem effectively [28].

The problem of HRA is a critical issue that requires further disquisition and attention. When resources are limited, and demand begins to overbalance the force, allocation becomes a serious problem, and racial issues arise. A comprehensive result that acknowledges the role of healthcare professionals is necessary to address the allocation problem effectively [26,27].

20.3.2.1 Advantages and Disadvantages

In healthcare, there are several styles used to allocate coffers effectively. These include approaches grounded on meeting population requirements, profitability-grounded, age-grounded, debate and dealing-grounded, and needs-grounded approaches. Each system has its advantages and disadvantages, which are listed below:

20.3.3 Meeting Population Needs Approach

Advantages: This approach focuses on meeting the conditions of the population to maximize their capability to profit from interventions. It ensures that coffers are allocated to meet the requirements of the larger population rather than just fastening on individual cases.

Disadvantages: One challenge is characterizing and measuring mass conditions directly, which can impact the out-of-line movement of coffers. In addition, it may be touchy to choose how imperative weight permits the necessities of assorted populaces in a given locale.

20.3.4 Profitability-Grounded Approaches

Advantages: This approach recognizes the most reasonable task of coffers to maximize prosperity benefits or other measures of social wealth. Prioritizing coffers grounded on cost-effectiveness can help ensure that compelled reserves are utilized efficiently.

Disadvantages: The catch-on charge of this approach is that it may lead to prioritization grounded solely on cost-effectiveness, which appears to neglect the prerequisites of certain calm groups. This might impact shaky efforts to care for defenceless populations.

20.3.5 Age-Grounded Approaches

Advantages: An age-grounded approach clearly and objectively demonstrates the resource task. It distinguishes between ensuring that specific age groups capitulate suitable thought and support.

Disadvantages: Ethical endeavours develop with regard to goodness and boundaries when allocating coffers grounded solely on age. Developed grown-ups may face challenges entering care if they do not fit into customary orders.

20.3.6 Debate and Logrolling-Grounded Approaches

Advantages: Accomplice consideration through concession licences for organized decision-making and resource designation. Propels collaboration between different parties in involved healthcare delivery.

Disadvantages: This approach can lead to inspiration due to contrasts in logrolling control among accomplices. Precedences might move depending on who holds the help effect during these talks. Conclusions may be less direct over time.

20.3.7 Requirements-Grounded Resource Allocation

Advantages: The advantage of progressing goodness and esteem by prioritizing qualification and populaces concurring to their prosperity requirements.

Disadvantages: It may fight to address complex conditions that bear distinctive mediations or, along the side, allocate coffers through calm volume or possibly than need.

20.3.8 The Supportability Runs the Show-Grounded Approach

Advantages: The complements are guidelines while tending to the long-term diminish of healthcare values.

Disadvantages: Striking an alter between this rule and others is basic to avoid unintended consequences.

In layout, each approach has pros and cons when considering the master, correspondence, and ethical components affecting healthcare resource task assumptions. Striking a fitting balance among these basics will remain challenging as healthcare systems continue to evolve.

20.4 SOLUTION APPROACH

Solution

Healthcare resources are a complex issue requiring serious examination and thought. Pressing disclosures about healthcare resource designation include:

- The development of a comprehensive frame for medicine that recognizes the role of healthcare professionals in resource allocation is imperative for successfully addressing the allocation challenges. Various perspectives on medicine delegate varying approaches to allocation, taking a holistic approach that incorporates their perceptivity.
- Operation of resource scheduling software using technology through resource scheduling software can help manage the complexity of HRA more efficiently. This can give lower translucence and delicacy in documentation, contributing to better decision-timber.
- An innovative allocation system called RARN has been proposed. RARN considers patient conditions, sanitarium responses, and profitable factors while striking a balance between functional effectiveness and the delivery of applicable care.
- Attention to the deficiency of good medical professionals in multitudinous nations, including the United States, the United Kingdom, Australia, and India, faces a severe dearth of trained medical professionals. Components identical to rapid-fire-fire improvement, uneven movement of resources, and constrained teacher openings contribute to this dissatisfaction. Settling this issue is significant to optimizing healthcare resource assignment.
- Optimizing resource sharing amid heads in circumstances like tribulations and resource designation in healthcare gets to be in truth development burning. By controlling methods to share resources effectively, we can palliate the impact of these events on healthcare systems. Figure 20.6 shows RARN Illustration.

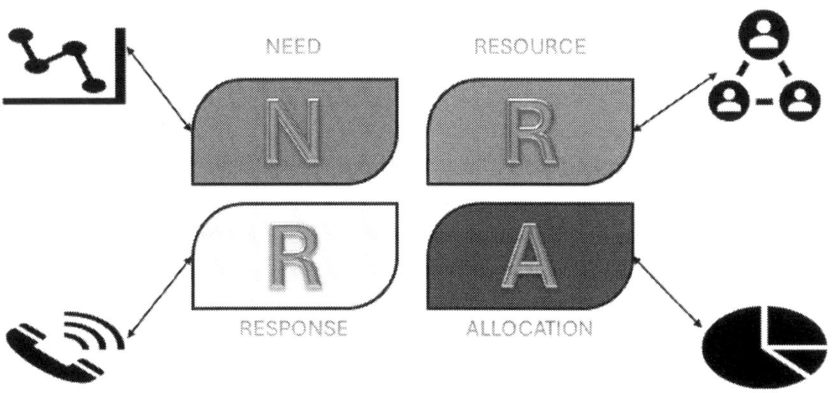

FIGURE 20.6 RARN illustration.

In the diagram, apportioning the complex issues of bracing healthcare resource scattering requires an all-encompassing strategy that counts distinctive essentials. This incorporates making an all-encompassing layout for pharmaceuticals, getting a handle on cutting-edge task styles, bridging the gap in the number of authorized restorative pros, and reevaluating how resources are shared among individuals amid inconveniences. By regulating these measures, we can improve both the viability and decency of healthcare asset assignment, guaranteeing that everybody gets appropriate care predicated on their conditions without any predisposition or segregation.

20.4.1 Roles of Ethics in Resource Allocation? Why Does It Matter?

Ethics plays a pivotal part in HRA. It provides a frame for examining and ordering values, ensuring that opinions are made considering ethical principles such as autonomy, beneficence, and justice [29]. The place of ethics in resource allocation is multifaceted and essential for several reasons.

- **Fairness and Justice**: Ethical principles accompany opinions to ensure fairness and justice in allocating scarce coffers. This is particularly important in healthcare, where resource allocation opinions can impact and end people's lives [30].
- **Cost-Effectiveness and Value**: Moral contemplations in asset allotment emphasize the centrality of cost-effectiveness and value. Designating coffers to maximize well-being benefits for the populace served is an ethical concern, and an allotment that isn't cost-effective produces smaller benefits than would have been conceivable with a diverse allotment [31].
- **Alignment with Societal Precedences**: Ethical morals in resource allocation opinions reflect societal values and precedences. Understanding how well a particular resource allocation aligns with a society's precedence can help decision-makers hand its adequacy to the community [32].
- **Ethical Trade-Offs**: Ethics provides a methodical way to navigate trade-offs between effectiveness and other important values. While effectiveness is valued, ethical considerations help decision-makers tease out rudiments that may be more important in specific surroundings, like funding preventative measures versus cures or allocating coffers grounded on age or health issues [32].
- **Equitable Access to Coffers**: Ethical resource allocation ensures effective and indifferent access to coffers, which is essential for good health for all. It impacts the equity and effectiveness of healthcare and public health goods and services, impacting the entire experience within the healthcare and public health systems [33].

In conclusion, ethics in resource allocation are essential for ensuring fairness, justice, and cost-effectiveness, aligning opinions with societal precedents, and navigating ethical trade-offs. Ethics plays a critical part in shaping resource allocation opinions in healthcare, impacting the equity and effectiveness of health services and goods and eventually impacting individuality within the healthcare system [29,30].

20.5 CONCLUSION

HRA is a complex and critical aspect of healthcare management, encompassing the distribution of limited resources to meet the population's diverse needs. The discussion around this topic emphasizes the material aspects and the nature and status of the available resources [34]. Coordination and efficiency in allocation play a vital role in overcoming barriers and ensuring optimal utilization of resources [35]. Alternative approaches and evaluations based on efficiency metrics, such as data envelopment analysis (DEA), provide insights into improving resource allocation strategies [36]. Fair allocation that prioritizes maximizing benefits for all patients remains a guiding principle in this context [35]. Results for HRA include developing a comprehensive model of medicine, espousing new allocation styles, addressing the insufficiency of professed medical professionals, and changing the voguish result for participating coffers during an epidemic.

REFERENCES

1. https://www.ncbi.nlm.nih.gov/pmc/articles/PMC8268397/
2. https://pubmed.ncbi.nlm.nih.gov/33817679/
3. https://www.commonwealthfund.org/publications/issue-briefs/2023/jan/us-health-care-global-perspective-2022
4. Gou, X., Xu, X., Deng, F. et al. Medical health resources allocation evaluation in public health emergencies by an improved ORESTE method with linguistic preference orderings. *Fuzzy Optim Decis Making*, 2023. https://doi.org/10.1007/s10700-023-09409-3
5. https://www.who.int/docs/default-source/blue-print/ethics-and-covid-19-resource-allocation-and-priority-setting.pdf?sfvrsn=4c14e95c_1
6. Yip, J. Y. C. Healthcare resource allocation in the COVID-19 pandemic: Ethical considerations from the perspective of distributive justice within public health. *Public Health in Practice (Oxf)*. 100111, 2021. https://doi.org/10.1016/j.puhip.2021.100111. Epub 2021 Mar 28. PMID: 33817679; PMCID: PMC8005252.
7. Carter, D., Gordon, J., Watt, A. M. Competing principles for allocating health care resources. *The Journal of Medicine and Philosophy: A Forum for Bioethics and Philosophy of Medicine*, 41(5), 558–583, 2016. https://doi.org/10.1093/jmp/jhw017
8. https://www.ncbi.nlm.nih.gov/pmc/articles/PMC8005252/
9. https://bmjopen.bmj.com/content/13/3/e065204
10. https://www.ncbi.nlm.nih.gov/pmc/articles/PMC5886160/
11. Raghupathi, V., Raghupathi, W. The association between healthcare resource allocation and health status: an empirical insight with visual analytics. *Journal of Public Health*, 31, 2021. https://doi.org/10.1007/s10389-021-01651-6
12. https://www.ncbi.nlm.nih.gov/books/NBK435786/
13. https://www.ncbi.nlm.nih.gov/pmc/articles/PMC1925021/
14. https://scholarworks.gvsu.edu/cgi/viewcontent.cgi?article=1800&context=honorsprojects
15. Ordu, M., Demir, E., Tofallis, C., Gunal, M. M. (2023). A comprehensive and integrated hospital decision support system for efficient and effective healthcare services delivery using discrete event simulation. *Healthcare Analytics*, 4, 100248, 2023. ISSN 2772-4425. https://doi.org/10.1016/j.health.2023.100248
16. Bodina, A., Pavan, A., Castaldi, S. Resource allocation criteria in a hospital. *Journal of Preventive Medicine and Hygiene*, 58(2), E184–E189, 2017. PMID: 28900360; PMCID: PMC5584089.

17. Fauci, A. J., Latina, R., Iacorossi, L., Coclite, D., D'Angelo, D., Napoletano, A., Terrenato, I., Iannone, P. Allocation of scarce critical care resources during public health emergencies: which ethical principles support decision making. *Clinical Therapeutics*, 173(4), 384–395, 2022. PMID: 35857058. https://doi.org/10.7417/CT.2022.2450
18. Fattahi, M., Keyvanshokooh, E., Kannan, D., Govindan, K. Resource planning strategies for healthcare systems during a pandemic. *European Journal of Operational Research*, 304(1), 192–206, 2023. ISSN 0377-2217. https://doi.org/10.1016/j.ejor.2022.01.023
19. Baker, T., Baker, P. Ethical criteria for allocating healthcare resources. *Lancet*, 373, 1424–1425, 2009; author reply 1425–6.
20. Asthana, S., Gibson, A., Moon, G., Brigham, P. Allocating resources for health and social care: the significance of rurality. *Health & Social Care in the Community*, 11, 486–493, 2003. https://doi.org/10.1046/j.1365-2524.2003.00454.x
21. Barasa, E. W., Molyneux, S., English, M., Clearly, S. Setting healthcare priorities in hospitals: a review of empirical studies. *Health Policy and Planning*, 30(3), 386–396, 2015.
22. Zohny, H., Davies, B., Wilkinson, D. Affirmative action in healthcare resource allocation: vaccines, ventilators and race. *Bioethics*, 36(9), 970–977, 2022. https://doi.org/10.1111/bioe.13067
23. https://www.ncbi.nlm.nih.gov/pmc/articles/PMC1925021/
24. Redondo, E., Nicoletta, V., Bélanger, V., Garcia-Sabater, J. P., Landa, P., Maheut, J., Marin-Garcia, J. A., Ruiz, A. A simulation model for predicting hospital occupancy for Covid-19 using archetype analysis. *Healthcare Analytics*, 3, 100197, 2023. ISSN 2772 4425. https://doi.org/10.1016/j.health.2023.100197
25. Radinmanesh, M., Ebadifard Azar, F., Hashjin, A. et al. A review of appropriate indicators for need-based financial resource allocation in health systems. *BMC Health Services Research*, 21, 674, 2021. https://doi.org/10.1186/s12913-021-06522-0
26. Stafinski, T., Menon, D., Marshall, D. et al. Societal values in the allocation of healthcare resources. *Patient-Patient-Centered-Outcomes-Research*, 4, 207–225, 2011. https://doi.org/10.2165/11588880-000000000-00000
27. Maharajan, M., Rajiah, K., Sivanandy, P. Use of health economic information in the management of health care resource allocation. *Value in Health*, 19(7), A836, 2016. https://doi.org/10.1016/j.jval.2016.08.557; https://www.valueinhealthjournal.com/article/S1098-3015(16)31137-8/fulltext
28. https://ojin.nursingworld.org/table-of-contents/volume-3-1998/number-3-december-1998/scarce-resources/
29. O'Sullivan, L., Aldasoro, E., O'Brien, Á., Nolan, M., McGovern, C., Carroll, Á. Ethical values and principles to guide the fair allocation of resources in response to a pandemic: a rapid systematic review. *BMC Medical Ethics*, 23(1), 70, 7. https://doi.org/10.1186/s12910-022-00806-8. PMID: 35799187; PMCID: PMC9261249.31. https://www.ncbi.nlm.nih.gov/books/NBK11739/
30. https://journalofethics.ama-assn.org/article/teaching-resource-allocation-and-why-it-matters/2011-04
31. Yip, Y. C., Yip, K. H., Tsui, W. K. When rationing becomes inevitable in a pandemic: A discussion on the ethical considerations from a public health perspective. *Public Health in Practice (Oxf)*, 4, 100294, 2022. https://doi.org/10.1016/j.puhip.2022.100294. Epub 2022 Jul 8. PMID: 35822188; PMCID: PMC9265141.
32. https://www.ncbi.nlm.nih.gov/pmc/articles/PMC1925021/
33. https://scholarworks.gvsu.edu/cgi/viewcontent.cgi?article=1800&context=honorsprojects
34. Liu, L., Xu, W., Su, Y., Zhou, X. Evaluation of health resource allocation efficiency based on data envelopment analysis 2014–2018 in two dimensions of time-region. *Discrete Dynamics in Nature and Society*, 2021, 10, 2021. Article ID 8273415. https://doi.org/10.1155/2021/8273415

35. https://www.researchgate.net/publication/24113478_The_advantages_and_disadvantages_of_needs-based_resource_allocation_in_integrated_health_systems_and_market_systems_of_health_care_provider_reimbursement
36. Sibbald, S. L., Gibson, J. L., Singer, P., et al. Evaluating priority setting success in healthcare: a pilot study. *BMC Health Services Research*, 10, 131, 2010.

Index

Note: **Bold** page numbers refer to tables and *italic* page numbers refer to figures.

Made in the USA
Monee, IL
12 November 2026

cb0b64f2-71d5-4f8c-9b6a-429d7728bb09R01